Pearson Nursing Reviews & Rationales

Maternal-Newborn Nursing

Third Edition

SERIES EDITOR

MaryAnn Hogan, MSN, RN

Clinical Assistant Professor
School of Nursing
University of Massachusetts–Amherst
Amherst, Massachusetts

CONSULTING EDITORS

Mary M. Tarbell, MS, RN

Dean, School of Nursing
Springfield Technical Community College
Springfield, Massachusetts

Maud Low, RNC, MSN, CLNC

Clinical Assistant Professor
School of Nursing
University of Massachusetts–Amherst
Amherst, Massachusetts

PEARSON

Boston Columbus Indianapolis New York San Francisco Upper Saddle River
Amsterdam Cape Town Dubai London Madrid Milan Munich Paris Montréal Toronto
Delhi Mexico City São Paulo Sydney Hong Kong Seoul Singapore Taipei Tokyo

Cataloging-in-Publication Data on File with the Library of Congress

Director of Readypoint™: Maura Connor
Executive Editor: Jennifer Farthing
Developmental Editor: Rachael Zipperlen
Editorial Assistant: Deirdre MacKnight
Director, Digital Product Development: Alex Marciante
Media Product Manager: Travis Moses-Westphal
Vice President, Director Sales & Marketing: David Gesell
Senior Marketing Manager: Phoenix Harvey
Marketing Coordinator: Michael Sirinides
Director of Media Production: Allyson Graesser
Media Project Manager: Rachel Collett
Managing Editor, Production: Patrick Walsh
Production Editor: GEX Publishing Services
Manufacturing Manager: Ilene Sanford
Art Director/Cover Designer: Mary Siener
Composition: GEX Publishing Services
Printer/Binder: Edwards Brothers Malloy
Cover Printer: Lehigh/Phoenix Color Hagerstown

10 9 8 7 6 5 4 3

PEARSON

ISBN 10: 0-13-295686-1
ISBN 13: 978-0-13-295686-4

Contents

Welcome to the Pearson Nursing Reviews & Rationales Series!

This series has been specifically designed to provide a clear and concentrated review of important nursing knowledge in the following content areas:

- Anatomy & Physiology
- Nursing Fundamentals
- Nutrition & Diet Therapy
- Fluids, Electrolytes, & Acid–Base Balance
- Medical-Surgical Nursing
- Pathophysiology
- Pharmacology
- Maternal-Newborn Nursing
- Child Health Nursing
- Mental Health Nursing
- Health & Physical Assessment
- Community Health Nursing
- Leadership & Management

The books in this series are designed for use either by current nursing students as a study aid for nursing course work, for NCLEX-RN® exam preparation, or by practicing nurses seeking a comprehensive yet concise review of a nursing specialty or subject area.

This series is truly unique. One of its most special features is that it has been developed and reviewed by a large team of nurse educators from across the United States and Canada to ensure that each chapter is edited by a nurse expert in the content area under study. The series editor, MaryAnn Hogan, designed the overall series in collaboration with a core Pearson team to take full advantage of Pearson's cutting edge technology. The consulting editors for each book, also experts in that specialty area, then reviewed all chapters and test questions submitted for comprehensiveness and accuracy. Finally, MaryAnn Hogan reviewed the chapters in each book for consistency, accuracy, and applicability to the NCLEX-RN® Test Plan.

All books in the series are identical in their overall design for your convenience. As an added value, each book comes with a comprehensive support package, including access to additional questions online, complete eText, and a tear-out ***NursingNotes*** card for clinical reference and quick review.

Study Tips

Use of this book should help simplify your review. To make the most of your valuable study time, also follow these simple but important suggestions:

1. Use a weekly calendar to schedule study sessions.
   - Outline the time frames for all of your activities (home, school, appointments, etc.) on a weekly calendar.
   - Find the "holes" in your calendar, which are the times when you can plan to study. Add study sessions to the calendar at times when you can expect to be mentally alert and follow your plan!
2. Create the optimal study environment.
   - Eliminate external sources of distraction, such as television, telephone, etc.
   - Eliminate internal sources of distraction, such as hunger, thirst, or dwelling on items or problems that cannot be worked on at the moment.
   - Take a break for 10 minutes or so after each hour of concentrated study, both as a reward and an incentive to keep studying.
3. Use prereading strategies to increase comprehension of chapter material.
   - Skim the headings in the chapter (because they identify chapter content).
   - Read the definitions of key terms, which will help you learn new words to comprehend chapter information.
   - Review all graphic aids (figures, tables, boxes) because they are often used to explain important points in the chapter.

4. Read the chapter thoroughly but at a reasonable speed.
   - Comprehension and retention are actually enhanced by not reading too slowly.
   - Do take the time to reread any section that is unclear to you.
5. Summarize what you have learned.
   - Use the accompanying online resource, NursingReviewsandRationales.com, to test yourself with hundreds of NCLEX-RN®-style practice questions.
   - Review again any sections that correspond to questions you answered incorrectly or incompletely.

Test-Taking Strategies

Test-taking strategies accompany the rationales for every question in the series. These strategies will assist you to select the correct answer by breaking down the question, even if you do not know the correct response. Use the following strategies to increase your success on nursing tests or examinations:

- Get sufficient sleep and have something to eat before taking a test. Avoid eating concentrated sweets, though, to prevent rapid upward and then downward surges in your blood glucose. Avoid also high-fat foods that will make you sleepy.
- Take deep breaths during the test as needed. Remember, the brain requires both oxygen and glucose as fuel.
- Read the question carefully, identifying the stem, all the options, and any critical words or phrases in either the stem or options.
  - Critical words in the stem such as *most important* indicate the need to set priorities, because more than one option is likely to contain a statement that is technically correct.
  - Remember that the presence of red flag words such as *never* or *only* in an answer option is more likely to make that option incorrect.
- Determine who is the client in the question; often this is the person with the health problem, but it may also be a significant other, relative, friend, or another nurse.
- Decide whether the stem is a true response stem or a false response stem. With a true response stem, the correct answer will be a true statement, and vice versa.
- Determine what the question is really asking, sometimes referred to as the core issue of the question. Evaluate all answer options in relation to this issue, and not strictly to the "correctness" of the statement in each individual option.
- Eliminate options that are obviously incorrect, then go back and reread the stem. Evaluate those remaining options against the stem once more to make a final selection.
- If two answers seem similar and correct, try to decide whether one of them is more global or comprehensive. If one option includes the alternative option within it, it is likely that the more global option is the correct answer.

The NCLEX-RN® Licensing Examination

Upon graduation from a nursing program, successful completion of the NCLEX-RN® licensing examination is required to begin professional nursing practice. The NCLEX-RN® exam is a Computer Adaptive Test (CAT) that ranges in length from 75 to 265 individual (stand-alone) test items, depending on your performance during the examination. The blueprint for the exam is reviewed and revised every three years by the National Council of State Boards of Nursing using the results of a job analysis study of new graduate nurses practicing within the first six months after graduation. Each question on the exam is coded to a *Client Need Category* and an *Integrated Process.*

Client Need Categories There are four categories of client needs, and each exam will contain a minimum and maximum percent of questions from each category. Each major category has subcategories within it. The *Client Need* categories according to the NCLEX-RN® Test Plan effective April 2010 are as follows:

- Safe Effective Care Environment
  - Management of Care (16–22%)
  - Safety and Infection Control (8–14%)
- Health Promotion and Maintenance (6–12%)
- Psychosocial Integrity (6–12%)
- Physiological Integrity
  - Basic Care and Comfort (6–12%)
  - Pharmacological and Parenteral Therapies (13–19%)
  - Reduction of Risk Potential (10–16%)
  - Physiological Adaptation (11–17%)

Integrated Processes The integrated processes identified on the NCLEX-RN® Test Plan effective April 2010, with condensed definitions, are as follows:

- Nursing Process: a scientific problem-solving approach used in nursing practice; consisting of assessment, analysis, planning, implementation, and evaluation.
- Caring: client–nurse interaction(s) characterized by mutual respect and trust and that are directed toward achieving desired client outcomes.
- Communication and Documentation: verbal and/or non-verbal interactions between nurse and others (client, family, health care team); a written or electronic recording of activities or events that occur during client care.
- Teaching and Learning: facilitating client's acquisition of knowledge, skills, and attitudes that lead to behavior change.

More detailed information about this examination may be obtained by visiting the National Council of State Boards of Nursing website at http://www.ncsbn.org and viewing the *2010 NCLEX-RN® Detailed Test Plan.*[1]

[1]Reference: National Council of State Boards of Nursing, Inc. *2010 NCLEX-RN® Test Plan.* Effective April, 2010. Retrieved from http://www.ncsbn.org/2010_NCLEX_RN_TestPlan.pdf.

HOW TO GET THE MOST OUT OF THIS BOOK

Each chapter has the following elements to guide you during review and study:

Chapter Objectives describe what you will be able to know or do after learning the material covered in the chapter.

Objectives

- Discuss legal considerations related to maternity nursing.
- Delineate ethical issues that influence maternal-newborn nursing practice.
- Identify culturally diverse health beliefs that impact the maternity cycle.
- Describe a philosophy of care that maintains maternal–newborn safety and fosters family unity.

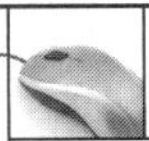

NCLEX-RN® Test Prep

Use the accompanying online resource, NursingReviewsandRationales, to test yourself with hundreds of NCLEX®-style practice questions.

Review at a Glance contains a glossary of critical terms used in the chapter, with definitions provided up-front and available at your fingertips, to help you stay focused and make the best use of your study time.

Review at a Glance

artificial insemination treatment of infertility where sperm are directly inserted into uterus

anovulatory menstrual cycles menstrual cycles that are not preceded by ovulation

basal body temperature (BBT) resting body temperature, taken daily prior to arising from bed; when graphed will assist in detecting ovulation

tube; spermatozoa that have been collected are also inserted via a large-bore needle under ultrasound guidance into fallopian tube; fertilization occurs in fallopian tube

hysterosalpingogram (HSG) a diagnostic test in which radiopaque dye is instilled into uterus and fallopian tubes via a catheter inserted through cervix; used to detect uterine or tubal anomalies

micro-epididymal sperm aspiration (MESA) is a microsurgical technique to obtain a sperm specimen from the epididymis; performed as an outpatient procedure under sedation and/or local anesthesia

pelvic inflammatory disease (PID) inflammation of uterus and fallopian tubes, usually caused by an infectious agent such as *Chlamydia trachomatis* or *Gonorrhea Neisseria*

Pretest provides a 10-question quiz as a sample overview of the material covered in the chapter and helps you decide in what areas you need the most—or the least—review.

PRETEST

1. The client is making her first visit to the contraceptive clinic to discuss her options for birth control. When teaching the client about family planning, the nurse should include information on which of the following? Select all that apply.

   1. Male condoms and spermicide should be used together
   2. Depomedroxyprogesterone acetate (DMPA)
   3. Oral contraceptives
   4. Screening for possible birth defects
   5. Semen analysis

Practice to Pass questions are open ended, stimulate critical thinking, and reinforce mastery of the chapter information.

Practice to Pass

A client reveals that she has PKU. She asks what the chances are for passing on the disease if the father does not have PKU. Knowing that this is an autosomal recessive trait, how would the nurse respond?

NCLEX Alert identifies concepts that are likely to be tested on the NCLEX-RN® examination. Be sure to learn the information highlighted wherever you see this icon.

!

Case Study, found at the end of the chapter, provides an opportunity for you to use your critical thinking and clinical reasoning skills to "put it all together." It describes a true-to-life client case situation and asks you open-ended questions about how you would provide care for that client and/or family.

Case Study

The client, who is a primigravida in her second trimester, has come in for a scheduled prenatal visit. When the nurse asks how things are going, the client replies, "Not very well. It seems like I'm just falling apart. I have heartburn after I eat, my ankles swell, I'm constipated all the time, and I think I may be getting hemorrhoids."

1. What questions should the nurse ask the client regarding the problems described?
2. What objective data should the nurse collect regarding the problems described?
3. What nursing diagnoses are appropriate for this client?
4. What teaching is needed in this situation?
5. How should the nurse followup with this client?

For suggested responses, see page 303.

Posttest provides an additional 10-question quiz at the end of the chapter. It provides you with feedback about mastery of the chapter material following review and study. All pretest and posttest questions contain comprehensive rationales for the correct and incorrect answers, and are coded according to cognitive level of difficulty, and the NCLEX-RN® Test Plan categories of client need and integrated processes.

POSTTEST

1 The results have been returned from a complete blood count for a pregnant client who came to the clinic for her initial prenatal visit. Which result would indicate a possible problem with oxygen-carrying capacity?

1. Decreased white blood cell count
2. Decreased red blood cell count
3. Decreased polymorphonuclear cell count
4. Decreased platelet count

NCLEX-RN® Test Prep: NursingReviewsandRationales.com

For those who want to prepare for the NCLEX-RN®, practicing online will help you become more familiar with the computer-based testing experience, especially for the new alternate item formats such as audio, media-enhanced, hot spot, and exhibit questions. With this new edition, use the code printed inside the front cover of the book to access Nursing Reviews & Rationales, which offers 700 practice questions using all NCLEX®-style formats. This includes the practice questions found in all chapters of the book as well as 30 additional questions per chapter. Nursing Reviews & Rationales allows you to choose two ways to prepare for the NCLEX-RN®. Both approaches personalize your practice experience according to what stage you are at in your NCLEX® preparation.

Nursing Reviews & Rationales includes the eText version of *Pearson Nursing Maternal-Newborn Nursing Reviews and Rationales*, Third Edition. This eText is fully searchable and includes features like note-taking, highlighting, and more. The eText allows you to take your review with you anywhere you have an internet connection to NursingReviewsandRationales.com.

NursingNotes Card

This tear-out card provides a reference for frequently used facts and information related to the subject matter of the book. These are designed to be useful in the clinical setting, when quick and easy access to information is so important!

About the Maternal-Newborn Nursing Book

Chapters in this book cover "need-to-know" information about maternal-newborn nursing, including family-centered care during normal and complicated experiences in the prenatal, labor and delivery, postpartal, and neonatal periods. Additional chapters focus on special topics such as ethical, legal, and cultural considerations; reproduction, fertility, and infertility; family planning and contraception; fetal development; and laboratory and diagnostic testing. The final chapter includes issues of loss and grief in childbearing. The term *parent* or *parents* has been used in this book to indicate the primary caretaker(s) for the newborn. The author understands and appreciates that there are a variety of family configurations in which a child can grow and thrive.

Acknowledgments

This book is a monumental effort of collaboration. Without the contributions of many individuals, this edition of *Maternal-Newborn Nursing: Reviews and Rationales* would not have been possible. Thank you to all the contributors and reviewers who devoted their time and talents to the third edition. The contributors are Mary Tarbell MS, RN, Springfield Technical Community College, Springfield, Massachusetts; and Maud Low, RNC, MSN, CLNC, University of Massachusetts–Amherst, Amherst, Massachusetts. The reviewers are Traci McDonald-Holmquist, RN MSN, University of South Dakota; and Jane Ragozine, MSN, WHNP-BC, CLC, Kent State University.

Thanks also to the contributors and reviewers who assisted with the previous editions of this book: Rita S. Glazebrook, RNC, PhD, ANP, Minnesota Intercollegiate Nursing Consortium, Northfield, Minnesota; Vera Brancato, EdD, MSH, RN, BC, Kurtztown University, Kutztown, Pennsylvania; Jean Rodgers, RN, MN, Hesston College, Hesston, Kansas; Deb Bartnick, RN, MSN, Indiana State University, Terre Haute, Indiana; Pamela Hamre, MS, RN, CNM, College of St. Catherine, St. Paul, Minnesota; A. Jenny

Harkey, RNC, MSN, ACCE, Southeast Missouri State University, Cape Girardeau, Missouri; Anita Kyle, MS, CNS-MCH, RNC, Texas Woman's University, Houston, Texas; Karla Luxner, RNC, MSN, Millikin University, Decatur, Illinois; Molly Meighan, RNC, PhD, Carson-Newman College, Jefferson City, Tennessee; Barbara Morrison, PhD, RN, FNP, CNM, Millikin University, Decatur, Illinois; Patricia Posey-Goodwin, MN, RN, Pensacola Junior College, Pensacola, Florida; Pamela Pranke, MSN, RNC, Jamestown College, Jamestown, North Dakota; and Angela Wood, PhD, RNC, Carson-Newman College, Jefferson City, Tennessee; Judy F. Barnes, RN, MSN, East Carolina University, Kinston, North Carolina; Irene Gonzales, PhD, RN, CNP, CLNC, San Francisco State University, San Francisco, California; Judith Johnson Hilton, MSN, RNC, Lenoir-Rhyne College, Hickory, North Carolina; Katherine A. Howe, RNC, MSN, MEd, WHNP, Henry Ford Community College, Dearborn, Michigan; Janet T. Ihlenfeld, RN, BSN, MSN, PhD, D'Youville College, Buffalo, NY; Anne Katz, RN, PhD, University of Manitoba, Winnipeg, Canada; Patricia A. Mynaugh, PhD, RN, Villanova University, Villanova, Pennsylvania; Carol S. Roane, RNC, MS, Cecil Community College, North East, Maryland; Stephanie Stewart, RN, PhD, University of Wisconsin-Oshkosh, Oshkosh, Wisconsin; Marcie Weissner, MSN, RNC, University of Saint Francis, Fort Wayne, Indiana; and Susan Wilhelm, RNC, PhD, UNMC, West Nebraska Division, Scottsbluff, Nebraska. Their work will surely assist both students and practicing nurses alike to extend their knowledge in the area of maternal-newborn health.

I owe a special debt of gratitude to the wonderful team at Pearson Nursing for their enthusiasm for this project, as well as their good humor, expertise, and encouragement as the series developed. Maura Connor, Director of Readypoint™, was unending in her creativity, support, encouragement, and belief in the need for this series. Jennifer Farthing, Executive Editor, Readypoint™, coordinated this revision with insight, talent, and zeal, and fostered a culture of true collaboration and teamwork. Rachael Zipperlen, Developmental Editor, devoted many long hours to coordinating different facets of this project. Her high standards and attention to detail contributed greatly to the final "look" of this book. Editorial Assistant, Deirdre MacKnight, helped to keep the project moving forward on a day-to-day basis, and I am grateful for her efforts as well. A very special thank you goes to the designers of the book and the production team, led by Patrick Walsh, Managing Editor, who brought the ideas and manuscript into final form.

Thank you to the team at GEX Publishing Services, led by Ashley Lewis and Kelly Morrison, Project Managers, for the detail-oriented work of creating this book. I greatly appreciate their hard work, attention to detail, and spirit of collaboration.

Finally, I would like to acknowledge and gratefully thank my children Michael Jr., Kathryn, Kristen, and William, who sacrificed precious hours of family time so this book could be revised. I would also like to thank my students, past and present, for continuing to inspire me with their quest for knowledge and passion for nursing. You are the future!

–MaryAnn Hogan

Introduction to Maternity Nursing 1

Chapter Outline

Legal Considerations
Ethical Issues
Cultural Health Beliefs and Cultural Competence
Family-Centered Maternity Care

Objectives

- ➤ Discuss legal considerations related to maternity nursing.
- ➤ Delineate ethical issues that influence maternal-newborn nursing practice.
- ➤ Identify culturally diverse health beliefs that impact the maternity cycle.
- ➤ Describe a philosophy of care that maintains maternal–newborn safety and fosters family unity.

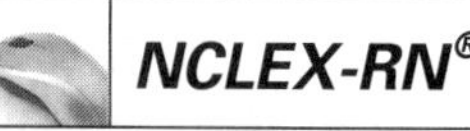

NCLEX-RN® Test Prep

Use the accompanying online resource, NursingReviewsandRationales, to test yourself with hundreds of NCLEX®-style practice questions.

Review at a Glance

belief something accepted as true, especially as a tenet or a body of tenets accepted by an ethnocultural group

cultural competency the awareness, knowledge, and skills necessary to appreciate, understand, and communicate with people of diverse cultural backgrounds

cultural imposition imposition of one's own values, beliefs, and practices on the client, family, or community in the belief that one's own lifeways are "best"; often arises from ignorance of others' cultural practices

diversity differences in race, ethnicity, national origin, religion, age, gender, sexual orientation, ability/disability, social and economic status or class, education, and related attributes of groups of people in society

ethnocentrism assumption that one's own beliefs and ways of doing things are best or superior

family a group of individuals related by blood, marriage, or mutual goals

family-centered maternity care maternity care that is family oriented and views childbirth as a vital, natural life event rather than an illness

infant mortality rate the number of deaths of infants under one year of age per 1000 live births in a given population

malpractice the failure of a professional person to act in accordance with the prevailing professional standards or failure to foresee consequences that a professional person, having the necessary skill and education, should foresee

maternity care health care provided to the childbearing family that involves physiologic, psychosocial, and cultural aspects of care

negligence omitting or committing an act that a reasonable prudent person, particularly a person with the same level of duty, would not omit or commit under the same or similar circumstances

scope of practice legally refers to permissible boundaries of practice and is defined by state statute (written law), rules and regulations, or a combination of the two

standards of care documents describing the minimal requirements that define an acceptable level of care, which is to exercise ordinary and reasonable effort to see that client experiences no harm during care

unlicensed assistive personnel health care workers who have no defined body of knowledge or educational preparation upon which to base their practice and who are uncredentialed

PRETEST

1 A client who is 38 weeks pregnant with a history of hypertension and proteinuria is admitted with severe upper abdominal pain, nausea, and a persistent headache. The nurse notes an elevated blood pressure (BP) on two readings 20 minutes apart. When notifying the physician 20 minutes after the second BP reading, the nurse reported the elevated BP, abdominal pain, nausea, and inability to void. The nurse did not report the client's headache, so the physician concluded the client had gastric disturbance from the flu. Later, the client had a grand mal seizure. Why would the nurse be considered negligent in this situation?

1. The nurse did not maintain clear, concise, and accurate documentation of the client's condition.
2. The nurse was not thorough in reporting assessment data to the physician.
3. The nurse did not develop a positive empowering relationship with the client.
4. The nurse told another nurse of not knowing that headache was a symptom of preeclampsia.

2 The newborn nursery nurse is working with a client who has given birth and is planning on placing the infant for adoption. When considering the legal issues of this situation rather than the ethical aspects, the nurse would look to which of the following?

1. Values and beliefs
2. Motives, attitudes, and culture
3. What is good for the individual
4. Rules and regulations

3 An unlicensed assistant asks the maternal-newborn nurse why the nurse needs to sign a client's consent form as a witness. The nurse responds that the signature affirms which of the following?

1. That the client agreeing to the procedure was the person who signed the consent.
2. That the client understood the information about the procedure before making a decision.
3. That the physician explained all components of the informed consent.
4. That the nurse explained all the components of the informed consent.

4 When picking up the dinner tray, the maternal-newborn nurse notices that a Vietnamese client did not eat any roast beef or mashed potatoes. Later, her family members brought in some steamed fish and vegetables with rice, which she ate. The nurse draws which conclusion about why the client prefers the food the family brought in?

1. The client is acculturated to American foods and prefers hamburgers and french fries.
2. Eating culturally desired foods is preferable to eating strange or taboo foods.
3. The foods on the dinner tray are considered hot foods and should be avoided.
4. The client's appetite was decreased because of her recent delivery.

5 The mother of a client who delivered a healthy infant four hours ago tells the nurse that the labor and delivery unit "is nothing like when I had my children 20-plus years ago." The nurse expects that this family will have increased satisfaction with the birth experience because of which changes in the care setting over the last few decades?

1. The expectant mother is transferred to multiple rooms during the birth process.
2. The father of the baby is allowed to be present for the delivery.
3. The infant will remain in the room with the family as long as it is well.
4. Newborns are routinely separated from their parents immediately after birth.

6 A pregnant client who is trying to select a health care provider during pregnancy asks the antenatal clinic nurse to explain the difference between midwifery and obstetrics. What should the nurse tell the client?

1. Midwifery and obstetrics have always been practiced simultaneously.
2. Midwifery is practiced in the home while obstetrics is practiced in the hospital.
3. The focus of midwifery is being with women and assisting the family in childbirth.
4. The primary focus of obstetrics is the management of low-risk pregnancies.

7 Several ethnic groups advise expectant mothers not to reach over the head because the umbilical cord will wrap around the infant's neck. What should the nurse tell a client about this type of belief?

1. This is a health promotion belief and may be a concern at this time in her pregnancy.
2. This is a prescriptive belief and may be a worry but it is not really true.
3. This is a restrictive belief and may reflect cultural beliefs about what to avoid to have a positive pregnancy outcome.
4. This is a taboo belief and you may regret doing this later if you have problems during the pregnancy.

8 A 26-year-old client who is pregnant for the first time is low risk and is very interested in being involved with care decisions and learning all she can about pregnancy and childbirth. Which type of health care provider would the nurse recommend for prenatal care and birth?

1. An obstetrician
2. A family practice resident
3. A physician's assistant
4. A certified nurse-midwife

9 The nurse manager of the maternal-child unit is evaluating how well the unit met the ACOG (American College of Obstetrics and Gynecology) standard of starting a cesarean section within 30 minutes of the decision for surgery. What is the best way for the nurse manager to assess if the standard is met?

1. Do a chart review for documentation of time of decision and time surgery began and compare to the national standard.
2. Interview the nurses involved in the case as to how long it took from decision to surgery.
3. Assume that all emergency cesarean sections are done within the recommended 30 minutes.
4. Ask the obstetricians how long it took from the time they ordered the surgery until they made the first cut.

10 The nurse notices that a fetus, which is a footling breech, is showing signs of fetal distress. The nurse notifies the obstetrician and expresses concern about the fetus's well-being. The obstetrician does not take any action. What should the nurse do next to remain legally accountable?

1. Rely on the obstetrician's judgment and remain with the client until delivery.
2. Ask another physician to review the fetal heart monitor strip.
3. Notify the nursing supervisor promptly about the nurse's concern and the obstetrician's inaction.
4. Tell the client that lack of action by the obstetrician warrants legal action.

➤ *See pages 23–25 for Answers and Rationales.*

I. LEGAL CONSIDERATIONS

A. Two arenas for consideration of legal implications
  1. Personal professional practice
  2. Client care and advocacy

B. Legal considerations in personal professional practice

! 1. **Scope of practice:** the Nurse Practice Act
  - **a.** Is a broad definition of permissible boundaries of practice within a state
  - **b.** Distinguishes nursing practice from practice of other health professionals
  - **c.** Specifies authorized activities of advanced practice nurses, such as certified nurse-midwives and nurse practitioners (women's health, perinatal, or neonatal)
  - **d.** Excludes untrained or unlicensed individuals from practicing nursing
  - **e.** Rules and regulations promulgated by state boards of nursing provide official interpretation of nurse practice acts
  - **f.** Correct interpretation and understanding of state practice acts enables the nurse
    - **1)** To provide safe care within the limits of nursing practice
    - **2)** To avoid risk of being accused of practicing medicine without a license

! 2. **Standards of care**
  - **a.** Description
    - **1)** Minimum criteria for competent, proficient delivery of nursing care
    - **2)** Are designed to protect the public
    - **3)** Used to evaluate quality of care provided
    - **4)** Formulated from skills and knowledge commonly possessed by members of a profession
    - **5)** Identify health, demographic, environmental, and psychosocial parameters of care
    - **6)** Reflect current knowledge in the field and, therefore, are dynamic and subject to change
  - **b.** Uses of standards of care
    - **1)** Criteria to determine if a nurse has violated a state Nurse Practice Act
    - **2)** Criteria to determine if a nurse has violated state or city criminal codes
    - **3)** Criteria to elevate nursing practice to a professional level
  - **c.** Internal standards of care: individual and institutional
    - **1)** Set by role and education of the nurse: job description, education, and expertise
    - **2)** Set by individual institutions via policies and procedures
  - **d.** External or national standards of care
    - **1)** External because they supersede individual practitioners and single institutions
    - **2)** Broader than *locality rules*: standards of care viewed from the perspective of care within a geographic area
    - **3)** Based on what is reasonable, and on the average degree of skill, care, and diligence practiced by members of the profession nationally
    - **4)** Nurses in a variety of settings and locales must meet same standards
      - **a)** Apply to homes, alternative birthing centers, hospitals, and ambulatory-care settings
      - **b)** Apply equally in urban, suburban, and rural localities
    - **5)** Standards established by various groups
      - **a)** State boards of nursing through nurse practice acts or promulgated rules and regulations
      - **b)** Professional organizations: e.g., American Nurses Association (ANA); Congress for Nursing Practice; and International Council of Nursing (ICN)

c) Specialty nursing organizations: e.g., Association of Women's Health, Obstetric, and Neonatal Nurses (AWHONN); National Association of Neonatal Nurses (NANN); and American College of Nurse-Midwives (ACNM)
d) Federal organizations and guidelines: e.g., the Joint Commission (formerly JCAHO)

!

e. Standards of care and negligence and malpractice
1) **Negligence** is omitting an act or deviating from the standard of care when carrying out an act that a reasonably prudent person with the same level of duty would not omit or commit under similar circumstances
a) Examples of omission: failing to give a medication, failing to assess properly, failing to notify a physician of a change in a client's condition
b) Examples of commission: giving medication to wrong client, placing an infant in wrong crib
2) Elements of negligence
a) There was a duty to provide care
b) Duty was breached
c) Injury occurred
d) Breach of duty caused injury
3) **Malpractice**: negligent action of a professional person
4) Nurses not meeting appropriate standards of care could be subject to allegations of negligence or malpractice

f. Nurse's responsibility in preventing negligence and malpractice
1) Obtain and maintain current information regarding state Nurse Practice Act
2) Obtain and maintain current information on internal and external standards of practice
3) Seek continuing education to remain current in specialty area
4) Develop a positive, empowering relationship with clients; see clients as important members of the health care team
5) Be thorough in completing and reporting assessments and implementing care
6) Maintain clear, concise, accurate, and complete documentation
7) Question appropriateness of care when harm to a client could occur

Practice to Pass

A nurse waited until the end of the shift to chart the medications given while on duty. The nurse also gave pain medications based on knowledge of the health care provider's routine orders without looking at the medication record, relying on information passed on during shift report. Inadvertently the nurse gave a pain medication an hour after the previous dose had been given. Discuss why the nurse should or should not be terminated by the employer.

C. Legal considerations for client care

1. Health care reform
a. The United States leads the world in health care spending, yet has one of the highest **infant mortality rates** (infant death rates) among all industrialized countries
b. A primary factor related to infant mortality (deaths under one year of age per 1000 live births) is an increase in delivery of low birth weight infants, which is linked to the lack of prenatal care
c. Barriers to access to prenatal care
1) Costs of health care, which continue to increase
2) Limited financial resources
3) Uncoordinated service systems
4) Individual behaviors and **beliefs** (things accepted as true, especially as a tenet or a body of tenets accepted by an ethnocultural group) concerning health care
5) Bureaucratic obstacles, such as complicated, lengthy application forms for Medicaid
6) Lack of availability of maternal services in certain parts of the country
7) Underfunded and overcrowded publicly supervised clinics
8) Difficulty in recruiting and retaining health care providers in publicly subsidized clinics

9) Lack of coordinated services for needy individuals
10) Inaccessibility to prenatal services because of transportation, location, and lack of child care facilities

d. Federal and state governments, through policies and legislation, have implemented strategies to resolve these barriers by
1) Broadening health insurance coverage for childbearing women and infants
2) Improving coordination and funding of public programs
3) Simplifying bureaucratic procedures
4) Increasing number of maternity care providers
5) Establishing a national council on children and health
6) Raising public awareness nationally

e. Need to continue to seek reform to further control costs, improve access to care, and improve quality of health care
1) Develop novel ways of thinking about and providing health care services with primary health care services as a foundation upon which all other secondary and tertiary services are built
2) Provide primary health care to all segments of population, focusing on
a) Health promotion
b) Prevention
c) Individual responsibility for one's own health

2. Managed care: private sector solution for decreasing health care costs

a. Health insurance plans that combine
1) Delivery of health care services
2) Financing of those services
3) Controlling use of services

b. Philosophy of managed care organizations includes
1) Health promotion and disease prevention
2) Desire to avoid serious disease and costly treatment services

c. To meet expenses and make reasonable profits, companies are reimbursing providers with less money per client served while increasing case loads

d. Creates a climate in which providers have
1) Little time and few resources with which to provide care
2) Financial disincentives for providers to give adequate services to their clients

e. Consequences
1) Fewer expensive tests or costly procedures performed, even if provider believes they are justified
2) Shortened hospital stays
3) Increased use of unlicensed assistive health care workers

3. Shortened hospital stays

a. During early- to mid-1990s, hospital stays after birth were shortened to 24 hours or less

b. Consequently, there was not enough time for maternal and parental teaching regarding infant and self-care
1) Cases of infant dehydration with harmful consequences were reported
2) First-time mothers unable to master breastfeeding before discharge
3) Some mothers not able to recognize signs of jaundice that may lead to brain damage

c. Several states passed laws requiring longer stays

d. U.S. Congress passed Senate Bill 969, the Newborns' and Mothers' Health Protection Act of 1996
1) Set a national standard requiring health insurance and employer-provided benefit plans to cover minimum hospital stays of
a) 48 hours after a vaginal delivery

b) 96 hours after delivery by cesarean section
c) Physicians can write an early discharge order after consulting with mother and if health plan provides postdelivery follow-up care, including home care, within 24 to 72 hours of discharge

2) Even with federal law mandating a longer postpartum stay, nurses are still responsible for
a) Verbal and written instructions about infant and self-care, and signs and symptoms indicating a problem
b) Evaluation of parents' learning
c) Recommending timely follow-up care, including a home visit, when mother seems at risk after a longer stay

4. Unlicensed assistive personnel (UAPs)

a. UAPs are health care workers who have no defined body of knowledge or educational preparation upon which to base their practice
1) Uncredentialed
2) No state or federal regulatory body to validate their competence

! **b.** Nurses are responsible for delegation of tasks to UAPs
1) UAPs can perform repetitive tasks, which are clearly defined and for which they have been trained
2) Nurses should obtain information on UAPs' training and skills prior to delegating tasks
3) Inappropriate delegation to UAPs increases nurse's liability and may jeopardize nurse's license
4) Nurses retain accountability for outcomes of care delegated to UAPs

c. What cannot be delegated to UAPs
1) Essential nursing processes of assessing, diagnosing a problem, planning client care, and evaluating outcomes of care
2) UAPs specifically do not perform assessments
3) Judgments about client status
4) Client teaching, including discharge instructions

5. Nurse's role as client advocate
a. Maintain current information about issues critical to client care
b. Educate clients and other significant persons about such issues
c. Become involved in the political process as an advocate for quality health care for all health care recipients
d. Ensure that interpreter services are used when necessary and in an appropriate fashion

II. ETHICAL ISSUES

A. Ethics and legal issues are interrelated as shown in Table 1-1

1. Law is based on a rights model establishing rules of conduct to define
a. Relationships among individuals
b. Relationships to impersonal entities such as agencies or hospitals
c. Formal and binding relationships

2. Ethics is based on a responsibility or duty model examining what our behavior ought to be in relation to ourselves, other human beings, and the environment
a. Incorporates factors such as
1) Risks
2) Benefits
3) Other relationships
4) Concerns
5) Needs and abilities of persons affected by and affecting decisions
b. Subject to philosophical, moral, and individual interpretations

Table 1-1 Differences between Law and Ethics

	Law	Ethics
Origin	Social rules and regulations; external to the individual	Individual values, beliefs, and interpretations; internal to the individual
Focus	Society as a whole; behavior of individuals; acts committed or omitted	Individual in society; relationship of attitudes and motives to behavior; desired behavior to achieve goodness
Regulation	Boards of nursing, statutes, courts	Professional organizations, ethics committees

B. Some ethical principles used in clinical practice

1. Respect: recognition of dignity of each person and his or her right to make decisions and to live or die by those decisions
2. Autonomy: recognition of an individual's personal freedom and self-determination; the right to choose what will happen to one's own person
3. Beneficence: duty to do good
4. Nonmaleficence: duty to do no harm
5. Veracity: duty to tell the truth
6. Fidelity: duty to keep one's promise or word
7. Justice: equitable distribution of risks and benefits, obligation to be fair to everyone

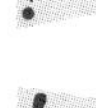

8. Confidentiality: holding information entrusted in the context of special relationships as private; protection of individual's right to privacy
9. Informed consent: contains four elements—disclosure or information, comprehension, voluntary agreement, competency to make decisions
10. Universality: same principle must apply for everyone regardless of time, place, or person involved

C. Ethical decision-making framework (similar to the nursing process); use acronym MORAL

1. M: Massage the dilemma
   a. Identify and define issues in dilemma
   b. Determine who owns the problem, information, decision, and its consequences
   c. Establish facts as best possible
   d. Consider opinions, values, and moral position of major players
   e. Identify value conflicts
2. O: Outline the options
   a. Examine all options fully, including less realistic and conflicting ones
   b. Identify pros and cons of all options
   c. Fully comprehend options and alternatives available
3. R: Resolve the dilemma
   a. Review issues and options
   b. Apply ethical principles to each option
   c. Decide best option for action based on views of all those concerned
4. A: Act by applying chosen option
5. L: Look back and evaluate entire process, including implementation
   a. Ensure that all those involved are able to follow through on final option
   b. Revise decision as indicated, starting process with initial step

D. Ways nurses can maintain legal rights within ethical dilemmas

1. Recognize difference between legal rights and ethical views; legal rights must be provided to client

2. Realize that nurse's personal ethical views and values may differ greatly from client's value system
   a. Understanding one's personal views and values provides nurse with objectivity when caring for clients and when serving as a consultant for decision making by the client
   b. The client's values are the focus of clinical work, rather than the nurse's values, unless the nurse is morally opposed to the client's values
   c. In this case, the nurse removes him- or herself from the client interaction and finds another nurse who is morally comfortable with the issue (e.g., abortion)
3. Remain current about recent judicial decisions in own jurisdiction and incorporate these standards and rights into nursing care
4. If a legal standard does not exist for a particular ethical issue, practice is guided by ethics of profession and by personal moral values
5. Follow established legal principles first when conflict occurs

E. "Clients' rights" intersect law and ethics in maternity nursing practice

1. Informed consent
   a. Designed to allow clients to make intelligent decisions regarding their own health care
   b. Information to be provided by individual who is ultimately responsible for treatment or procedure, generally the health care provider
   c. Information must be clearly and concisely presented in a manner understandable to client
   d. Components of informed consent
      1) Nature and purpose of treatment or procedure
      2) Risks and benefits
      3) Significant treatment alternatives
      4) Probabilities of success
      5) Consequences of receiving no treatment or procedure
      6) Right to refuse a specific treatment or procedure and that refusing a specific treatment will not result in withdrawal of all support or care
   e. Nurse's role in obtaining informed consent
      1) Preferably, be present during health care provider's conversation with client about informed consent
      2) Clarify information physician provides
      3) Determine that client understands information before making a decision
      4) Sign consent form as witness to client's signature, which indicates that client agreeing to treatment or procedure was the person who signed informed consent form
      5) Client may need to sign a form to release health care provider and agency from liability when treatment, medication, or procedure is refused after appropriate information has been provided
2. Right to privacy
   a. The right of clients to keep their person and property free from public scrutiny
   b. Only the health professional responsible for a client's care should examine client and share information about client's treatment, condition, and prognosis
   c. If information needs to be shared with others, such as insurance companies or referral health care professionals, an authorization for release of client information should be obtained from competent clients or their surrogate decision maker
   d. Whenever a situation requires release of information, client should be consulted regarding what information may be released and to whom
3. Confidentiality
   a. Maintaining confidentiality is crucial for development of a trusting relationship between client and provider
      1) Information requested of clients is highly personal and intimate
      2) Is considered privileged conversation

b. Right to confidentiality of medical records may be waived by action or word when
   1) Lawsuit is pursued and records are a source of evidence
   2) Consent is given for information to be released to insurance companies or employers
   3) Public good takes precedence and providers are required by law to report some findings (e.g., child abuse, gunshot wounds, some communicable diseases)

c. The Health Insurance Portability and Accountability Act (HIPAA) is a federal law providing protection of client confidentiality in medical records

F. Ethical considerations in maternity nursing

1. Assisted reproduction
   a. Artificial insemination
   b. In vitro fertilization and embryo transfer
   c. Gamete intrafallopian transfer
   d. Surrogate childbearing
2. Amniocentesis and chorionic villus sampling
3. Abortion
4. Fetal or embryo research
5. Cord blood banking
6. The Human Genome Project and genetic counseling
7. Fetal rights versus maternal rights
   a. Fetus is not viewed as a person by U.S. Supreme Court even if "viable"
   b. Advances in technology have enabled monitoring and treatment of fetus
   c. Fetus is given consideration as a client separate from mother
      1) Treatment of fetus involves the mother
      2) Leads to contradictory moral claims on ethical obligation to do good and avoid harm
      3) Fundamental right of expectant mothers to make informed, uncoerced decisions regarding medical intervention to themselves and fetus
      4) When maternal–fetal conflict occurs, it involves two clients, both of whom deserve respect and treatment
      5) Cases are best resolved through internal hospital mechanisms such as counseling, interventions of specialists, or ethics committees
      6) Judicial intervention should be a last resort

Practice to Pass

The recommended lifesaving treatment for a newborn's congenital anomaly is surgery. The parents refuse surgery for their newborn. When exploring the reasons for their refusal, the nurse finds the parents have strong beliefs that intentional cutting of the body will result in spiritual death. How can the nurse help resolve the conflict between the parents' convictions and the recommended medical treatment?

G. Nurses' responsibilities when preparing for ethical decision making in maternity nursing

1. Anticipate ethical dilemmas
2. Identify attitudes, values, and beliefs about ethical dilemmas taking into consideration the influence of cultural, religious, and social factors on development of values
3. Recognize influence of personal values on care provided to clients by engaging in values clarification activities
4. Review and update theoretical knowledge base
   a. Gather current information on technologic advances and changing trends in maternity nursing
   b. Review ethical principles and practice codes in regard to new technology and trends
   c. Become familiar with client's knowledge base by reading lay literature related to maternity advances
5. Attend continuing education programs related to ethical issues and decision making
   a. Participate in ethics committees with other health care professionals
   b. Provide inservice programs to peers on ethical issues and decision making
6. Review research journals regarding current trends in ethical decision making, comparing and contrasting the results with what is occurring in clinical practice

7. Evaluate current social norms by following social, legal, religious, and political debates that may influence clinical decision making and quality care for clients experiencing dilemmas
8. Avoid judgments about the life decisions of others
   a. Aim to accept values of others and their decisions regarding issues and provisions of care
   b. Do not allow personal beliefs and values to interfere with provision of quality care
9. Understand legal implications of issues
10. Develop appropriate strategies for ethical decision making

III. CULTURAL HEALTH BELIEFS AND CULTURAL COMPETENCE

A. **Beliefs about pregnancy and childbearing:** are significantly influenced by culture or cultures in which expectant family was raised and is now living
   1. Ideas about conception, pregnancy, and childbearing practices are passed down from generation to generation
   2. Beliefs are acculturated into society without validation or being completely understood
   3. Many societies do not consider pregnancy an illness
      a. May not seek advice from health care professionals or prenatal care
      b. May seek and follow advice from elders and family members

B. **National and global populations:** characterized by increasing diversity

! C. ***Diversity***: differences in race, ethnicity, national origin, religion, age, gender, sexual orientation, ability/disability, social and economic status or class, education, and related attributes of groups of people in society

D. **Every human being is *ethnocentric***
   1. Subconsciously view other people by using own group of customs as the standard for all judgments
   2. View others' ways as inferior to personal ways
   3. Need to avoid **cultural imposition**: imposing personal cultural beliefs and practices on clients while trivializing or disregarding theirs

E. **Developing *cultural competency***
   1. Concept of cultural competency
      ! a. A complex integration of knowledge, attitudes, and skills that enhance cross-cultural communication and appropriate, effective interaction with others
      b. A process in which one continuously strives to effectively work within cultural context of an individual, family, or community from a diverse cultural background
   2. Components of cultural competency
      a. Cultural awareness
      b. Cultural knowledge
      c. Cultural skill
      d. Cultural encounter
   3. To become culturally competent the nurse should:
      a. Critically examine one's own cultural beliefs
      b. Identify personal biases, attitudes, stereotypes, and prejudices
      c. Make a conscious decision to respect values and beliefs of others
      d. Use sensitive, current language when describing client's culture
      e. Learn rituals, customs, practices, values, and beliefs for major cultural and ethnic groups with whom one has contact
      f. Include cultural assessment and assessment of family's expectations of health care system as a routine part of perinatal nursing care
      g. Incorporate family's cultural practices into perinatal care as much as possible

Practice to Pass

As a new manager on the obstetric unit, the nurse quickly realizes that there are cultural conflicts between the nursery nurses, who are Filipino, and the new mothers, most of whom are African American or Latino and of low socioeconomic status. How can the nurse manager help to improve communication and cultural sensitivity between the nursery nurses and the new mothers?

- **h.** Foster an attitude of respect for and cooperation with alternative healers and caregivers whenever possible
- **i.** Provide for services of an interpreter if language barriers exist to assure accuracy of information obtained; family members or other lay people may or may not be skilled in medical terms; also, it is inappropriate to use untrained lay people when gathering information of a private and sensitive nature
- **j.** Learn the language (or at least key phrases) of at least one cultural group with whom one interacts
- **k.** Recognize that ultimately it is the expectant mother's right to make her own health care choices
- **l.** Evaluate whether client's health beliefs have any potential negative consequences for client's health

F. Incorporating cultural assessment and planning into perinatal care

1. Cultural assessment
   - **a.** Identify main beliefs, values, and behaviors that relate to pregnancy and childbearing
     - **1)** Ethnic background
     - **2)** Amount of affiliation with ethnic group
     - **3)** Patterns of decision making
     - **4)** Religious preferences
     - **5)** Language
     - **6)** Communication style
     - **7)** Common etiquette practices
   - **b.** Explore expectant mother's and family's expectation of health care system
2. Planning to meet cultural beliefs
   - **a.** Consider extent to which expectant mother's personal values, beliefs, and customs agree with the following:
     - **1)** Expectant family's identified cultural group
     - **2)** Nurse providing care
     - **3)** Health care agency
   - **b.** If there are discrepancies, determine whether expectant family's system is supportive, neutral, or harmful in relation to possible interventions
   - **c.** If supportive or neutral, incorporate cultural practices into plan of care
   - **d.** If cultural practices might pose a threat to health of expectant mother or fetus:
     - **1)** Discuss with client and understand reasons for refusal
     - **2)** Identify ways to persuade expectant mother to accept proposed interventions
     - **3)** Accept expectant mother's decision to refuse intervention if client is not willing to adapt her belief system
     - **4)** Explain alternative therapies that might be acceptable to expectant mother within her cultural beliefs

G. Cultural variation during pregnancy, labor, birth, and the postpartum

1. Support system
   - **a.** Formalized assistance from health care providers
     - **1)** Western medicine is perceived as having curative rather than preventive focus; pregnancy is a physiologic state that will become pathologic
     - **2)** Subcultures view pregnancy as a normal physiologic process, not an illness or condition requiring curative services of a health care provider, which may result in delay or neglect in seeking prenatal care
   - **b.** Nontraditional support systems
     - **1)** Traditionally, emphasis on female support and guidance
     - **2)** Some ethnic/cultural groups, such as Orthodox Jews, Muslims, Chinese, or Asian Indians, have strict religious and cultural prohibitions against husbands or any man viewing a woman's body during labor and birth

3) Family and social network, especially grandmother or other maternal relatives, are of primary importance in advising and supporting expectant mother
4) Traditional healers

2. Prescriptive, restrictive, and taboo beliefs and practices
   a. Prescriptive beliefs and practices: describe expectancies of behavior, those things that an expectant mother should do to have a healthy pregnancy and baby (phrased positively)
   b. Restrictive beliefs and practices: limit choices and behaviors, describe things that mother should not do in order to achieve a positive outcome (phrased negatively)
   c. Taboo beliefs and practices: restrictions with supernatural consequences, those things that are likely to harm mother or baby
   d. Box 1-1 provides examples of prescriptive, restrictive, and taboo beliefs and practices
3. Expressions of labor pain
   a. Factors interacting to influence labor and perception of pain
      1) Cultural attitude toward normalcy and conduct of birth
      2) Expectations of how a woman should act in labor
      3) Role of significant others
      4) Physiologic processes involved
   b. Examples of responses to labor by many women of a cultural group
      1) Filipino women feel it is best to lie quietly
      2) Middle Eastern women are verbally expressive, sometimes crying and screaming loudly while refusing pain medication
      3) Samoan women believe that no verbal expressions of pain are permissible and only "spoiled" Caucasian women need any analgesia
      4) Hispanic women are instructed by their *parteras* to endure pain with patience and close the mouth, for opening it to cry out would cause uterus to rise
      5) Japanese, Chinese, Vietnamese, Laotian, and others of Asian descent maintain that screaming or crying out during labor or birth is shameful; birth is believed to be painful but something to be endured
   c. Culturally appropriate ways of preparing for labor and birth
      1) Assisting with or participating in birth from time of adolescence
      2) Listening to birth and baby stories told by respected elderly women
      3) Following special dietary and activity prescriptions in antepartal period
      4) Learning formal breathing and relaxation techniques
4. Postpartum
   a. Pregnancy and birth are considered most dangerous and vulnerable by those subscribing to Western medicine
   b. For many other cultures, postpartal period is a vulnerable time for mother and newborn and requires special practices that
      1) Serve to mobilize support for new mother
      2) May involve restrictive dietary customs or activity level, taboos, and rituals associated with purification and seclusion, all of which positively influence mother's mental health after delivery
   c. Concept of postpartum vulnerability is based on beliefs related to imbalance or pollution
      1) Imbalance: disharmony caused by processes of pregnancy and birth
      2) Pollution: caused by "unclean" bleeding associated with birth and postpartum period
      3) Ritual seclusion and activity restrictions may reduce risk of increasing personal vulnerability to spirit influence or risk of spreading evil and misfortune
      4) Restitution of physical balance and purification occur through mechanisms such as dietary restrictions, ritual baths, seclusion, restriction of activity, and other ceremonial events

Box 1-1

Examples of Prescriptive, Restrictive, and Taboo Practices during Pregnancy, Labor, Birth, and the Postpartum for a Variety of Cultural Groups

Prescriptive Practices

Navajo: During labor, wear a necklace made of juniper seeds and beads to assist with a safe birth; bury placenta after birth to symbolize child being tied to land; feed baby a mixture with juniper to cleanse baby's insides and rid it of mucus
Crow Indian: Remain active during pregnancy to aid baby's circulation
Polish Americans: To have a healthy pregnancy and baby, pregnant mothers are expected to seek preventive care, eat well, and get adequate rest
Latino: Wear a *muneco* (special article of clothing) to ensure a safe delivery and prevent morning sickness
Chinese: Add more meat to diet to make blood stronger for fetus
Mexican: Keep active during pregnancy to ensure a small baby and easy delivery
Filipino: Continue daily baths and frequent shampoos during pregnancy to produce a clean baby
Haitian, Mexican: Continue sexual intercourse to lubricate birth canal and prevent a dry labor
Hispanic: Bury placenta to prevent mother from having afterbirth pains

Restrictive Practices

Egyptian: Do not bathe during postpartum period as it could expose mother to colds and chills
Navajo: Clothes should not be purchased for infant before birth as preparing for infant is forbidden by Indian tradition, and newborn may not survive; do not tie knots or braids or allow baby's father to do so as it will cause difficult labor
African American, Latino, white, Asian: Do not reach above one's head as cord will wrap around baby's neck
Vietnamese: Avoid weddings and funerals or bad fortune will come to baby
Vietnamese, Filipino, Samoan: Do not continue sexual intercourse; harm will come to expectant mother and baby
Latino: Fathers are not allowed in delivery room or to see mother or baby before both have been cleaned as this can cause harm to baby

Taboo Practices

Navajo: Do not have a weaving comb (rug) with more than five points or baby will have extra fingers; do not jump around or ride a horse when pregnant or it will induce labor; do not cut a baby's hair when it is small or he or she will have cognitive problems later in life
Mexican: Avoid lunar eclipses and moonlight or baby may be born with a deformity
Haitian: Do not get involved with persons who cast spells or baby will be eaten in the womb
Orthodox Jewish: Do not say baby's name before the naming ceremony or harm might come to baby
African American: Do not have picture taken during pregnancy or it might cause stillbirth
Korean: Do not eat chicken, duck, rabbit, goat, crab, sparrow, pork, or blemished fruit to guard child from unwanted physical characteristics (chicken may cause bumpy skin, blemished fruit may cause an unpleasant child)

5. Hot and cold theory: humoral balance and imbalance
   a. Health is a state of balance among body humors or body fluids (blood, phlegm, black bile, and yellow bile) that manifests itself in a somewhat wet, warm body
   b. Illness results from a humoral imbalance causing body to become excessively dry, cold, hot, wet, or a combination of these states
   c. Natural balance can be restored by therapeutic use of food, herbs, and medications, which are also classified as wet or dry, hot or cold

d. To achieve balance, illnesses are treated with substances having the opposite property of the illness
e. Pregnancy is a "hot" state and a great deal of heat is thought to be lost during birth process
f. Postpartum practices focus on restoring balance between hot and cold
   1) Avoidance of cold: air or food
   2) Example: Haitians believe that exposure to cold air may cause a uterine "cold"; use of sanitary napkin is thought to prevent air from entering vagina
   3) Fruits and vegetables, milk products, and foods that are sour to taste may be considered "cold" foods; animal products, chilies, spices, and ginger may be considered hot foods

H. An example of cultural influences on an expectant family: an African-American family

1. Variations in African-American families
   a. Influenced by geographic location, level of acculturation, religious background, and socioeconomic status
   b. Socioeconomic status very significant to consider as persons of different cultural backgrounds who live in poverty share similar social problems
2. Adaptive strengths of African-American family that help bring about positive pregnancy outcomes
   a. Kinship bonds
      1) Kinship network important source of support
      2) Not always along "bloodlines"
      3) Based on complex patterns of co-residence and kinship-based exchange networks linking various domestic units
      4) Family units have broad household boundaries with strong bonds to three generations of households
      5) Individuals within network are involved in cooperative domestic exchanges
      6) May include a large number of people inside and outside nuclear family creating a complex family network: partner, parents, children, uncles, aunts, preachers, friends, siblings, cousins
      7) Networks are often well organized and provide lifelong relationships that offer stability
   b. Family roles
      1) Role of men may be inconsistent, but many men have a great investment in family
      2) Women and men may have significant role flexibility, especially in care of children, childrearing, and household responsibilities
      3) Members of kinship network may take on roles usually assumed by nuclear family members
         a) Maternal or paternal aunt or grandmother may share or assume responsibility for child care
         b) Infant may be adopted informally and reared by extended family members who have resources not available to child's parents
   c. Religion and church
      1) Religious system provides support in pastors, deacons, deaconesses, and other church members
      2) Spirituality influences health and well-being
      3) Religious beliefs provide spiritual comfort and support
      4) Church activities may provide a social life for members of entire family
      5) During pregnancy, church family may promote physical health of expectant mother by encouraging early prenatal care and maintaining a lifestyle that fosters healthy pregnancy outcomes

Practice to Pass

A nurse was caring for a 15-year-old African-American client on the day of discharge after the birth of her first infant. When the nurse entered the room, both the maternal and paternal grandmothers were present and continually made comments about the care and teaching the nurse was providing the client. How should the nurse handle the situation so the provision of care and education of the new mother can continue?

IV. FAMILY-CENTERED MATERNITY CARE

! **A. What is a *family*?**

1. A group of individuals related by blood, marriage, or mutual goals
2. A group of individuals who are bound by strong emotional ties, a sense of belonging, and a passion for being involved in one another's lives
3. Critical attributes of family
   - **a.** Family is a system or unit
   - **b.** Its members may or may not be related and may or may not live together
   - **c.** Unit may or may not contain children
   - **d.** There is a commitment and attachment among unit members that include future obligation
   - **e.** Unit caregiving functions consist of protection, nourishment, and socialization of its members
4. Types of families
   - **a.** Traditional forms
     - **1)** Nuclear family: father, mother, and child living together but apart from both sets of grandparents
     - **2)** Extended family: three generations, including grandparents, married brothers and sisters and their families
   - **b.** Nontraditional forms
     - **1)** Single-parent family: divorced, never married, separated, or widowed man or women and at least one child; considered at greatest risk for lack of support of all family types
     - **2)** Three-generational family: any combination of first-, second-, and third-generation members living within a household
     - **3)** Dyad family: husband and wife or other couple living alone without children
     - **4)** Step-parent family: one or both spouses have been divorced or widowed and have remarried into a family with at least one child
     - **5)** Blended or reconstituted family: a combination of two families with children from one or both families and sometimes children of newly married couple
     - **6)** Cohabiting family: an unmarried couple living together
     - **7)** Gay or lesbian family: a homosexual couple living together with or without children; children may be adopted, from previous relationships, or artificially conceived
     - **8)** Adoptive family: single persons or couples who have at least one child who is not biologically related to them and to whom they have legally become parents
5. Family is a system nested within and influenced by broader systems such as neighborhood, class, region, and country
6. These broader systems are the context that permeates and circumscribes individuals and their family, and include
   - **a.** Ethnicity
   - **b.** Race
   - **c.** Social class
   - **d.** Religion and spirituality
   - **e.** Environment

B. The family development theory of family life: there are eight stages in family development from leaving home as single young adult to aging families accepting shifting generational roles

1. Family stage identified by age of oldest child
2. Theories initially developed to describe middle-class North American family life

3. Developmental tasks for family during childbearing years
   a. Joining of families: couples without children
      1) Finding, furnishing, and maintaining a first home
      2) Establishing mutually satisfactory means of support
      3) Allocating responsibilities
      4) Establishing mutually acceptable personal, emotional, and sexual roles
      5) Interacting with in-laws, relatives, friends, and community
      6) Planning for children or no children
      7) Maintaining couple motivation and morale
   b. Families with young children: childbearing with oldest child under age 30 months
      1) Arranging space (territory) for child
      2) Financing childbearing and childrearing
      3) Assuming mutual responsibility for child care and nurturing
      4) Facilitating role learning of family members or defining and assuming maternal and paternal roles
      5) Adjusting to changed communication patterns to accommodate a newborn and young child
      6) Planning for subsequent children
      7) Realigning intergenerational patterns to establish grandparent roles and grandparent–grandchild subsystems
      8) Maintaining family members' motivation and morale
      9) Establishing family rituals and routines
4. Theory has been modified to describe a variety of family lifecycles including divorced families, remarried families, economically disadvantaged families, and adoptive families

C. **The childbearing family:** a family in crisis
1. Childbearing is a developmental crisis
   a. Normal and routinely experienced during process of growth and development
   b. Periods of marked physical, psychological, and social change characterized by disturbances in life's patterns or a sense of disorganization
   c. Certain tasks must be faced and mastered by individual or family to achieve next maturational stage and be ready for further growth and development
2. Situational crises are unexpected, stressful external events that may or may not coincide with a developmental crisis, such as a high-risk pregnancy

D. **Historical trends in moving toward family-centered *maternity care*** (health care provided to the childbearing family that involves physiologic, psychosocial, and cultural aspects of care)
1. Midwifery, originally a branch of medicine that deals with practice of assisting in childbirth, has been practiced since earliest of times
   a. Midwives are mentioned in Bible
   b. The midwife, meaning "with women," was responsible for delivery of infants
2. Obstetrics, as a branch of medicine, was introduced in late 19th century
   a. Branch of medicine that deals with phenomena and management of pregnancy, labor, and the postpartum in low- and high-risk circumstances
   b. Certified Nurse Midwifery is now used to delineate practice of nurses who are trained at the master's level, certified by examination, and responsible for managing childbearing women and neonates in collaboration with other providers
3. During 1920s and 1930s, childbirth moved from home to hospital
   a. Advances in medical services introduced various drugs and obstetric procedures to control pain and combat infection; these were provided by hospitals and superseded giving birth in home environment

- **b.** Mobility and urbanization minimized social network of female support for childbearing women
- **c.** Childbirth became viewed as a pathophysiologic, physician-centered process
- **d.** Traditional maternity care reorganized into subspecialties
- **e.** Intrapartum care became based on a surgical, multitransfer system
  - **1)** Mothers labored in one room, delivered in another, recovered in a third room, and spent remainder of hospital stay on a postpartum unit
  - **2)** Newborns were immediately separated from their mothers and kept in a separate nursery to be transported to their mothers for feedings on a predetermined schedule
- **f.** After World War II, focus of care shifted from provider of care to recipient of care, and then to a broader view involving psychosocial, cultural, and physiologic aspects of the childbearing family
- **g.** By the 1960s, professionals and consumers were concerned with a continuing assumption that every woman was a "disaster waiting to happen"
  - **1)** Traditional hospital care detracted from biophysical development of new family
  - **2)** Consumers sought to understand technology and to take interest in their own health and basic self-care skills, assuming many primary care functions
  - **3)** Focus of care needed to shift to promote health and well-being with family unit as recipient of care
  - **4)** Nurses became significant members of health care team
    - **a)** Foster self-care by readily providing information
    - **b)** Acknowledge family members' right to ask questions and become actively involved in their own care
    - **c)** Encourage family members to speak up for preferences in dealing with health care providers

E. Philosophy of family-centered maternity care: childbirth is a natural event

1. Components of **family-centered maternity care** philosophy
   - **a.** Childbearing is a family event
     - **1)** Family members need to be included in all aspects of care
     - **2)** Family members are capable of making decisions about childbearing care when provided education, support, and advocacy
   - **b.** The reproductive health of entire family is important to health of society
   - **c.** Childbirth is a normal physiologic process that generally requires few medical interventions and is a natural life event rather than an illness
     - **1)** Childbirth is generally an uncomplicated, joyful event for families
     - **2)** An understanding of social and psychological factors related to childbirth improves family satisfaction with and provision of nursing care
   - **d.** Parenting is learned
     - **1)** There are many physical, psychological, and social changes to be navigated during transition to parenthood
     - **2)** Nurses and health care professionals can help expectant families develop appropriate expectations, knowledge, and skills for good parenting
2. Goals of care
   - **a.** To assist expectant parents to make informed decisions about their own health care
   - **b.** To foster family unity while providing safe, quality, cost-effective care
3. Components of care
   - **a.** Collaboration with parents, siblings, and extended family members during entire childbearing experience
   - **b.** Childbirth preparation of both parents, siblings, and others as designated by mother

c. Involvement of significant other in entire birthing process
d. Choice of birthing environment when possible
e. Sibling visitation
f. Early discharge programs
g. Strategies to foster family members' attachment to newborn
h. Parental leave options for both parents
i. Nursing management for families throughout childbearing cycle

F. Prenatal care providers and expertise are presented in Table 1-2

1. Maternity health care providers differ in their philosophical approach to care
2. Expectant women and their families need to know their options and choose provider with whom they are most comfortable

G. Nursing members of health care team

1. Maternal/child nurses: nurse generalists who have graduated from an accredited basic nursing program and have additional continuing education in specialized area of maternity nursing
2. Lay midwife: provider of pregnancy, birth, and postpartum care for low-risk women in community settings; often are neither certified nor registered nurses; often not covered by insurance; often perform home deliveries; however, practice varies by region and state
3. Advanced practice nurses: professional nurses who have additional education preparation at least at the graduate level, certification in a specific advanced area of practice, expertise in a specific clinical area, and function in an expanded role
   a. Certified nurse-midwives (CNMs): individuals educated in the two disciplines of nursing and midwifery, and are certified by American College of Nurse-Midwives (ACNM)
      1) Prepared to manage independently care of women and families at low risk for complications during pregnancy and birth, routine gynecological services, and care of normal newborns
      2) Take a holistic approach in assessing and identifying needs of expectant mother and her family
      3) Provide cost-effective care that achieves outcomes that are consistently better than national statistical averages
   b. Nurse practitioners (NPs): primary care providers focusing on physical and psychosocial assessments leading to clinical diagnosis and treatment while seeking physician consultation when necessary; includes neonatal nurse practitioner, a nurse with a master's degree in nursing specializing in care of neonates, and who often provides care to hospitalized neonates in intensive care units

Table 1-2 Prenatal Care Providers and Expertise

Levels of Prenatal Care	Types of Care Provider	Prenatal Care Expertise
Low-risk pregnancy (basic care)	Family physician; nurse practitioner; certified nurse-midwife; obstetrician; lay midwife	Initial and ongoing risk assessment; routine physical and laboratory assessment; monitoring normal pregnancy progress; psychosocial support; childbirth education; consultation and referral
Moderate-risk pregnancy (specialty care)	Family physician; obstetrician	Basic care; basic fetal diagnostic testing (ultrasound, biophysical profile, amniotic fluid analysis); management of medical and obstetric complications; consultation and referral
High-risk pregnancy (subspecialty care)	Maternal-fetal medicine specialist or perinatologist; geneticist	Basic and specialty care; advanced fetal diagnostic testing (targeted ultrasound, echocardiogram); advanced fetal treatment (intrauterine transfusion, cardiac dysrhythmia management); medical, surgical, and genetic consultation; management of severe obstetric complications

Practice to Pass

Your best friend just discovered she is pregnant. She asks you, a nurse, who she should go to for prenatal care. How will you respond?

   c. Clinical nurse specialists (CNSs): assume a leadership role within their specialty, focus on improving client care by evaluating nursing practice, recommending improvements, establishing standards of care, and conducting research studies; includes maternal child health CNSs who often work with staff of labor and delivery units in hospitals
4. Unlicensed assistive personnel: carry out activities delegated by and under the supervision of the registered nurse; includes doulas (entry-level position; practitioners are trained by a combination of classroom and hands-on training to provide direct physical care to women in labor, usually from pregnancy through birth and/or postpartum; often reimbursed via fee-for-service as not often covered by insurance)

H. Environments for birth

1. Single-room maternity care (SRMC)
   a. Has replaced multitransfer system that characterized traditional childbirth care
   b. Labor/delivery/recovery and/or postpartum (LDR/LDRP) rooms
      1) Designed and equipped to accommodate entire birthing process, including complicated vaginal deliveries
      2) No screening criteria
      3) Equipment brought to expectant mother based on individual needs and different stages of childbearing process
      4) Newborns are not routinely separated from parents and family after birth
      5) Well infants may remain in room with family under care of maternity nurses who are proficient in both maternal and neonatal nursing
      6) Cesarean births occur in delivery/operating rooms
      7) Preterm and ill newborns are cared for in high-risk nurseries
   c. Advantages of single-room maternity care
      1) Clinical safety
         a) Increased effectiveness in responding to emergencies
         b) Improved communication and continuity of care
         c) Decreased risk of client exposure to many different areas and departmental staff
      2) Marketability
         a) Noninstitutional environment increases market share by attracting parents-to-be and promotes their use of facility for future family needs
         b) Continuity of care and comprehensive cross-training promote recruitment and retention of staff
      3) Cost efficiency
         a) Space is more efficient since SRMC eliminates need for duplication of support area (i.e., utility and linen rooms)
         b) Staffing for one area rather than three combined with increased flexibility of staff through cross-training reduces personnel costs
         c) Nontransfer of care and smaller space decreases cleaning and maintenance
         d) Combined practices of physiologic management with mother–baby nursing help to decrease use of technology and provide support needed for early discharge, thereby reducing operational costs
   d. Risk to implementing SRMC: inability to change culture, staff attrition, and loss of commitment
2. Birth centers
   a. Maternity unit that provides low-technology care in a homelike setting; families generally return home shortly after giving birth
   b. Types of birth centers
      1) Freestanding
         a) Separate from acute care hospital setting

- **b)** Has more autonomy in formulating policies and procedures for center operations and programs of care for clients
- **c)** Provide comprehensive maternity services including prenatal care, education and counseling, intrapartum and postpartum care with home visiting and family planning

2) In-hospital birth centers
- **a)** Located on hospital grounds or inside a hospital
- **b)** Generally provide only intrapartum and early postpartum care

3) Commonalties
- **a)** Both types of centers have capabilities of initiating emergency procedures
- **b)** Have contingency plans for in-hospital obstetric and newborn services
- **c)** Caregivers: CNMs, obstetricians, pediatricians, professional nurses

3. Home births

a. Some families choose to give birth at home as a rejection of physician-directed and hospital-based rituals
- **1)** Many of these expectant mothers are well educated, especially related to childbearing, and are middle- to upper-middle-class
- **2)** May be ideal for low-risk, healthy clients who are motivated to actively participate in the whole childbearing process
- **3)** May be attended by lay nurse-midwives

b. Some women give birth at home through lack of choice or access to health care system

Case Study

During the pregnancy with their second child, an Asian Indian Hindu couple discovered their son had Wiskott–Aldrich syndrome. This syndrome is an X-linked recessive disorder that leads to an early death from a super infection. At the birth of their daughter, the stem cells were harvested from the umbilical cord for a bone marrow transplant to their son.

1. What are the ethical issues involved in using stem cells from one child to improve the health and well-being of another?
2. Are there any cultural conflicts in harvesting stem cells for Hindus or Asian Indians?
3. What is the significance of having a son or daughter for an Asian Indian family?
4. Who might be available to support the family as it adapts to a new child and awaits the results of the compatibility test on the stem cells?
5. What steps should the nurses take to be able to support the family and give appropriate guidance in this situation?

For suggested responses, see page 301.

POSTTEST

POSTTEST

1 A client who has diabetes mellitus that is difficult to regulate is seeking to get pregnant. The nurse working in a primary care provider's office suggests that which health care provider would be an optimal choice?

1. A certified nurse-midwife
2. A family nurse practitioner
3. An obstetrician
4. A maternal-fetal medicine specialist

2 The nursery nurses prefer keep newborns in the nursery except for feeding times, saying they can monitor newborns better in the nursery. They justify this action by saying that the infants need to be available for pediatricians whenever they might make rounds. What type of views are the nursery nurses expressing?

1. Ethnocentric views
2. Culturally aware views
3. Culturally sensitive views
4. Culturally diverse views

3 A client, who is a gravida 14, para 10-3-0-16, gave birth to all her children vaginally. She presents in labor and upon vaginal examination the obstetrician discovers the infant is in footling breech position. The obstetrician plans to do a cesarean section immediately but the client adamantly refuses. How can the nurse help resolve the dilemma?

1. Follow the physician's orders and prepare the client for surgery.
2. Help identify all the options, taking action on the best option for all concerned.
3. Side with the client and refuse to prepare her for surgery.
4. Call the supervisor so she can mediate the dispute.

4 A 16-year-old female client who lives in a state without an emancipated minor law needs to have a dilatation and curettage (D&C) after manual delivery of the placenta. Who can legally give informed consent for the client to have this procedure?

1. The client herself
2. The client's physician
3. The client's mother
4. The client's best friend

5 The maternal-newborn nurse is making a home visit to a client who delivered an infant 48 hours ago. The other young children of the client address the woman who stays in their home three days a week as "Auntie." Why would she most likely be considered part of the family unit?

1. She may be the client's closest colleague.
2. She lives in the same neighborhood the other four days a week.
3. She has no children of her own.
4. She has strong emotional ties with the children.

6 A nursing student who is pregnant asks the antenatal nurse why childbearing is considered a developmental crisis for a family. What should be included in a response by the nurse?

1. It is an abnormal experience in the process of growth and development.
2. It is a period of physical, psychological, and social change causing a sense of disorganization.
3. It is a stressful, unexpected event caused by external factors.
4. The family has already mastered the tasks of this maturational stage.

7 A nurse is the defendant in a lawsuit brought by a client who had a postpartum hemorrhage requiring transfusion of 15 units of blood and a hysterectomy after delivery of her third child. The client had an epidural before delivery and had persistent uterine atony with heavy bleeding immediately after delivery of the placenta. In the immediate postpartum period, the client's uterus continued to get boggy and the client had a heavy, bright rubra lochial flow. The nurse is being sued for not providing appropriate care. Which of the following nursing actions would demonstrate upholding the standard of care for a client experiencing a postpartum hemorrhage?

1. Palpate the fundus every 10–15 minutes and if boggy, massage to expel clots.
2. Have the client empty her bladder only when she has the urge to void.
3. Discontinue the pitocin IV when the uterus is firm and 4 cm above the umbilicus.
4. Do assessments every 30 minutes as indicated on the postpartum flow sheet.

8 During labor the nurse notices that the husband of a Ukrainian client just sits beside the bed and is not actively involved with the client. While the nurse interprets this as not being very supportive, how might the client interpret her husband's actions?

1. The client would prefer more active involvement in coaching from her husband.
2. The client interprets her husband's presence in the labor room as caring.
3. The client would like him to leave the room so her mother could be there instead.
4. The client wants to labor alone with only the hospital staff present.

9 A newly employed public health nurse learns that the United States has a high infant mortality rate and that preterm labor and delivery of low-birth-weight infants (which lead to infant mortality) can be linked to the lack of prenatal care. The nurse suspects which of the following as a reason why many clients are unable to obtain prenatal care?

1. Health care and other services are well coordinated for needy clients.
2. All uninsured pregnant women are eligible for Medicaid.
3. Prenatal care services and providers are not available in certain areas.
4. Many health care providers are willing to provide care in subsidized clinics.

10 A client from the Gusii tribe in Kenya presents in active labor. As the nurse does a vaginal exam she realizes that the client has been circumcised and the vaginal opening is not large enough to admit two fingers. The nurse believes female circumcision is a type of mutilation. What should the nurse do to be able to continue to give appropriate, supportive care?

1. Recognize that her personal beliefs and values differ from those of the client.
2. Report the finding of the circumcision to the primary care provider.
3. Avoid entering the client's room and making further assessments.
4. Accept that personal values and beliefs will interfere with the provision of care.

➤ *See pages 25–26 for Answers and Rationales.*

POSTTEST

ANSWERS & RATIONALES

Pretest

1 **Answer: 2 Rationale:** Reporting all information gathered, such as the headache, may have heightened the physician's concern about progressing preeclampsia. It is the nurse's responsibility to report all information from an assessment. The nurse furthered the negligence by not recognizing all the signs of preeclampsia, an accepted standard of maternal-newborn practice, but the immediate concern of this situation was not reporting all information to the physician. There is no evidence that the nurse failed to document correctly or develop a positive relationship with the client. **Cognitive Level:** Analyzing **Client Need:** Management of Care **Integrated Process:** Nursing Process: Implementation **Content Area:** Fundamentals **Strategy:** The focus of the question is reporting of assessment data. Only the correct option addresses this nursing action. Critical words are *headache* and *elevated BP* and *proteinuria*, all indicating preeclampsia. Knowledge of signs and symptoms of preeclampsia would eliminate all incorrect options. Knowledge of the scope of practice and standards of care helps the nurse to practice within legal parameters. **Reference:** Ricci, S. (2009). *Essentials of maternity, newborn, and women's health nursing* (2nd ed.). Philadelphia, PA: Lippincott Williams & Wilkins, pp. 545–549.

2 **Answer: 4 Rationale:** The legal system is founded on rules and regulations that are external to oneself and that guide society in a formal and binding manner. Ethical issues are subject to an individual's values, beliefs, culture, and interpretation. What is good for a particular individual may vary from person to person, while the law contains rules that guide all who are in the same situation. **Cognitive Level:** Applying **Client Need:** Management of Care **Integrated Process:** Communication and Documentation **Content Area:** Fundamentals **Strategy:** The three incorrect options are individually and internally focused. The legal system is external to the nurse and only the correct option offers an external influence. **Reference:** Ladewig, P., London, M., & Davidson, M. (2009). *Contemporary maternal-newborn nursing care* (7th ed.). Upper Saddle River, NJ: Pearson Education, pp. 149–150.

ANSWERS & RATIONALES

3 **Answer: 1 Rationale:** A nurse signs the consent form as witness to the client's signature. The nurse's signature does not attest to the client's understanding of the procedure, or that the physician fully explained all aspects of the procedure. It is not the nurse's role to explain a procedure to the client, only to reinforce information provided by the physician and clarify any misunderstandings. **Cognitive Level:** Applying **Client Need:** Management of Care **Integrated Process:** Communication and Documentation **Content Area:** Fundamentals **Strategy:** The critical word is *witness*, which means validating the signature. The other answers all deal with understanding and explaining, which are not included in the details of the question or part of witnessing the event. **Reference:** Ricci, S. (2009). *Essentials of maternity, newborn, and women's health nursing* (2nd ed.). Philadelphia, PA: Lippincott Williams & Wilkins, p. 20.

4 **Answer: 2 Rationale:** When clients can eat the foods they prefer, they are more satisfied and recover more quickly. Foods that are provided by the hospital kitchen might be unknown to the client. When one is under stress or ill, there is a longing for foods that are known and liked and culturally accepted. There is no indication that the client wishes to avoid foods that are considered hot. There is no basis for assuming the client has a decreased appetite due to delivery or prefers hamburgers and french fries. **Cognitive Level:** Analyzing **Client Need:** Health Promotion and Maintenance **Integrated Process:** Nursing Process: Diagnosis **Content Area:** Maternal-Newborn **Strategy:** Try to eliminate incorrect options. The client did not eat beef so would be unlikely to prefer hamburger, a form of beef. The client did eat foods so decreased appetite is probably incorrect. Note that avoiding foods that are hot could be a part of the correct answer about preferring known and culturally accepted foods. **Reference:** Ricci, S. (2009). *Essentials of maternity, newborn, and women's health nursing* (2nd ed.). Philadelphia, PA: Lippincott Williams & Wilkins, p. 15.

5 **Answer: 3 Rationale:** As maternity care has become more family centered, efforts are made to keep the family together all the time. This is done by providing single-room maternity care, letting the client define her family and designate who she wants to have present at the birth, and encouraging the family to keep the infant with them in the room so they have more opportunity for bonding and learning about each other. **Cognitive Level:** Applying **Client Need:** Management of Care **Integrated Process:** Caring **Content Area:** Maternal-Newborn **Strategy:** The critical words are *satisfaction* and *changes in the care setting*. Use the knowledge of family-centered care and maternity care to choose the correct response. **Reference:** Ricci, S. (2009). *Essentials of maternity, newborn, and women's health nursing* (2nd ed.). Philadelphia, PA: Lippincott Williams & Wilkins, pp. 4–7.

6 **Answer: 3 Rationale:** Midwifery is the branch of nursing that deals with the practice of assisting women and their families in childbirth. It has been practiced since very early times. Obstetrics was not introduced to medicine until the late 1800s and primarily focuses on high-risk circumstances in pregnancy, labor, and postpartum. Only a small percentage of nurse-midwives currently practice in the home. **Cognitive Level:** Applying **Client Need:** Management of Care **Integrated Process:** Teaching and Learning **Content Area:** Maternal-Newborn **Strategy:** The critical word is *midwifery*, meaning "with women at childbirth." Eliminate the incorrect options because the history of midwifery is ancient, while obstetrics is relatively new to medicine, because midwives and obstetricians practice in the hospital with few births occurring at home, and because midwifery is focused on the normal childbirth experience. **Reference:** Ladewig, P., London, M., & Davidson, M. (2009). *Contemporary maternal-newborn nursing care* (7th ed.). Upper Saddle River, NJ: Pearson Education, p. 4.

7 **Answer: 3 Rationale:** Restrictive beliefs and practices are those things an expectant mother should not do or should avoid so that she will have a positive pregnancy outcome. This type of belief does not promote healthy outcomes, does not prescribe what to do, and does not represent a cultural taboo according to the usual definition of the word. **Cognitive Level:** Applying **Client Need:** Psychosocial Integrity **Integrated Process:** Teaching and Learning **Content Area:** Maternal-Newborn **Strategy:** The critical words are *concern* and *heard*. Use knowledge about different beliefs and practices that clients hear about from other nonprofessionals to choose a restrictive belief, which indicates something one should not do. **Reference:** Ladewig, P., London, M., & Davidson, M. (2009). *Contemporary maternal-newborn nursing care* (7th ed.). Upper Saddle River, NJ: Pearson Education, pp. 20–23.

8 **Answer: 4 Rationale:** Certified nurse-midwives are prepared to manage independently the care of women and their families who are at low risk for complications during pregnancy and birth. They take a holistic approach to assessment and identification of needs, providing education and information to empower the expectant mother and her family for active involvement during the reproductive years. An obstetrician, family practice resident, and physician's assistant practice using a medical model are examples in which the health care provider is a primary decision maker about care. **Cognitive Level:** Applying **Client Need:** Health Promotion and Maintenance **Integrated Process:** Nursing Process: Planning **Content Area:** Maternal-Newborn **Strategy:** The core issue of this question is identifying the health care provider that would emphasize education and counseling; these are nursing functions. Critical words are *low risk* and *interested in being involved*. Use knowledge of nurse-midwife's capabilities and focus to choose correctly. **Reference:** Ladewig, P., London, M., & Davidson, M. (2009). *Contemporary maternal-newborn nursing care* (7th ed.). Upper Saddle River, NJ: Pearson Education, p. 5.

9 **Answer: 1 Rationale:** Documentation needs to reflect the standards of care. If the nurses routinely chart time of the

decision and time surgery began, data can be collected to compare the unit's practice with national standards. Asking physicians or nurses after the fact will not give accurate data. One cannot assume that 30 minutes is always the time unless it is consistently documented. **Cognitive Level:** Applying **Client Need:** Management of Care **Integrated Process:** Nursing Process: Evaluation **Content Area:** Maternal-Newborn **Strategy:** This question focuses on collection of objective data about time. Only the client's chart would provide this information. The critical words are *evaluate* and *assess*. The other answers are incorrect because of subjective data involved and the type of data collection. **Reference:** Ladewig, P., London, M., & Davidson, M. (2009). *Contemporary maternal-newborn nursing care* (7th ed.). Upper Saddle River, NJ: Pearson Education, pp. 2–11.

10 **Answer: 3 Rationale:** It is the nurse's responsibility to report the situation to the nurse's supervisor when the physician does not act on information from the nurse regarding concerns about client safety. The nurse also needs to document that the obstetrician was notified, the obstetrician's response, and the nurse's further actions in reporting to the supervisor. Relying on the obstetrician's judgment fails to uphold the standard of care. Another physician is not responsible for the client's care and may have no influence over the decisions of another care provider. Telling the client to take legal action against the obstetrician is not part of maintaining own legal accountability. **Cognitive Level:** Applying **Client Need:** Management of Care **Integrated Process:** Nursing Process: Implementation **Content Area:** Maternal-Newborn **Strategy:** Critical words are *fetal distress* and *professionally accountable*. Use knowledge of professional standards and nurse's role in abnormal events to identify correct answer. Recall also that accountability includes reporting upward in the chain of command and ensuring client safety. **Reference:** Ladewig, P., London, M., & Davidson, M. (2009). *Contemporary maternal-newborn nursing care* (7th ed.). Upper Saddle River, NJ: Pearson Education, pp. 7–8.

Posttest

1 **Answer: 4 Rationale:** A person who has diabetes mellitus that is difficult to regulate is considered high risk and will need to be monitored closely. Family nurse practitioners and certified nurse-midwives do not have the expertise to manage complicated cases such as these. Many obstetricians have expertise in management of medical complications but will also recognize situations such as this when the client needs referral to a maternal-fetal medicine specialist. **Cognitive Level:** Applying **Client Need:** Management of Care **Integrated Process:** Nursing Process: Planning **Content Area:** Maternal-Newborn **Strategy:** Critical words are *diabetes mellitus that is difficult to regulate*, indicating a high-risk client. Eliminate certified nurse-midwives and family nurse practitioners first, because their services would be indicated during a normal pregnancy. Choose the maternal-fetal medicine specialist as the one who is a high-risk practitioner. **Reference:** Pilliteri, A. (2007). *Maternal and child health nursing* (5th ed.). Philadelphia: Lippincott Williams & Wilkins, pp. 22–23.

2 **Answer: 1 Rationale:** The views of the nursery nurses are ethnocentric and based on the culture of the Western health care system where convenience for the pediatricians is of primary importance and only the nurses can adequately monitor the clients. The terms *culturally aware*, *culturally sensitive*, and *culturally diverse* imply an appreciation of other cultures and their preferences surrounding childbirth. **Cognitive Level:** Applying **Client Need:** Management of Care **Integrated Process:** Nursing Process: Implementation **Content Area:** Maternal-Newborn **Strategy:** Emphasis in this situation is on the nurses' views and not the preferences of clients; therefore the correct option is ethnocentric. The other three options indicate appreciation of another's culture. **Reference:** Pilliteri, A. (2007). *Maternal and child health nursing* (5th ed.). Philadelphia: Lippincott Williams & Wilkins, pp. 52–54.

3 **Answer: 2 Rationale:** One step in an ethical decision-making framework is to identify the options. The next step is to resolve the dilemma by deciding on the best option for action based on the views of all concerned. Since this client has successfully delivered vaginally numerous times, there are options available to the client. Using an ethical decision-making framework is a good way to resolve the dilemma. Siding with either the client or physician does not respect the view of the other. Calling a nursing supervisor is unnecessary and does not hold the nurse accountable for participation in decision making. **Cognitive Level:** Applying **Client Need:** Management of Care **Integrated Process:** Communication and Documentation **Content Area:** Maternal-Newborn **Strategy:** Core concepts are high parity and how the nurse can "resolve the dilemma," indicating that an ethical decision-making process should be used to assist with looking at all alternative options. **Reference:** Ladewig, P., London, M., & Davidson, M. (2009). *Contemporary maternal-newborn nursing care* (7th ed.). Upper Saddle River, NJ: Pearson Education, p. 8.

4 **Answer: 3 Rationale:** In a state with no emancipated minor law, the client's parents are granted the authority and responsibility to give consent for their minor children. The client, physician, and best friend have no authority in this situation. **Cognitive Level:** Applying **Client Need:** Management of Care **Integrated Process:** Communication and Documentation **Content Area:** Maternal-Newborn **Strategy:** The core issue is determining who can give consent for a minor. Key words are *16-year-old*, *without emancipated minor law*, and *informed consent*, indicating the correct answer is the parent. **Reference:** Ladewig, P., London, M., & Davidson, M. (2009). *Contemporary maternal-newborn nursing care* (7th ed.). Upper Saddle River, NJ: Pearson Education, p. 12.

5 **Answer: 4 Rationale:** A family can be defined as a group of individuals who are bound by strong emotional ties, a

sense of belonging, and a passion for being involved in one another's lives. They may or may not be related or live together on a permanent basis. There is not enough information in the question to support the other conclusions. **Cognitive Level:** Analyzing **Client Need:** Health Promotion and Maintenance **Integrated Process:** Caring **Content Area:** Maternal-Newborn **Strategy:** Critical words are *Auntie* and *considered part of the family unit*. Think of the functions performed by a family to answer this question. Use knowledge of definition of family to make your selection. **Reference:** Wright, L. M., & Leahy, M. (2009). *Nurses and families: A guide to family assessment and intervention* (5th ed.). Philadelphia: F. A. Davis Company, p. 69.

6 **Answer: 2 Rationale:** Childbearing is a developmental crisis because it is a normal period of growth and development. As new roles are learned and assumed, the changes may cause disturbances in life's patterns and a sense of disorganization. External factors cause situational crises, not developmental crises. Family mastery of a task of a maturational stage does not indicate any type of crisis. **Cognitive Level:** Applying **Client Need:** Psychosocial Integrity **Integrated Process:** Teaching and Learning **Content Area:** Maternal-Newborn **Strategy:** Critical words are *developmental crisis*. Use knowledge of childbearing as a normal process, while two options deal with abnormal patterns. Eliminate the option indicating mastery because childbearing has not been mastered yet until after the pregnancy is completed with delivery, and the next stage of childrearing begins. **Reference:** Pilliteri, A. (2007). *Maternal and child health nursing* (5th ed.). Philadelphia: Lippincott Williams & Wilkins, pp. 911–912.

7 **Answer: 1 Rationale:** Standard of care for clients experiencing a postpartum hemorrhage requires frequent assessments (every 10–15 minutes) of vital signs, uterine tone and placement, characteristics and amount of lochia, condition of the perineum, urinary elimination, and level of pain. Massaging the uterus helps to ensure that the uterus stays firm, empty, and involutes toward the umbilicus. Immediately after delivery the client might not have an urge to void and needs to be encouraged to do so, especially when the uterus is rising above the umbilicus. The IV should be maintained until there is no further risk of postpartum hemorrhage. **Cognitive Level:** Applying **Client Need:** Physiological Adaptation **Integrated Process:** Nursing Process: Implementation **Content Area:** Maternal-Newborn **Strategy:** Critical words are *uterine atony and with heavy bleeding*, indicating a postpartum hemorrhage. Eliminate the option regarding voiding, which states *only* when the client has the urge. Discontinuing the IV is incorrect because the uterus is still above the umbilicus, and assessments done every 30 minutes is incorrect because it is not routine for postpartum hemorrhage. Use knowledge of postpartum hemorrhage to answer question **Reference:** Ricci, S. (2009). *Essentials of maternity, newborn, and women's health nursing* (2nd ed.). Philadelphia, PA: Lippincott Williams & Wilkins, pp. 648–651.

8 **Answer: 2 Rationale:** As Ukrainian men become more acculturated they are learning to be supportive of and involved with their wives during pregnancy and labor. The women tend to interpret the presence of their spouses as an indication of care. The other options indicate a client preference rather than an interpretation of the husband's behavior. **Cognitive Level:** Analyzing **Client Need:** Psychosocial Integrity **Integrated Process:** Caring **Content Area:** Maternal-Newborn **Strategy:** A critical word is *Ukrainian*, cueing you to the potential for another perspective from this culture and difference in interpretation of behaviors. The nurse's response indicates a negative perception of the husband's behavior; the correct option is the only one that is a positive interpretation of the behavior. **Reference:** Pilliteri, A. (2007). *Maternal and child health nursing* (5th ed.). Philadelphia: Lippincott Williams & Wilkins, pp. 49–59.

9 **Answer: 3 Rationale:** Many barriers to prenatal care have been identified including the lack of available prenatal care services and providers in many areas of the country. The other options would likely help improve the infant mortality rate over time. **Cognitive Level:** Analyzing **Client Need:** Management of Care **Integrated Process:** Nursing Process: Diagnosis **Content Area:** Maternal-Newborn **Strategy:** Critical words are *unable to obtain prenatal care*, indicating a reason for this lack of care. The incorrect options indicate positive reasons why there should be the availability of care, making the correct option the only plausible reason for the lack of care for clients. **Reference:** Ricci, S. (2009). *Essentials of maternity, newborn, and women's health nursing* (2nd ed.). Philadelphia, PA: Lippincott Williams & Wilkins, pp. 11–18.

10 **Answer: 1 Rationale:** Personal values and beliefs clarification is the first step in appreciating that personal ethical views may differ greatly from the client's value system. Understanding the differences allows the nurse to remain objective when providing care and when serving as a consultant for decision making by the client. Reporting the finding to the physician focuses on physiological needs. Avoiding entering the room does not address the need to provide the appropriate standard of care. Assuming that personal values and beliefs will interfere with care does not address the need to provide appropriate supportive care. **Cognitive Level:** Applying **Client Need:** Psychosocial Integrity **Integrated Process:** Caring **Content Area:** Maternal-Newborn **Strategy:** Critical words are *Gusii*, *circumcised*, and *appropriate and supportive care*. Because of the difference in culture, recall that it is necessary for the nurse to clarify personal values and beliefs to perhaps understand the differences and continue to provide the standard of care. **Reference:** Ladewig, P., London, M., & Davidson, M. (2009). *Contemporary maternal-newborn nursing care* (7th ed.). Upper Saddle River, NJ: Pearson Education, pp. 17–26.

References

Andrews, M. M., & Boyle, J. S. (2007). *Transcultural concepts in nursing care* (5th ed.). Philadelphia: Lippincott Williams & Wilkins.

Bohay, I. Z. (2001). Culture care meanings and experiences of pregnancy and childbirth of Ukrainians. In M. M. Leininger (Ed.), *Culture care diversity and universality: A theory of nursing*. Boston: Jones and Bartlett, pp. 203–229.

Davidson, M., London, M., & Ladewig, P. (2012). *Olds' maternal newborn nursing & women's health across the lifespan* (9th ed.). Upper Saddle River, NJ: Prentice Hall.

Guido, G. W. (2010). *Legal and ethical issues in nursing* (5th ed.). Upper Saddle River, NJ: Pearson Education, pp. 52–58.

Ladewig, P., London, M., & Davidson, M. (2010). *Contemporary maternal-newborn nursing care* (7th ed.). Upper Saddle River, NJ: Pearson Education.

Leininger, M., & McFarland, M. R. (2002). *Transcultural nursing: Concepts, theories, research & practices* (3rd ed.). New York: McGraw-Hill, p. 199.

London, M., Ladewig, P., Ball, J., Bindler, R., & Cowen, K. (2011). *Maternal & child nursing care* (3rd ed.). Upper Saddle River, NJ: Pearson Education.

Murray, M., & Huelsmann, G. (2009). *Labor and delivery nursing: A guide to evidence-based practice.* New York: Springer Publishing Company.

NANDA Nursing Diagnosis (2009). Retrieved January 29, 2011, from http://www.scribd.com/doc/11885949/NANDA-2009

Perry, S., Hockenberry, M., Lowdermilk, D., & Wilson, D. (2010). *Maternal child nursing care* (4th ed.). St. Louis, MO: Elsevier.

Pilliteri, A. (2009). *Maternal and child health nursing* (6th ed.). Philadelphia: Lippincott Williams & Wilkins.

Ricci, S. (2009). *Essentials of maternity, newborn, and women's health nursing* (2nd ed.). Philadelphia: Lippincott Williams & Wilkins.

Streltzer, J. M., & Tseng, W. S. (2008). *Cultural competence in health care: A guide for professionals.* New York: Springer-Verlag.

Wright, L. M., & Leahey, M. (2009). *Nurses and families: A guide to family assessment and intervention* (5th ed.). Philadelphia: F. A. Davis Company.

2 Reproduction, Fertility, and Infertility

Chapter Outline

The Reproductive System
Fertility
Nursing Care of the Infertile Couple

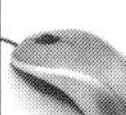

NCLEX-RN® Test Prep

Use the accompanying online resource, NursingReviewsandRationales, to test yourself with hundreds of NCLEX®-style practice questions.

Objectives

- Describe the structure and function of the female and male reproductive systems.
- Summarize the components essential for fertility.
- Describe possible psychological reactions of an infertile couple.
- Explain common diagnostic studies used to evaluate fertility.
- Describe nursing care of clients receiving treatment for infertility.

Review at a Glance

artificial insemination treatment of infertility where sperm are directly inserted into uterus

anovulatory menstrual cycles menstrual cycles that are not preceded by ovulation

basal body temperature (BBT) resting body temperature, taken daily prior to arising from bed; when graphed will assist in detecting ovulation

endometrial biopsy a diagnostic test whereby endometrium is sampled via a catheter inserted through cervix and into body of uterus, and a small amount of endometrium is suctioned and sent to a laboratory for analysis

fertility awareness use of BBT graphing and daily cervical mucus examination to detect ovulation, and therefore determine optimal day to have intercourse to achieve pregnancy or days to avoid intercourse if the goal is avoiding conception

gamete intrafallopian transfer (GIFT) multiple ova are harvested via large-bore needle under ultrasound guidance and are inserted into fallopian tube; spermatozoa that have been collected are also inserted via a large-bore needle under ultrasound guidance into fallopian tube; fertilization occurs in fallopian tube

hysterosalpingogram (HSG) a diagnostic test in which radiopaque dye is instilled into uterus and fallopian tubes via a catheter inserted through cervix; used to detect uterine or tubal anomalies

intracytoplasmic sperm injection (ICSI) a micro-surgical procedure where an individual sperm is selected and then injected into cytoplasm of a chosen oocyte

in vitro fertilization (IVF) multiple ova are harvested via large-bore needle under ultrasound guidance and mixed with sperm in laboratory; gametes or embryos are either reinserted into fallopian tubes or uterus, or frozen for later use

laparoscopy procedure carried out under general or epidural anesthesia; abdomen is insufflated with carbon dioxide, one or more trochars are inserted into peritoneum near umbilicus and symphysis pubis; laparoscope is then used to visualize pelvic structures or perform surgical procedures

micro-epididymal sperm aspiration (MESA) is a microsurgical technique to obtain a sperm specimen from the epididymis; performed as an outpatient procedure under sedation and/or local anesthesia

pelvic inflammatory disease (PID) inflammation of uterus and fallopian tubes, usually caused by an infectious agent such as *Chlamydia trachomatis* or *Gonorrhea Neisseria*

percutaneous epididymal sperm aspiration (PESA) a procedure that uses a small needle under local anesthesia to aspirate sperm from epididymis

postcoital exam exam that occurs 8 to 12 hours post-intercourse, which should be scheduled one to two days before expected ovulation; mucus from endocervical canal is aspirated into a catheter and examined microscopically for infection, consistency and ferning of cervical mucus, and number and type of active and nonmotile sperm

semen analysis client ejaculates into a specimen container, and ejaculate is examined microscopically for number, morphology, and motility of sperm

tubal embryo transfer (TET) multiple ova are harvested via large-bore needle under ultrasound guidance and fertilized in vitro (in the laboratory); up to four of the subsequent embryos are reinserted into fallopian tube

zygote intrafallopian transfer (ZIFT) multiple ova are harvested via large-bore needle under ultrasound guidance and fertilized in vitro (in laboratory); a select number of subsequent fertilized ova (zygotes) are reinserted into fallopian tube

PRETEST

1 The client brings her basal body temperature (BBT) chart to the clinic. In evaluating the chart, the nurse suspects that ovulation has occurred. Indicate the area on the chart that supports the nurse's judgment.

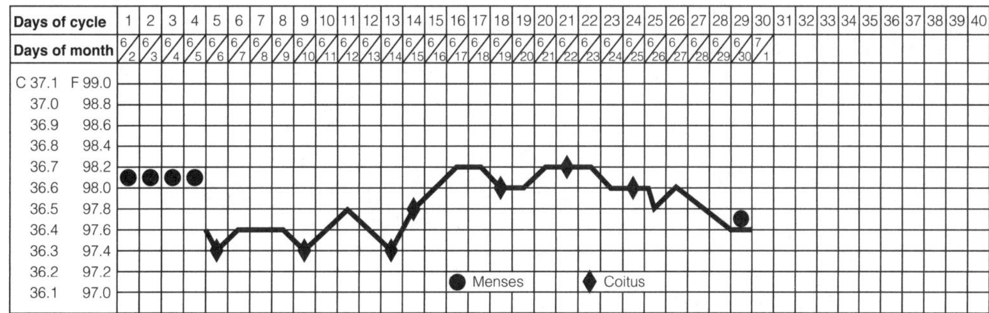

2 A client who has had pelvic inflammatory disease (PID) caused by *Chlamydia trachomatis* is at risk for which of the following?

1. Anovulatory menstrual cycles
2. Ectopic pregnancy
3. Multifetal pregnancy
4. Cervical dysplasia

3 The nurse explains to a male client with a vas deferens blockage to expect which of the following problems?

1. Frequent urination
2. Decreased sperm in seminal fluid
3. Inability to achieve or maintain an erection
4. Decreased sexual drive

4 The nurse concludes that a client being treated for infertility needs further teaching when the client makes which statement about what the couple needs to do to achieve pregnancy?

1. Have intercourse on the 14th day of the menstrual cycle.
2. Have intercourse when basal body temperature rises.
3. Have intercourse every other day during the week before and after ovulation.
4. Abstain from intercourse for the month prior to the month they want to conceive.

5 The nurse working in an infertility clinic explains to an infertile couple that they will likely have which tests ordered as a part of their original work-up? Select all that apply.

1. Semen analysis
2. Mammogram
3. Colposcopy
4. Nonstress test
5. Hysterosalpingogram

PRETEST

6. The nurse would include which nursing intervention when planning care for an infertile couple?

1. Assistance in dealing with feelings of guilt and shame
2. Helping to determine which partner is to blame
3. Referral to a financial counselor to plan for their child's future
4. Discussion of the advantages of adoption instead of infertility treatment

7. The nurse reinforces the physician's explanation that a client with fallopian tube blockage would be a candidate for which method of achieving pregnancy?

1. Natural family planning
2. In vitro fertilization
3. Tubal ligation
4. Sperm washing

8. The client has been scheduled to have a hysterosalpingogram. Which question does the nurse need to ask?

1. "Do you douche?"
2. "Have you used any type of lubricant with intercourse?"
3. "When was the first day of your last menstrual cycle?"
4. "What was your age at menarche?"

9. Which statement made by the client scheduled for in vitro fertilization would indicate the need for additional teaching?

1. "The egg retrieval procedure may be uncomfortable, but medication will be available for me."
2. "The fertilized eggs will be implanted into my uterus two to three days after the egg retrieval."
3. "I will need to limit my activities the day of the egg retrieval and the day of implantation."
4. "I will have 10 embryos implanted to maximize my chance of carrying a baby to term."

10. The nurse interprets that partner sperm intrauterine insemination is likely to be indicated for a couple when which of the following has occurred?

1. The male partner has a varicocele.
2. The female partner has irregular menses.
3. The female partner produces anti-sperm antibodies.
4. The male partner has human immunodeficiency virus.

➤ *See pages 39–40 for Answers and Rationales.*

I. THE REPRODUCTIVE SYSTEM

A. Female structures

1. External structures
   - **a.** Labia majora: fleshy longitudinal folds of tissue that cover and protect underlying structures
   - **b.** Labia minora: small, soft folds of tissue beneath labia majora that directly cover vaginal introitus
   - **c.** Clitoris: small (6 mm × 6 mm) erectile tissue with rich blood and nerve supply covered by labia minora
2. Internal structures (Figure 2-1)
   - **a.** Vagina: muscular, membranous tube with side walls covered with rugae that connect external genitalia with cervix and uterus; also called birth canal; provides a passageway for sperm for conception, menstrual flow during menstruation, and fetus during childbirth
   - **b.** Cervix: neck of uterus, extends down into vagina; consists of fibrous tissue that dilates and shortens during labor

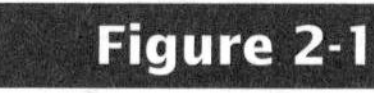
Figure 2-1

Structures of the uterus

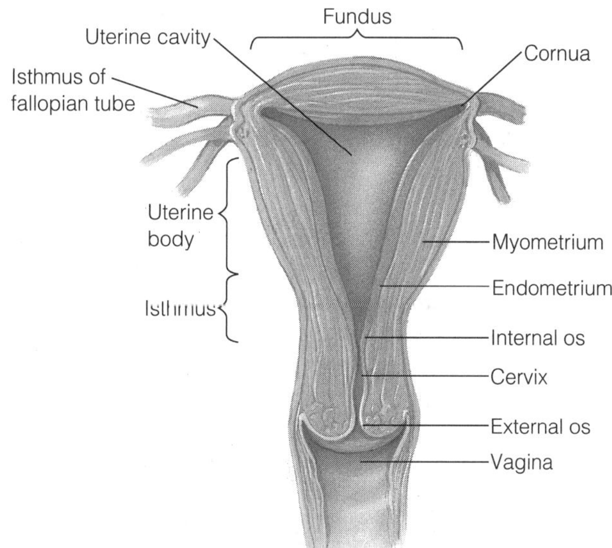

   - **c.** Uterus: hollow muscular organ at superior end of vagina; also called womb; sheds its lining (called endometrium) during menstrual cycles and holds fetus during pregnancy; superior portion is known as fundus; inferior portion ends in cervix
   - **d.** Fallopian tubes: connect each ovary with uterine body; these hollow tubes are ciliated to transport ovum or zygote; portion that attaches to uterus is isthmus; middle section is ampulla; ends at ovary in funnel-shaped infundibulum, which has finger-like fimbriae reaching towards ovary
   - **e.** Ovaries: almond-sized endocrine functioning glands that secrete estrogen and progesterone; usually mature one follicle and ovum during each menstrual cycle from menarche to menopause, except during pregnancy

B. Male structures

- **1.** External
   - **a.** Foreskin: circular fold of skin that covers glans, frequently removed via circumcision
   - **b.** Penis: vascular shaft that contains urethra and erectile tissue, which lengthens and elongates through stasis of blood in blood vessels; glans is tip of penis and has urethral meatus centered in it; shaft is midportion, and base attaches to scrotum and groin
   - **c.** Scrotum: rugated covering of testes composed of muscle tissue that raises and lowers testes to control their temperature for optimal sperm production
- **2.** Internal
   - **a.** Testes: two lobular oval glands located within scrotum where spermatogenesis takes place via meiosis
   - **b.** Epididymis: tubelike duct arising from top of each testis and ending in vas deferens
   - **c.** Vas deferens: connects epididymis to prostate gland
   - **d.** Prostate gland: encircles urethra just below bladder, producing alkaline fluid that is released during ejaculation
   - **e.** Seminal vesicles: lobular glands located just superior to prostate, produce seminal fluid that is secreted during ejaculation to support sperm metabolism and motility

f. Urethra: tube that passes through prostate gland and connects bladder and urethral meatus; also is passage for ejaculate
g. Semen: male ejaculate comprised of spermatozoa and glandular secretions; milky white in color; average volume from 2 to 5 mL

C. Functions of female structures

1. Oogenesis: all oocytes are present at birth; meiosis leads to maturation of an individual ovum under influence of follicle stimulating hormone (FSH); luteinizing hormone (LH) transforms follicle into corpus luteum, which maintains pregnancy through production of progesterone; ovaries produce estrogen and progesterone in both pregnant and nonpregnant states
2. Menstruation occurs if ovum is not fertilized and corpus luteum disintegrates; endometrium becomes ischemic as progesterone and estrogen levels drop during last week of menstrual cycle, leading to sloughing of myometrium
3. Conception occurs in fallopian tube when a 23 chromosome-containing spermatozoon enters a 23 chromosome-containing ovum and produces a 46 chromosome zygote arranged as 23 chromosomal pairs
4. Pregnancy: cleavage (rapid mitotic division of zygote) creates a blastocyst, which in turn becomes a multicellular solid ball of 16 cells (morula); further division leads to trophoblast stage, when it implants within endometrium
5. Secretion production: cervical secretions become thin and elastic in consistency during ovulation to facilitate sperm transport towards ovum; endometrial secretions are rich in glycogen to nourish developing embryo until placental circulation is in place

D. Age-related changes of female reproductive system

1. Menses begin during puberty, stimulated by release of estrogen and progesterone
2. Menopause is characterized by one year of amenorrhea, and occurs on average at age 50; postmenopausal changes of reproductive tract include thinning and atrophy of external and internal structures

E. Functions of male structures

1. Spermatogenesis takes place in the testes; spermatozoa then proceed through tubules of epididymis where motility and fertility develop, finally being stored in the reservoir of the epididymis
2. Ejaculation is a series of muscular contractions that release spermatozoa and seminal fluid through urethral meatus of penis
3. Urination also takes place through male urethra
4. Secretion production: prostate gland and seminal glands create a milky-white fluid that nourishes spermatozoa during and after ejaculation

F. Age-related changes of male reproductive system

1. Puberty is characterized by greatly increased serum levels of testosterone, which in turn stimulate elongation and thickening of penile shaft, spermatozoa production, and enlargement of testes and scrotum
2. Spermatozoa count, motility, and morphology begin to decrease in middle age
3. External organs atrophy in older adults

II. FERTILITY

A. Female components

1. Infertility: situation in which a couple is unsuccessful in achieving pregnancy following at least 12 months of trying to conceive; length of time is adjusted downward as maternal age increases
   a. Primary infertility is that which occurs prior to ever having conceived
   b. Secondary infertility occurs after at least one pregnancy

2. Menstrual cycle: changes that occur in normal female reproductive system on an approximately 28-day cycle; this cycle enables pregnancy to occur
   a. Follicular phase: occurs during days 1 to 14 of the cycle; variations in length of menstrual cycle are caused by variations in length of follicular phase; within this phase the following occur:
      1) Menstrual phase: period of time when the woman sheds lining of uterus
      2) Proliferative phase: beginning of endometrial thickening
   b. Luteal phase: occurs from days 15 to 28 of menstrual cycle, and is always 12 to 14 days in length; within luteal phase the following occur:
      1) Secretory phase: plush endometrium secretes glycogen in preparation for implantation of a fertilized ovum
      2) Ischemic phase: beginning of breakdown of endometrium when fertilization has not occurred

! 3. Ovulation: an ovum begins to mature during follicular phase as a result of FSH production; at onset of luteal phase, a blisterlike graafian follicle appears and enlarges on ovarian surface under influence of FSH and LH; ovum is released from follicle at time of ovulation; ruptured follicle becomes corpus luteum, which disintegrates if fertilization does not occur or creates progesterone if fertilization occurs; a body fat percentage of 14% or more is needed to support ovulation (estrogen is stored in body fat); lower than 14% body fat will result in irregular menses or amenorrhea
4. Cervical mucus: becomes more plentiful, with thinner and more elastic consistency, and forms columns during ovulation to facilitate sperm transport into uterus; cervical mucus production can be impeded by surgical treatments for abnormal Pap smears
5. Uterine structure: a septum (fibrous, vertical, wall-like structure in center of uterine body), a unicornuate uterus (one-sided, banana-shaped uterus) or a bicornuate uterus (two banana-shaped uteri side by side, curving away from each other; may end at one cervix, or have two cervices and vaginas) will have less normal myometrium and fewer healthy places for an embryo to implant successfully; a bicornuate uterus may have one underdeveloped horn and ovary and be ovulating and fertile every other cycle; a complete bicornuate uterus with double vagina may result in sperm being present in horn of uterus, which is underdeveloped or not ovulating (see Figure 2-2)
6. Hormones
   a. Estrogen: produced by ovaries, especially ovarian follicle during ovulation; responsible for development of secondary sex characteristics at puberty; peaks during follicular phase of menstrual cycle; inhibits FSH and LH production
   b. Progesterone: secreted by corpus luteum; peaks during luteal phase; stimulates FSH and LH secretion; responsible for endometrial thickening

Figure 2-2

Uterine structures

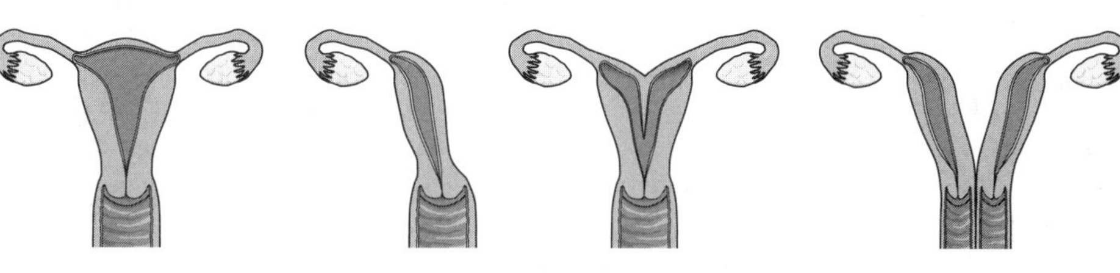

c. FSH: anterior pituitary hormone that normally matures one ovarian follicle each cycle
d. LH: anterior pituitary hormone that completes maturation of ovarian follicle; ovulation occurs 10 to 12 hours after LH peaks

7. Fallopian tube(s) must be patent for sperm to reach ovum and for fertilized ovum to reach uterus; scarring can occur from an infection, such as a ruptured appendix during adolescence or **pelvic inflammatory disease (PID)**, an infection of uterus and fallopian tubes; cilia in fallopian tubes, which propel ovum toward oncoming sperm, will have decreased motility in cigarette smokers, thereby decreasing fertility

B. Male components

!

1. Sperm production
   a. Morphology: at least 50% of sperm must have normal form to achieve optimal fertility
   b. Count: normal levels are >20 million sperm per milliliter of ejaculate
   c. Motility: at least 50% of sperm should have normal motion patterns
   d. Decreased sperm count and motility can be caused by increased scrotal temperature resulting from frequent hot tub or sauna use, tight clothing, or varicocele; heavy alcohol, marijuana, or cocaine use; trauma to scrotum; mumps during adulthood; developmental factors; and cigarette smoking
2. Testosterone is primary hormone responsible for libido, sperm production, ability to have and maintain an erection, and ejaculation
3. Erections must be able to be maintained long enough for ejaculation to occur in vagina and near cervix for optimal fertility
4. Ejaculation must occur and contain sufficient numbers of normally formed and motile sperm to achieve fertility

III. NURSING CARE OF THE INFERTILE COUPLE

A. Assessment

1. Common diagnostic studies to detect physiological factors associated with infertility
   a. Female
      1) **Basal body temperature (BBT)**, or resting body temperature, is obtained by woman measuring her oral temperature each day before arising from bed and graphing results on a month-long graph; a sudden dip occurs the day prior to ovulation and is followed by a rise of 0.5 to 1.0°F, which indicates ovulation; this rise will remain until menstruation begins; **fertility awareness** includes monitoring BBT and cervical mucus changes to detect ovulation
      2) Serum hormone testing: venous blood is drawn from infertile women to assess levels of FSH and LH, which are indicators of ovarian function
      3) **Postcoital exam**: exam that occurs 8 to 12 hours post-intercourse, one or two days before expected ovulation; a 10-mL syringe with catheter attached is used to collect a specimen of secretions from vagina; secretions are examined for signs of infection, number of active and nonmotile spermatozoa, sperm–mucus interaction, and consistency of cervical mucus; cervical mucus and ejaculate are tested for agglutination, an indication that secretory immunological reactions are occurring between cervical mucus and spermatozoa
      4) **Endometrial biopsy** (obtaining an endometrial tissue sample for examination) is achieved by positioning client on exam table with her feet in stirrups; provider inserts a vaginal speculum to visualize cervix; an endometrial sample is obtained by inserting a sharp-tipped stiff catheter attached to a syringe for suction; sample is then biopsied to check for a luteal phase defect (lack of progesterone);

Practice to Pass

The client has been instructed to start taking her basal body temperature and graph the results. She tells you that she works the night shift. When is the best time for her to take her daily temperatures?

Practice to Pass

The client scheduled for a hysterosalpingogram reports an allergy to iodine. What should the nurse do?

preprocedure care includes assisting client (after undressing below waist and given proper drape) onto exam table with feet in stirrups and advising client that she will feel crampy discomfort during aspiration; postprocedure care includes providing sanitary napkins, as vaginal bleeding will occur, and assessing client for a vasovagal response (sudden fainting caused by hypotension induced by vagus nerve stimulation) prior to arising from exam table

! 5) **Hysterosalpingogram (HSG)** detects uterine anomalies, such as septate, unicornuate, or bicornuate structures, and tubal anomalies or blockage; iodine-based radiopaque dye is instilled through a catheter into uterus and tubes to outline these structures and x-rays are taken to document findings

6) **Laparoscopy** is carried out under general or epidural anesthesia; abdomen is insufflated with carbon dioxide, one or more trochars are inserted into peritoneum near umbilicus and symphysis pubis; laparoscope is then used to visualize structures in pelvis or perform surgical procedures

b. **Semen analysis**: client ejaculates into a specimen container, and ejaculate is examined microscopically for number, morphology, and motility of sperm; Table 2-1 presents normal results of semen analysis

! 2. Psychological factors associated with infertility: many couples experience shame, guilt, blame, or stages of grief when diagnosed with infertility as well as during treatment for infertility

Practice to Pass

The semen analysis of the male client indicates that he is ejaculating no sperm. What options exist for this couple to achieve pregnancy?

a. Each partner brings his or her own baseline psychological health to the situation and will experience individual emotional reactions to infertility as well

b. Most often, each member of couple processes infertility experience differently; thus, disharmony may result

c. Facilitate communication between couple and provide information on resources for coping with infertility, such as support groups, or individual or marital counseling

d. Most infertility services include a social worker on interdisciplinary team specifically to assess and treat any psychosocial issues related to infertility

e. Same sex couples may also be seen for infertility care, utilizing available technologies and sometimes surrogates to enable them to parent

1) Just as heterosexual couples are challenged emotionally by infertility, so are same sex couples

2) It is important to treat these couples with same respect and caring as any other couple trying to conceive

B. **Possible nursing diagnoses:** Deficient Knowledge; Anxiety; Low Self-Esteem: Situational; Disturbed Body Image; Ineffective Coping; Hopelessness; Powerlessness; Grieving; Compromised Family Coping; Ineffective Sexuality Patterns; Interrupted Family Processes; Risk for Impaired Parenting

Table 2–1 Normal Semen Analysis Results

Factor	Value
Volume	>2.0 mL
pH	7.0 to 8.0
Total sperm count	>20 million per mL
Motility	50% or greater
Normal forms	50% or greater

Practice to Pass

An infertile couple reports marital difficulty caused by the stress of the infertility treatments the couple is undergoing. How should the nurse respond to this information?

C. Implementation and collaborative care

1. Educational needs of infertile couple will be extensive; couple will need education on how to do the following:
   - **a.** Perform various procedures (e.g., semen collection for analysis or postcoital exam)
   - **b.** Interpret meaning of results of tests and assessments
   - **c.** Perform self-monitoring during medication administration, and understand how assisted reproductive technologies (ART) are performed
2. Hormonal therapy is used for induction of ovulation in preparation for in vitro fertilization; client and/or partner must learn how to give subcutaneous (subQ) and/or intramuscular (IM) injections
3. Medications are used to achieve induction of ovulation in cases of **anovulatory menstrual cycles** (menstrual cycles without ovulation) or to achieve multiple ova prior to in vitro fertilization
   - **a.** Clomiphene citrate (Clomid, Serophene) is often used to increase FSH and LH secretion, thereby stimulating ovulation
   - **b.** If clomiphene is not effective, other medications may be prescribed to induce ovulation or for use during follow-up procedures
     - **1)** Human menopausal gonadotropins (hMG) such as menotropin (Repronex) or urofollitropin (Bravelle)
     - **2)** Recombinant FSH (Gonal-F, Follistim)
     - **3)** Recombinent LH (Luveris)
     - **4)** Human chorionic gonadotropin (hCG) (Pregnyl, Novarel)
     - **5)** GnRh analogs such as leuprolide (Lupron), nafarelin (Synarel), or goserelin (Zoladex)
   - **c.** Risks of ovulation induction include multiple births and ovarian hyperstimulation, which can result in enlarged ovaries, abdominal distention, pain, and ovarian cysts
4. Sperm washing for intrauterine insemination (IUI): client's ejaculate is centrifuged to concentrate spermatozoa, which are then rinsed in saline to remove seminal fluid; spermatozoa are again centrifuged, and then used for either in vitro or intrauterine artificial insemination

5. Intrauterine insemination is a form of **artificial insemination**, whereby
   - **a.** Sperm that are no more than three hours old are inserted via a catheter into uterus
   - **b.** Donor sperm may be used if male partner's sperm count or motility is low or for single women who desire to become pregnant
   - **c.** Identity of the sperm donor is kept confidential

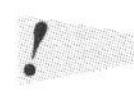

6. **In vitro fertilization (IVF)**: multiple ova are harvested transvaginally via a large-bore needle and syringe under ultrasound guidance; ova are then mixed with spermatozoa, and a specific agreed upon number of resultant embryos are returned to uterus two to three days later; extra embryos can be frozen for implantation at a later date; side effects include ovarian cysts, multiple births related to multiple embryos, and ovarian hyperstimulation
   - **a.** Nursing care before and during procedure includes instructing client to self-administer synthetic FSH injections to stimulate ovary to produce multiple ova for five to six days before procedure, giving sedation for ova retrieval procedure, observing client for about two hours after egg retrieval, and instructing woman to limit activity for 24 hours after procedure
   - **b.** Postprocedure care following embryo placement in uterus includes instructing client to have minimal activity for 24 hours; progesterone supplementation is commonly prescribed
7. **Gamete intrafallopian transfer (GIFT)**: harvested ova and sperm are mixed and placed via large-bore needle and syringe under ultrasound guidance into ovarian end of fallopian tube

Practice to Pass

The client is undergoing ovulation induction in preparation for IVF. She has business commitments and wants to know when to schedule her meetings around the IVF procedure. What should the nurse tell her?

8. **Tubal embryo transfer (TET)**: in vitro fertilized embryos are placed into fallopian tube via large-bore needle and syringe under ultrasound guidance; performed 42 to 72 hours after egg retrieval
9. **Zygote intrafallopian transfer (ZIFT)**: ova fertilized in vitro are placed into fallopian tube via large-bore needle and syringe under ultrasound guidance; performed 18 to 24 hours after egg retrieval
10. **Micro-epididymal sperm aspiration (MESA)** is a micro-surgical technique to obtain a sperm specimen from the epididymis; it is done as an outpatient procedure under sedation and/or local anesthesia
11. **Percutaneous epididymal sperm aspiration (PESA)** utilizes a small needle under local anesthesia to aspirate sperm from the epididymis
12. **Intracytoplasmic sperm injection (ICSI)** is a micro-surgical procedure where an individual sperm is selected and then injected into cytoplasm of a chosen oocyte
13. Methods involving a third individual
    a. Surrogacy: use of a third-party female to provide eggs for conception and to carry pregnancy through delivery—when infertile couple receives infant
    b. Gestational carrier: use of a third-party female who is implanted with genetic material (sperm and egg) from either infertile couple or a donor; she carries pregnancy through delivery when infertile couple receives infant

D. **Evaluation:** couple's knowledge is increased regarding diagnostic studies, their infertility problem(s), and infertility treatment options; clients experience decreased anxiety regarding infertility, share their feelings openly, and make an informed decision to pursue or not pursue treatment for infertility

Case Study

The client is a 38-year-old woman with primary infertility. The client and her husband are in today for a first appointment at the infertility clinic where you work.

1. What medical and surgical history questions will you ask of the woman?
2. What medical and surgical history questions will you ask of the client's husband?
3. When the client asks you what to expect in the initial assessment of her infertility, how will you answer?
4. What information about the couple's sexual activity do you need to obtain?
5. How will the woman's age affect the couple's probable infertility treatment?

For suggested responses, see pages 301–302.

POSTTEST

1 Which of the following should the nurse include when developing the plan of care for an infertile client?

1. Assistance in resolving feelings of guilt
2. Past year medical and surgical history of both partners
3. Brief answers to questions asked and issues raised
4. Referral to another clinic for a second opinion

2. The client is scheduled for a hysterosalpingogram (HSG). What information should the nurse obtain during the preoperative assessment?

1. History of pelvic inflammatory disease (PID)
2. Allergy to peanuts
3. Presence of metal implants
4. Difficulty swallowing

3. A female client is considering in vitro fertilization and gamete intrafallopian transfer (GIFT). Which statement indicates the client needs additional information?

1. "I will give myself injections of medications to cause my ovaries to ripen more than one egg."
2. "My husband will need to produce a sample of his sperm the day my eggs are retrieved."
3. "I will be in the hospital overnight for this procedure."
4. "I can expect to have some discomfort after the procedure."

4. The client is seeking to become pregnant through artificial insemination using donor sperm. In teaching the client about this procedure, which information should the nurse plan to include?

1. Processing procedures to prevent transmission of genetic defects or infectious disease are optional.
2. There is an unlimited number of pregnancies per donor.
3. Donor sperm need to be frozen and quarantined for a year to prevent risk of disease transmission.
4. Informed consent must be obtained from all parties.

5. Which statement made by a female client indicates that she and her husband are having difficulty coping with their infertility regimen?

1. "I am never going to consider pregnancy a spontaneous event again."
2. "I don't like giving myself shots, but I'll do it to get pregnant."
3. "We had to take out a home equity loan to pay for these treatments."
4. "My husband just hates having to plan when we make love."

POSTTEST

6. What interpretation should the nurse make about a client who has a complete bicornate uterus with two vaginas? Select all that apply.

1. She will be unable to ever achieve pregnancy.
2. She will be at increased risk for preterm labor.
3. She will need artificial insemination to conceive.
4. She will need to have a cesarean delivery.
5. She will be at risk for multiple pregnancy loss.

7. The nurse determines that which of the following clients in the infertility clinic needs to be seen first?

1. A 27-year-old woman being seen for an initial infertility exam
2. A 34-year-old man in for semen analysis results
3. A 32-year-old woman taking human chorionic gonadotropin (hCG) who reports severe abdominal pain
4. A 30-year-old woman in for a pregnancy test following implantation as part of in vitro fertilization

8. The nurse has explained to the client that the results of her hysterosalpingogram revealed bilateral tubal blockage. The nurse realizes that further education about the results of the hysterosalpingogram is needed when the client asks which question?

1. "Will the surgery to unblock my tubes be done in the hospital or the surgery center?"
2. "Will the acupuncture treatments I am getting interfere with the surgical procedure?"
3. "Will this plug in my fallopian tubes go away forever after I become pregnant?"
4. "Will long-distance running and a low percentage of body fat affect the success of the surgery?"

9 The client is a long-distance runner, with 9.0% body fat. Which findings would the nurse expect to assess in this client?

1. Regular menses, and a BBT that indicates ovulation
2. Irregular menses, and a BBT that shows ovulation
3. Regular menses, and a BBT that indicates lack of ovulation
4. Irregular menses, and a BBT that indicates lack of ovulation

10 The client is a 43-year-old nullipara who is in for her first intrauterine insemination of her partner's washed semen. The nurse determines that client teaching has been effective when the client makes which statement about basal body temperature (BBT)?

1. "If I get pregnant, I'll see an increase in my BBT."
2. "If I do not become pregnant, I'll see an increase in my BBT."
3. "If I get pregnant, I'll see a decrease in my BBT."
4. "If I do not get pregnant, I'll see a dip and an increase in my BBT."

➤ *See pages 40–42 for Answers and Rationales.*

ANSWERS & RATIONALES

Pretest

1 **Answer:**

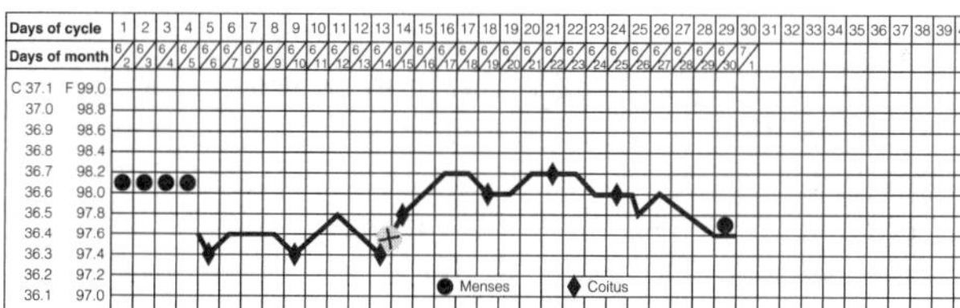

Rationale: An ovulatory cycle is biphasic. The basal body temperature drops slightly then rises 0.5-1.0°F 24 to 48 hours after ovulation. Progesterone is thermogenic (heat producing), thereby maintaining the temperature increase during the second half of the menstrual cycle. **Cognitive Level:** Analyzing **Client Need:** Health Promotion and Maintenance **Integrated Process:** Nursing Process: Assessment **Content Area:** Maternal-Newborn **Strategy:** Recall the timing of ovulation at about the midpoint of the menstrual cycle and the changes in basal body temperature to help choose correctly. **Reference:** Ladewig, P., London, M., & Davidson, M. (2009). *Contemporary maternal-newborn nursing care* (7th ed.). Upper Saddle River, NJ: Pearson Education, p. 138.

2 **Answer: 2 Rationale:** Chlamydial PID causes scarring of the fallopian tubes, thus increasing the incidence of ectopic pregnancy. Anovulatory menstrual cycles, multifetal pregnancy, and cervical dysplasia do not reflect the true possible consequence of chlamydial PID. **Cognitive Level:** Applying **Client Need:** Physiological Adaptation **Integrated Process:** Nursing Process: Assessment **Content Area:** Maternal-Newborn **Strategy:** Critical words are *PID* and *Chlamydia trachomatis*. Use knowledge of residual effects of STI to determine correct answer. Recognize the option with the greatest risk to client safety: ectopic pregnancy with tubal rupture and hemorrhage. **Reference:** Ladewig, P., London, M., & Davidson, M. (2009). *Contemporary maternal-newborn nursing care* (7th ed.). Upper Saddle River, NJ: Pearson Education, p.119.

3 **Answer: 2 Rationale:** A vas deferens blockage will prevent the sperm from being ejaculated, resulting in a deficiency of sperm in the seminal fluid (oligospermia). Frequent urination, the inability to achieve or maintain an erection, and decreased sexual drive do not occur as a result of the blockage. **Cognitive Level:** Applying **Client Need:** Physiological Adaptation **Integrated Process:** Teaching and Learning **Content Area:** Maternal-Newborn **Strategy:** Critical words are *vas deferens* and *blockage*. Use knowledge of normal anatomy and physiology to determine correct answer. This is a positively worded question, so the correct answer would be a true statement about the client with this condition. **Reference:** Ladewig, P., London, M., & Davidson, M. (2009). *Contemporary maternal-newborn nursing care* (7th ed.). Upper Saddle River, NJ: Pearson Education, p. 143.

4 **Answer: 4 Rationale:** Having intercourse on the 14th day of the menstrual cycle, when the basal body temperature rises, and every other day during the weeks before and after ovulation increase the likelihood of conception by timing intercourse around the expected time of ovulation. Abstaining from intercourse for the month prior to planned conception does not increase the likelihood of becoming pregnant and indicates a need for further teaching. **Cognitive Level:** Analyzing **Client Need:** Health Promotion and Maintenance **Integrated Process:** Teaching and Learning **Content Area:** Maternal-Newborn **Strategy:** Critical words are *needs further teaching*, indicating that an incorrect response from the client is the correct answer to the question. Use knowledge of the normal menstrual cycle to eliminate the three incorrect options. **Reference:** Ladewig, P., London, M., & Davidson, M. (2009). *Contemporary maternal-newborn nursing care* (7th ed.). Upper Saddle River, NJ: Pearson Education, p. 142.

5 **Answer: 1, 5 Rationale:** Inadequate number or motility of sperm and tubal anomaly or blockage are the most common causes of infertility. Semen analysis will provide information on number of and motility of sperm, and hysterosalpingogram will detect uterine or tubal anomalies or blockage. Mammogram, colposcopy, and a nonstress test do not diagnose infertility problems. **Cognitive Level:** Applying **Client Need:** Health Promotion and Maintenance **Integrated Process:** Nursing Process: Planning **Content Area:** Maternal-Newborn **Strategy:** Critical words are *infertile* and *tests*, which eliminate those tests not pertinent to infertility diagnosis. The focus of the question is testing for the couple, so the correct responses will include tests for both the male and the female. **Reference:** Ladewig, P., London, M., & Davidson, M. (2009). *Contemporary maternal-newborn nursing care* (7th ed.). Upper Saddle River: Pearson Education, pp. 140–147.

6 **Answer: 1 Rationale:** Infertile couples must deal with guilt, shame, and other psychosocial issues. The nurse's role is to be supportive, facilitate sharing of feelings between the couple, and provide guidance through the infertility assessment and treatment process. Although it can occur, it is not helpful to blame one partner or the other for the infertility problem. There is no indication that the couple needs financial counseling. There is no evidence that the couple is ready to talk about other parenting options such as adoption. **Cognitive Level:** Applying **Client Need:** Health Promotion and Maintenance **Integrated Process:** Nursing Process: Planning **Content Area:** Maternal-Newborn **Strategy:** Critical words are *nursing care* and *infertile couple*. Use knowledge of appropriate psychosocial support and response to loss of childbearing capability to choose the correct answer and eliminate others. **Reference:** Ladewig, P., London, M., & Davidson, M. (2009). *Contemporary maternal-newborn nursing care* (7th ed.). Upper Saddle River, NJ: Pearson Education, pp. 135–136.

7 **Answer: 2 Rationale:** Tubal blockage will prohibit sperm from traveling through the fallopian tubes to reach an ovum and fertilize it. In vitro fertilization involves harvesting ova and placing them with sperm in a petri dish. The resultant embryos are then returned to the uterus. Natural family planning and sperm washing would not help this couple to achieve pregnancy because of the tubal blockage. Tubal ligation is used to stop pregnancy from occurring. **Cognitive Level:** Applying **Client Need:** Health Promotion and Maintenance **Integrated Process:** Nursing Process: Planning **Content Area:** Maternal-Newborn **Strategy:** Critical words in the stem of the question are *fallopian tube blockage* and *achieve pregnancy*. Use knowledge of anatomy and physiology and methods of artificial insemination to choose correctly. **Reference:** Ladewig, P., London, M., & Davidson, M. (2009). *Contemporary maternal-newborn nursing care* (7th ed.). Upper Saddle River, NJ: Pearson Education, p. 146.

8 **Answer: 3 Rationale:** Hysterosalpingograms are performed in the follicular phase of the cycle to avoid interrupting an early pregnancy, so the nurse needs to establish the client's phase of the menstrual cycle. Douching, using lubricant during intercourse, and the age at the start of menarche do not address the need to become familiar with the client's menstrual cycle. **Cognitive Level:** Applying **Client Need:** Reduction of Risk Potential **Integrated Process:** Nursing Process: Assessment **Content Area:** Maternal-Newborn **Strategy:** The core issue of the question is an assessment that could reduce the risk associated with hypersalpingogram. Recalling that interruption of pregnancy is a risk, use knowledge of the test and timing of the menstrual cycle to choose correctly. **Reference:** Ladewig, P., London, M., & Davidson, M. (2009). *Contemporary maternal-newborn nursing care* (7th ed.). Upper Saddle River, NJ: Pearson Education, p. 148.

9 **Answer: 4 Rationale:** A large number of embryos implanted in the uterus or fallopian tube following IVF increases the chance of achieving pregnancy; however, it also increases the risk of multifetal pregnancy. Placing 10 embryos via IVF would be unethical because of the possibility of high multiples. Understanding discomfort of egg retrieval procedure, that the fertilized eggs will be implanted two to three days after egg retrieval, and the need to limit physical activity on the days of the egg retrieval and implantation are items of correct information and do not require follow-up by the nurse. **Cognitive Level:** Applying **Client Need:** Reduction of Risk Potential **Integrated Process:** Teaching and Learning **Content Area:** Maternal-Newborn **Strategy:** Critical words are *in vitro fertilization* and *need for additional teaching*, indicating the correct answer is one that is a wrong statement from the client, which deals with the number of eggs implanted. **Reference:** Ladewig, P., London, M., & Davidson, M. (2009). *Contemporary maternal-newborn nursing care* (7th ed.). Upper Saddle River, NJ: Pearson Education, p. 149.

10 **Answer: 3 Rationale:** Anti-sperm antibodies can develop in the vaginal and cervical secretions. Inserting the sperm directly into the uterus via intrauterine insemination bypasses the secretions so that the sperm are not destroyed. Sperm intrauterine insemination will not necessarily increase the chances of the couple getting pregnant when the male partner has a varicocele or the human immunodeficiency virus, or the female partner has irregular menses. **Cognitive Level:** Analyzing **Client Need:** Health Promotion and Maintenance **Integrated Process:** Nursing Process: Assessment **Content Area:** Maternal-Newborn **Strategy:** The critical phrase is *intrauterine insemination*, which indicates the process of bypassing the vagina and cervical secretions. Compare each option to this phrase to determine which option has the closest association with this process. **Reference:** Ladewig, P., London, M., & Davidson, M. (2009). *Contemporary maternal-newborn nursing care* (7th ed.). Upper Saddle River, NJ: Pearson Education, p. 149.

Posttest

1 **Answer: 1 Rationale:** Either partner may experience feelings of guilt when faced with infertility. If the problem is with

one partner, that partner's feelings of guilt are often more intense. Taking a medical and surgical history of both partners relates to the clients' histories, not the plan of care. Only giving brief answers to questions asked and raised is nontherapeutic. Referring the clients to another clinic for a second opinion is not the role of the nurse. **Cognitive Level:** Applying **Client Need:** Psychosocial Integrity **Integrated Process:** Nursing Process: Planning **Content Area:** Maternal-Newborn **Strategy:** Critical words are *infertile client* and *plan of care*. Only one option deals with the feelings of loss. Remember that infertility has a large emotional component and it is important to remember to address the emotional needs of the client. **Reference:** Ladewig, P., London, M., & Davidson, M. (2009). *Contemporary maternal-newborn nursing care* (7th ed.). Upper Saddle River, NJ: Pearson Education, p. 136.

2 **Answer: 1** **Rationale:** A recurrence of PID can occur following HSG, so this data should be assessed before the procedure so that prophylactic antibiotics can be prescribed. A water- or oil-based dye is instilled into the uterus and watched on x-ray to detect uterine anomalies or lack of tubal patency; however, a peanut allergy is of no concern with the use of contrast media. The presence of metal implants or difficulty swallowing will not affect the test. **Cognitive Level:** Analyzing **Client Need:** Reduction of Risk Potential **Integrated Process:** Nursing Process: Assessment **Content Area:** Maternal-Newborn **Strategy:** A critical word in the stem is *hysterosalpingogram*, which is a diagnostic test. Recall that invasive procedures carry a risk of infection, so clients already at high risk for recurrence of infection will need prophylactic treatment. **Reference:** Ladewig, P., London, M., & Davidson, M. (2010). *Contemporary maternal-newborn nursing care* (7th ed.). Upper Saddle River, NJ: Pearson Education, p. 142.

3 **Answer: 3** **Rationale:** Ova retrieval and GIFT are outpatient procedures. The client will not be hospitalized overnight. The other statements are correct and do not require any follow-up by the nurse. **Cognitive Level:** Analyzing **Client Need:** Physiological Adaptation **Integrated Process:** Teaching and Learning **Content Area:** Maternal-Newborn **Strategy:** The wording of the question has a negative stem, which leads you to look for an option that contains a false statement about a point of client teaching. Specific knowledge of this procedure is necessary to answer this question, so review it carefully if you chose incorrectly. **Reference:** Ladewig, P., London, M., & Davidson, M. (2010). *Contemporary maternal-newborn nursing care* (7th ed.). Upper Saddle River, NJ: Pearson Education, p. 149.

4 **Answer: 4** **Rationale:** When sperm are donated for use in artificial insemination, informed consent must be obtained from all parties. Processing procedures to prevent transmission of genetic defects or infectious disease are mandatory. Guidelines have been established to limit the number of pregnancies per donor. Donor sperm must be frozen and quarantined for six months to prevent risk of disease transmission. **Cognitive Level:** Applying **Client Need:** Health Promotion and Maintenance **Integrated Process:** Teaching and Learning **Content Area:** Maternal-Newborn **Strategy:** Critical words in the stem are *artificial insemination* and *donor sperm*. Use knowledge of donor sperm processes to choose correctly. **Reference:** Ladewig, P., London, M., & Davidson, M. (2010). *Contemporary maternal-newborn nursing care* (7th ed.). Upper Saddle River, NJ: Pearson Education, p. 147.

5 **Answer: 4** **Rationale:** To maximize the chances of conception through achieving the greatest number of motile sperm, couples must abstain for two to three days prior to expected ovulation and then have intercourse on the day of ovulation or the date of artificial insemination or in vitro fertilization. Because of this, the client's husband must be a willing participant in the infertility regimen. The other statements indicate the client has motivation and a realistic view of the fertility regimen. **Cognitive Level:** Applying **Client Need:** Psychosocial Integrity **Integrated Process:** Communication and Documentation **Content Area:** Maternal-Newborn **Strategy:** Critical words in the stem are *difficulty coping* with *infertility regimen*. Only one option contains a response about finding the process difficult; the other three options are typical responses to the cost and procedures involved. **Reference:** Ricci, S. (2009). *Essentials of maternity, newborn, and women's health nursing* (2nd ed.). Philadelphia, PA: Lippincott Williams & Wilkins, pp. 74–78.

6 **Answer: 2, 5** **Rationale:** A complete bicornate uterus is two complete and separate unicornate uteri. Because of the shape of the uteri being long and narrow (instead of pear-shaped), the maximum uterine volume is often less than a normally shaped uterus. Risks of bicornate uterus include multiple pregnancy losses, preterm labor, and breech presentation. Becoming pregnant is not an issue; carrying the pregnancy to term is the problem. A cesarean delivery may or may not be needed. **Cognitive Level:** Applying **Client Need:** Physiological Adaptation **Integrated Process:** Nursing Process: Diagnosis **Content Area:** Maternal-Newborn **Strategy:** The critical words are *bicornuate uterus*. Use knowledge of the anatomy of the uterus and bicornuate uterus to answer the question, keeping in mind that the risks involve carrying a pregnancy due to the altered anatomy. **Reference:** Ladewig, P., London, M., & Davidson, M. (2010). *Contemporary maternal-newborn nursing care* (7th ed.). Upper Saddle River, NJ: Pearson Education, p. 135.

7 **Answer: 3** **Rationale:** Severe abdominal pain during a cycle of induced ovulation may indicate hyperstimulation of the ovaries. The ovaries could potentially rupture, leading to death. The risk of this complication takes precedence over any clients requiring routine care. The woman being seen for an initial infertility exam, the man waiting for semen analysis results and the woman coming in for a pregnancy test require routine care. **Cognitive Level:** Analyzing **Client Need:** Management of Care **Integrated Process:** Nursing Process: Planning **Content Area:** Maternal-Newborn **Strategy:** The critical word in the question is *first*. This indicates that the correct option is the one where the client is most at risk. Use knowledge of hCG side effects to determine that this client might be at highest risk. Using Maslow's hierarchy of needs would also allow you to choose correctly, because this client has the greatest physiological need over those with needs for routine care. **Reference:** Ladewig, P., London, M., & Davidson, M. (2009). *Contemporary maternal-newborn nursing care* (7th ed.). Upper Saddle River, NJ: Pearson Education, p. 145.

8 **Answer: 3 Rationale:** Bilateral tubal blockage requires surgical intervention. The client will not become pregnant until the tubes are cleared surgically; a pregnancy cannot occur and "unblock" the tube. This statement indicates that the client does not understand her situation and requires further education. The other options contain statements that indicate understanding of the need for surgical treatment. **Cognitive Level:** Analyzing **Client Need:** Physiological Adaptation **Integrated Process:** Teaching and Learning **Content Area:** Maternal-Newborn **Strategy:** Critical words are *bilateral tubal blockage* and *further education*. The correct option is the one that indicates a faulty understanding on the part of the client. Use nursing knowledge of this condition and the process of elimination to select correctly. **Reference:** Ladewig, P., London, M., & Davidson, M. (2010). *Contemporary maternal-newborn nursing care* (7th ed.). Upper Saddle River, NJ: Pearson Education, p.145.

9 **Answer: 4 Rationale:** Fourteen percent body fat is considered adequate to have regular menses and regular ovulation. A client with less than 10% body fat will ovulate and menstruate very irregularly if at all. **Cognitive Level:** Applying **Client Need:** Health Promotion and Maintenance **Integrated Process:** Nursing Process: Assessment **Content Area:** Maternal-Newborn **Strategy:** Critical words are *long-distance runner* and *9.0% body fat*. Use knowledge of physiology of menstrual cycle and ovulation to answer the question. **Reference:** Ladewig, P., London, M., & Davidson, M. (2010). *Contemporary maternal-newborn nursing care* (7th ed.). Upper Saddle River, NJ: Pearson Education, p. 137.

10 **Answer: 1 Rationale:** Pregnancy is characterized by a 0.5 to 1.0°F persistent increase in BBT. The incorrect responses do not follow this trend. **Cognitive Level:** Applying **Client Need:** Health Promotion and Maintenance **Integrated Process:** Teaching and Learning **Content Area:** Maternal-Newborn **Strategy:** Critical words are *intrauterine insemination* and *effective* teaching. These tell you that the correct option is also a correct statement. Use knowledge of pregnancy and its effect on body temperature to answer the question. **Reference:** Ladewig, P., London, M., & Davidson, M. (2010). *Contemporary maternal-newborn nursing care* (7th ed.). Upper Saddle River, NJ: Pearson Education, p. 139.

References

Davidson, M., London, M., & Ladewig, P. (2012). *Olds' maternal newborn nursing & women's health across the lifespan* (9th ed.). Upper Saddle River, NJ: Pearson Education.

Ladewig, P., London, M., & Davidson, M. (2010). *Contemporary maternal-newborn nursing care* (7th ed.). Upper Saddle River, NJ: Pearson Education.

Morris, R. (n.d.). *IVF1 reproductive medicine*. Retrieved January 28, 2011, from http://www.ivf1.com

NANDA Nursing Diagnosis (2009). Retrieved January 29, 2011, from http://www.scribd.com/doc/11885949/NANDA-2009

Pilliteri, A. (2009). *Maternal and child health nursing* (6th ed.). Philadelphia: Lippincott Williams & Wilkins.

Ricci, S. (2009). *Essentials of maternity, newborn, and women's health nursing* (2nd ed.). Philadelphia: Lippincott Williams & Wilkins.

Family Planning and Contraception 3

Chapter Outline

Overview of Family Planning and Contraception
Nursing Process in Family Planning and Contraception
Natural Methods of Family Planning and Contraception
Fertility Awareness Methods of Family Planning and Contraception
Barrier Methods of Family Planning and Contraception
Hormonal Methods of Family Planning and Contraception
Surgical Methods of Contraception

Objectives

- Identify the goals of family planning.
- Compare the advantages, disadvantages, and effectiveness of various contraceptives.
- Describe nursing responsibilities related to client education regarding contraception.

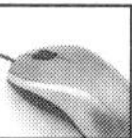

NCLEX-RN® Test Prep

Use the accompanying online resource, NursingReviewsandRationales, to test yourself with hundreds of NCLEX®-style practice questions.

Review at a Glance

abstinence refraining voluntarily from sexual intercourse

calendar method method of contraception in which a woman abstains from intercourse during fertile period; also known as rhythm method

cervical cap a small cap made of soft rubber that is placed over cervix to block entry of sperm into cervix

coitus interruptus withdrawal of penis and ejaculation away from vagina

contraceptive sponge a small, round polyurethane sponge containing a spermicide

Depo-Provera long-acting progestin administered by injection every three months for contraception

diaphragm flexible, dome-shaped rubber device to cover the cervix and prevent conception

female condom disposable, polyurethane sheath with a flexible ring at each end; closed end is placed into vagina to prevent sperm from entering vagina

intrauterine device (IUD) a plastic or metal device placed into the uterus for long periods of time to prevent implantation of a fertilized egg or cause changes in lining of endometrium

male condom sheath made of latex, plastic, or natural membranes and placed on an erect penis prior to inserting into vagina to collect contents of ejaculation

mittelschmerz old term for midcycle pain experienced at time of ovulation; may last from one to two days and may be accompanied by pressure, aching felt into rectum, or distention

oral contraceptives birth control pills that contain estrogen and progestin, or progestin alone, to prevent ovulation and promote thinning of endometrium

emergency contraception a method of contraception initiated within 72 hours of unprotected intercourse or contraceptive failure to prevent pregnancy

spermicide chemical agent contained in a variety of forms that is used to kill sperm or neutralize vaginal secretions to immobilize sperm; commonly nonoxynol-9 and oxynol-9

subdermal implant a single rod filled with synthetic progestin etonogestrel (Implanon), which is surgically inserted on inner side of a woman's upper arm to prevent pregnancy for three years by thickening cervical mucus, altering endometrium, and suppressing ovulation

symptothermal method a fertility awareness method of contraception that assesses and records daily the primary and secondary signs of ovulation and a coital history on a menstrual cycle calendar and includes abstinence from intercourse during period of fertility

tubal ligation surgical intervention to cut, tie, cauterize, or band fallopian tubes to block passage of eggs from ovary to uterus

vasectomy resection of vas deferens to prevent sperm from being ejaculated outside body

PRETEST

1 The client is making her first visit to the contraceptive clinic to discuss her options for birth control. When teaching the client about family planning, the nurse should include information on which of the following? Select all that apply.

1. Male condoms and spermicide should be used together
2. Depomedroxyprogesterone acetate (DMPA)
3. Oral contraceptives
4. Screening for possible birth defects
5. Semen analysis

2 The client has come to the family planning clinic to discuss the use of contraceptives. The nurse should do which of the following to facilitate a productive discussion?

1. Discuss contraceptive options with the married client only if her partner is present.
2. Instruct the client in which contraceptive option she should use.
3. Inform the client about use, side effects, and effectiveness of different contraceptive options so that the client can select one that meets her needs.
4. Avoid discussion of side effects as this might frighten the client and result in her not using a contraceptive.

3 The client, who has been married for three years and is sexually active but not yet ready to begin having children, has expressed a desire to use a natural method of family planning. Based on this information, which of the following would be the best choice for this client?

1. Total abstinence
2. Basal body temperature method
3. Male condoms
4. Female condoms with a spermicide

4 Which statement by a male client would indicate that he understands the instructions for use of a condom?

1. "I should lubricate the condom with an oil-based product to avoid friction that could rupture the condom."
2. "I should unroll the condom and check it for holes before applying it."
3. "I should hold the rim of the condom while withdrawing my penis from the vagina to avoid leakage."
4. "I should begin sexual intercourse without the condom and don the condom just before ejaculation."

5 After counseling a client about several contraception options, the client tells the nurse that she has decided to use female condoms. The nurse evaluates that the client understood the information when the client makes which statement?

1. "I understand that I shouldn't apply the condom more than one hour before having sex."
2. "I understand that if I develop a latex allergy I will need to find a different type of birth control."
3. "I understand that this will provide protection against sexually transmitted diseases for me and my partner."
4. "I understand that my doctor will measure me for the condoms, and then I will purchase them at the drug store."

6 In planning education for a client who has decided to use a diaphragm for contraception, the nurse should include which items of information in the teaching plan? Select all that apply.

1. An oil-based lubricant should be used to facilitate insertion.
2. The diaphragm should be washed with mild soap and water after each use.
3. One teaspoonful of spermicidal cream or jelly should be applied around the rim and inside the cup.
4. The diaphragm may be used during the menstrual period.
5. The diaphragm should remain in place for at least six hours after coitus.

7 When reviewing the assessment data of the client, what data would lead the nurse to recommend a method of contraception other than oral contraceptives?

1. Family history of ovarian cancer
2. Type 1 diabetes mellitus
3. History of iron-deficiency anemia
4. Fibrocystic breast disease

8 The client is interested in having an intrauterine device (IUD) inserted. As part of maintaining a standard of quality care, the nurse would ensure that the client is aware of which side effect of this therapy?

1. Fewer episodes of dysmenorrhea
2. Increased risk of pelvic inflammatory disease
3. Increased production of thin cervical and vaginal mucus
4. Incomplete emptying of the bladder

9 A male client has come to the clinic to discuss having a vasectomy. Which client statement indicates the client understands the procedure?

1. "I will be able to return to my job as a construction worker immediately following the procedure."
2. "The procedure should be performed in a hospital, preferably under general anesthesia."
3. "It will be safe for me to have unprotected sex one week following the procedure."
4. "The procedure will not affect my sexual function."

10 A pregnant client, who is considering a tubal ligation following her delivery, asks the nurse about the effectiveness of the method. What is the best response by the nurse?

1. "Like all methods of contraception, the effectiveness depends on client compliance."
2. "Effectiveness depends on whether the tubes are clipped, banded, or plugged."
3. "The method is very effective. Only 1 to 4 women per 1000 get pregnant after a tubal ligation."
4. "If you have a tubal ligation, you won't ever have to worry about getting pregnant again because the procedure is 100% effective."

➤ *See pages 64–65 for Answers and Rationales.*

I. OVERVIEW OF FAMILY PLANNING AND CONTRACEPTION

A. **Goal of family planning**: to assist clients with reproductive decision making, enabling client to have control in preventing pregnancy, limiting number of children, spacing time between children, and voluntarily interrupting pregnancy as desired

B. **Decision to use a contraceptive:** may be made individually by a man or woman, or jointly by a couple

C. **Legal issues related to family planning and contraception**

1. Laws pertaining to provision of contraceptives to minors without parental consent vary from state to state
2. Some states may require consent from client's spouse regarding sterilization and voluntary interruption of pregnancy

3. Because of potentially serious complications associated with many contraceptive methods, informed consent is obtained
   a. Document information provided and client understanding of information
   b. The mnemonic BRAIDED shown in Box 3-1 may be useful to when counseling a client about family planning and contraceptive methods
4. Decisions about family planning and contraception should be made voluntarily with knowledge of advantages, disadvantages, effectiveness, side effects, risks, contraindications, and long-term effects of a method

Box 3-1

Acronym for Informed Consent with Contraception: BRAIDED

B = Benefits: information about advantages
R = Risks: information about disadvantages
A = Alternatives: information about other methods available
I = Inquiries: opportunity for the client to ask questions
D = Decisions: opportunity for the client to decide or change mind
E = Explanations: information about the selected method and how to use it
D = Documentation: information given and client's understanding of the information

5. Emancipated minor statutes are legal mandates where minors, under age 18, may hold legal decision-making rights usually reserved for adults based upon privacy issues; in most states this statute goes into effect for minors seeking birth control or pregnancy services

II. NURSING PROCESS IN FAMILY PLANNING AND CONTRACEPTION

A. Assessment

1. Obtain a history to identify client's past and current health status and potential risk factors, including risk of a current pregnancy
2. Obtain additional information through a sexual history regarding client's reproductive health and future plans for childbearing
3. Psychosocial data provides information regarding client's lifestyle, motivation, religious beliefs, cultural influences, and financial factors that may affect selection, access, and use of a particular method; do not assume client is heterosexual
4. Knowledge of and concerns about contraceptive methods need to be determined and are necessary to identify potential deficits and need for accurate or additional information

B. Priority nursing diagnoses: Health-Seeking Behaviors; Deficient Knowledge; Risk for Disturbed Self-Concept; Disturbed Body Image; Anxiety; Risk for Ineffective Sexuality Patterns

C. Planning and implementation

1. Identify actual or potential problems from client assessment
2. Provide privacy to facilitate discussion; include partner, if desired
3. Establish mutual goals that facilitate client understanding, compliance, and method effectiveness
4. Provide information about risks, benefits, use, side effects, and cost to facilitate decision making
5. Utilize educational materials designed at client's level of comprehension; provide information that progresses from simple to complex
6. Assist client to select a contraceptive method that meets both physiological and psychosocial needs

Practice to Pass

How might a nurse modify a teaching plan for a client with low literacy skills?

D. Evaluation

1. Client expresses satisfaction and willingness to comply with selected method of contraception
2. Client demonstrates desired changes in knowledge or behavior
3. Pregnancy is prevented

III. NATURAL METHODS OF FAMILY PLANNING AND CONTRACEPTION

A. Natural methods: safe, situational methods requiring increased self-awareness and self-control to be effective

B. Types of natural family planning methods

1. **Abstinence** is the practice of avoiding sexual intercourse
   a. Advantages
      1) Method is safe, free, and available to all clients

2) 100% effective in preventing pregnancy and sexually transmitted infections (STIs) when consistently practiced
3) Can be initiated at any time
4) Encourages communication between partners
5) Often is the only method that is endorsed by conservative religions such as Roman Catholic Church

b. A disadvantage is that both participants must practice self-control

c. Client education

1) Teach alternative methods of obtaining sexual pleasure
2) Provide positive feedback to clients who desire and maintain abstinence

2. **Coitus interruptus** (withdrawal)

a. Coitus interruptus requires male to withdraw penis from female's vagina when urge to ejaculate occurs and to ejaculate away from external female genitalia

b. Clients who choose this method must utilize self-control, as the most pleasurable moment during sexual intercourse may coincide with time to withdraw penis

c. Advantages

1) Coitus interruptus can be practiced at any time during menstrual cycle
2) Method is free

d. Disadvantages

1) It is one of the oldest but least reliable contraceptive methods; 80% effective with typical use
2) Some pre-ejaculatory fluid, which may contain sperm, may escape from penis during excitement phase prior to ejaculation
3) At peak of sexual excitement, exercising self-control may be difficult

e. Client education

1) Before engaging in sexual intercourse, male should urinate and wipe off tip of penis to decrease potential of introducing sperm into vagina
2) Conception may occur if pre-ejaculatory fluid containing sperm enters introitus
3) A spermicide or postcoital contraceptive may be needed if female partner is exposed to sperm

IV. FERTILITY AWARENESS METHODS OF FAMILY PLANNING AND CONTRACEPTION

A. Overview

1. These methods are based on an understanding of woman's ovulation cycle and timing of sexual intercourse
2. All methods attempt to identify period of female fertility and to avoid unprotected intercourse during that time period

B. Advantages of fertility awareness methods

1. Free, safe, and acceptable to couples whose religious beliefs prohibit other methods, such as Roman Catholics
2. Increases awareness of woman's body
3. Encourages couple communication
4. Can be used to prevent or plan a pregnancy

C. Disadvantages of fertility awareness methods

1. Requires extensive initial counseling and education
2. May interfere with sexual spontaneity
3. May be difficult or impossible for women with irregular menstrual cycles
4. Used alone, they offer no protection against STIs
5. Are theoretically reliable, but less effective in actual use

D. Calendar method

1. Also known as rhythm method, is based on assumptions that ovulation occurs 14 days (plus or minus 2 days) prior to next menses, sperm are viable for 5 days, and the ovum is capable of being fertilized for 24 hours
2. **Calendar method** is least reliable of fertility awareness methods, being 91% effective with perfect use and 75% effective with typical use
3. Client education
   a. Teach woman to maintain a menstrual calendar for six to eight months to identify shortest and longest cycles
   b. With first day of menstruation as first day of cycle, calculate fertile period by subtracting 18 days from length of shortest cycle through length of longest cycle minus 11 days
   c. Counsel woman to avoid intercourse during fertile period

E. Basal body temperature (BBT) method

1. Based on thermal shift in menstrual cycle, client's temperature drops just prior to ovulation, rises and fluctuates at a higher level until two to four days prior to next menses, then falls if no conception occurs; best used after gathering three to six months worth of cycle charting to evaluate for regular or predictable temperature fluctuations; is 97% effective with perfect use, and 75% effective with typical use
2. Client education
   a. Instruct woman to measure temperature with a basal body thermometer, which shows 10ths of a degree, and record findings on a temperature chart
   ! b. Teach client to measure temperature each morning before getting out of bed or beginning activity
   ! c. Counsel client to avoid intercourse on day temperature drops and for three days thereafter
   d. Inform client that reliability of method can be affected by
      1) A decrease in BBT that is too small to detect
      2) Factors that may raise or lower BBT such as illness, stress, fatigue, consumption of alcohol the prior evening, or sleeping in a heated waterbed
      3) Intercourse just prior to drop in temperature may result in pregnancy

F. Cervical mucus method

1. Also known as ovulation or Billings method, this method is based on cervical mucus changes that occur during menstrual cycle; effectiveness is same as BBT method
2. Changes in cervical mucus in response to levels of estrogen and progesterone are shown in Table 3-1
3. Client education
   a. Teach woman to assess her cervical mucus daily for amount, color, consistency, and viscosity
   ! b. Counsel woman to avoid intercourse when she first notices cervical mucus becoming more clear, elastic, and slippery and for about four days
   c. Convey sensitivity because women who are uncomfortable touching their genitals may find this method unacceptable
   d. Instruct client that cervical mucus can be affected by
      1) Douches and vaginal deodorants
      2) Semen
      3) Blood and discharge from vaginal infections
      4) Contraceptive gels, foams, film, or suppositories
      5) Antihistamine drugs

Table 3–1 Cervical Mucus Assessment

Factors to assess	Menstrual Cycle Phase	
	Luteal phase (infertile period)	***Follicular phase/ovulation (fertile period)***
Dominant hormone	Progesterone	Estrogen
Vaginal characteristics	Dryness	Wetness
Cervical mucus characteristics		
Amount	Scant	Profuse
Color	Cloudy, white to yellow	Clear
Consistency	Thick, sticky	Thin, watery, slippery
Viscosity	None	Stretchable, spinnbarkheit
		Present at ovulation
Microscopic appearance	No ferning	Ferning

G. Symptothermal method

1. The **symptothermal method** incorporates assessment of multiple indicators of ovulation, recording findings and coital history on a menstrual calendar, and then abstaining from intercourse during fertile period; effectiveness is 98% with perfect use and 75% with typical use
2. Client education
   a. Instruct client to assess and record the primary indicators of ovulation
      1) Basal body temperature
      2) Cervical mucus
   b. Teach client to become self-aware of and record secondary indicators of ovulation
      1) Increased libido
      2) Abdominal bloating
      3) **Mittelschmerz**: midcycle abdominal pain
      4) Breast or pelvic tenderness
      5) Pelvic or vulvar fullness
      6) Slight dilatation of cervical os
      7) Softer cervix located higher in vagina
   c. Counsel client to avoid unprotected sexual intercourse during fertile period
   d. Teach client that this method provides no protection against STIs

Practice to Pass

Discuss the changes that occur during ovulation to be included in a teaching plan for a client who wants to use a fertility awareness method.

V. BARRIER METHODS OF FAMILY PLANNING AND CONTRACEPTION

A. Barrier methods: provide a physical or chemical barrier to block sperm from entering cervix; some barrier devices are made from latex and should be avoided by those with latex allergies

B. Male condom

1. The **male condom** is a sheath made of latex, plastic, or natural membranes, which is placed over an erect penis to collect semen; effectiveness is 97% with perfect use and 86% with typical use
2. Client education
   a. Instruct client to check expiration date on package, and if it is past date, obtain another condom
   b. ! Teach client to avoid using oil-based lubricants, although contraceptive foam or water-based lubricants may be used

c. Instruct client to put on a condom by placing unrolled condom on tip of erect penis, leaving enough room at tip to collect sperm, then unrolling condom from tip of erect penis to base
d. Counsel client that after intercourse, erect penis should be withdrawn from vagina while holding rim of condom to prevent leakage
e. Advise client to inspect used condom for tears or holes, as a break in integrity of sheath will decrease effectiveness
f. Teach client to discard used condom in a disposable waste container; do not flush in toilet

3. Advantages
   a. Males are able to participate in contraception
   b. Sexual intercourse may be prolonged
   c. Condoms are available in a variety of sizes and styles at low cost
   d. Partners can participate in placing condom to enhance enjoyment
   e. All condoms except those made of natural skins offer protection against pregnancy and STIs; natural skin condoms have pores that can allow passage of viruses
4. Disadvantages
   a. Penis must be erect before placing condom
   b. To prevent spillage of semen, male must withdraw after ejaculating, while penis is still erect
   c. Condoms can rupture or leak, increasing potential for semen to escape into vagina
   d. Oil-based lubricants can decrease effectiveness of condom
   e. Condoms are for single use only
   f. Misplacement, perineal or vaginal irritation, or dulled penile sensation are possible

C. Female condom

1. The **female condom** is a thin, polyurethane sheath with flexible rings at each end, which covers cervix, lines vagina, and partially shields perineum; effectiveness is 95% with perfect use and 79% with typical use
2. Client education
   a. Instruct client to insert closed end of condom into vagina so ring fits loosely against cervix
   b. Counsel client to have partner insert penis into open end, leaving approximately one inch of sheath from flexible ring outside of introitus

   c. Advise client that after intercourse, remove condom before standing up by squeezing and twisting outer ring to close sheath while gently pulling it out of vagina
3. Advantages
   a. Condom may be inserted up to eight hours before intercourse
   b. Clients who are sensitive to latex can use female condom
   c. Both partners are protected against STIs during intercourse
   d. Female condoms are available without a prescription
   e. Use of lubricants will not decrease effectiveness
   f. Breastfeeding women can safely use condoms
4. Disadvantages
   a. These condoms may twist or slip during intercourse
   b. If penis is placed outside of condom, effectiveness is jeopardized
   c. Improper removal results in risk of ejaculate leaking out of condom
   d. Outer ring may irritate external genitalia
   e. The high cost, noise produced with intercourse, or altered sensation are unacceptable for some couples
   f. Initially, insertion may be difficult or awkward

D. Spermicides

1. **Spermicides** form a chemical barrier preventing pregnancy by killing sperm or neutralizing vaginal secretions and are available in a variety of forms including creams, gels, melting suppositories, foaming tablets, aerosol foams, and vaginal contraceptive film
2. When used alone, effectiveness is 94% with perfect use and 74% with typical use; when spermicides and other methods are combined, contraceptive and antimicrobial benefits are increased
3. Nonoxynol-9 and octoxynol-9 are most common spermicidal agents; allergic response is possible
4. Client education
   - **a.** Instruct client to apply spermicide inside vagina and close to cervix before penis is placed near introitus
   - ! **b.** Advise that spermicides must be applied with each act of sexual intercourse
   - ! **c.** Teach client that onset of spermicidal action varies; when used alone effectiveness lasts no longer than one hour
   - **d.** Counsel client that contraceptive foams, creams, and gels are effective immediately
   - **e.** Counsel client that vaginal contraceptive film and suppositories become effective 15 minutes after insertion into vagina
5. Advantages
   - **a.** No prescription is required to purchase spermicides
   - **b.** Spermicides may be used alone, with a diaphragm, or with a condom
   - **c.** Foams, gels, and suppositories may add additional lubrication and moisture
   - **d.** Penis can remain in vagina following ejaculation
   - **e.** Method is safe for breastfeeding women
   - **f.** The availability of a variety of forms offers clients additional choices in selecting a spermicide
6. Disadvantages
   - **a.** Spermicide may be irritating to one or both clients
   - **b.** Some forms may be perceived as messy
   - **c.** This method may interfere with spontaneity, as it is inserted before each act of intercourse and may require an interval of time before onset of action

E. Diaphragm

1. The **diaphragm** is a dome-shaped appliance made of rubber with a flexible rim that fits over cervix, is used with spermicidal cream or jelly, and prevents sperm from entering cervix; effectiveness is 94% with perfect use and 80% with typical use
2. Client education
   - **a.** Use models and visual aids when demonstrating insertion and removal of diaphragm
   - **b.** Teach client to insert and remove diaphragm (Figure 3-1)
     - **1)** Apply about a teaspoon of spermicidal cream or jelly around rim and inside cup
     - **2)** Squeeze sides of diaphragm together, insert through vagina, place side of device containing spermicide over cervix, and push upper edge under symphysis pubis
     - **3)** Remove diaphragm by grasping rim to dislodge from cervix and pull down to remove through vagina
   - **c.** Encourage client to practice insertion and removal when health care provider is present to check for proper placement in vagina
   - ! **d.** Teach client that diaphragm remains effective if inserted up to four hours before sexual intercourse and should be left in place at least six hours after coitus
   - ! **e.** Counsel client that if diaphragm is placed more than four hours before intercourse or coitus is desired again within six hours, a condom should be used or additional spermicide should be inserted into vagina without disturbing diaphragm

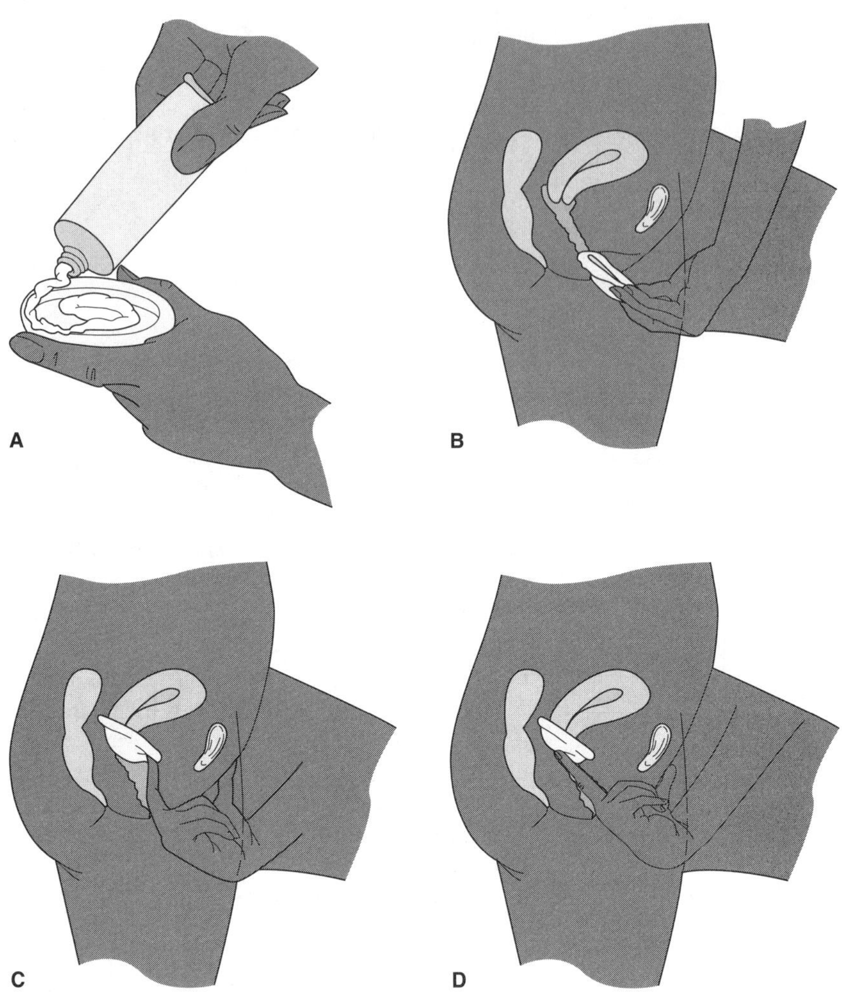

Figure 3–1

Inserting the diaphragm. A. Apply jelly to rim and center, B. Insert diaphragm, C. Push diaphragm rim under symphysis pubis, D. Check placement; cervix should be felt through diaphragm.

! **f.** Instruct client that device should be removed at least once during a 24-hour period to decrease risk of toxic shock syndrome

g. Advise client to clean diaphragm with mild soap and water and inspect for tears, punctures, and thinning, avoid use of oil-based lubricants, which weaken the rubber, and replace diaphragm if any damage is observed

h. Teach client to dry device thoroughly, dust with cornstarch, and store in carrying case away from light and heat

i. Advise client to avoid use during menstrual period or when abnormal vaginal discharge is present to decrease risk of toxic shock syndrome

! **j.** Instruct client to contact health care provider if experiencing any warning signs as shown in Table 3-2

3. Advantages

a. Using a diaphragm gives the woman control

b. Barrier provides some protection against STIs

c. A partner may insert diaphragm if client has trouble with placement or as part of foreplay

d. Diaphragm contains no hormones and is safe for breastfeeding client

e. Penis can remain inside vagina after ejaculation

Table 3–2 Warning Signs and Symptoms Associated with Various Methods of Contraception

Method	Warning Signs and Symptoms
Cervical cap, diaphragm, and contraceptive sponge	Toxic Shock Syndrome • Elevation of temperature >101.4°F • Diarrhea and vomiting • Weakness and faintness • Muscle aches • Sore throat • Sunburn-type rash • Difficult or painful urination • Abdominal or pelvic fullness • Foul-smelling vaginal discharge
Intrauterine device (IUD)	Acronym **PAINS** **P** = Period late (pregnancy), abnormal spotting or bleeding **A** = Abdominal pain, pain with intercourse **I** = Infection exposure (STI), abnormal vaginal discharge **N** = Not feeling well, fever >100.4°F, chills **S** = String missing, shorter or longer than usually felt
Oral contraceptives	Acronym **ACHES** **A** = Abdominal pain **C** = Chest pain, cough, and/or shortness of breath **H** = Headaches, dizziness, weakness or numbness **E** = Eye problems (blurring or change in vision) and speech problems **S** = Severe leg, calf, and/or thigh pain
Vasectomy	Fever >100.4°F Excessive pain Difficulty urinating Redness, swelling, bruising, drainage, or skin edges of the incision that are not closed Bleeding at the site
Tubal ligation	Fever >100.4°F Excessive pain Difficulty with defecation or urination Nausea or vomiting Redness, swelling, bruising, drainage, or skin edges of the incision that are not closed

4. Disadvantages
   a. Diaphragm must be fitted by a qualified health care provider and replaced annually
   b. Refitting or replacement may be needed following pregnancy or a 15-pound weight gain or loss
   c. Some clients may have difficulty learning to correctly place diaphragm
5. Contraindications
   a. A history of urinary tract infections; pressure from diaphragm on urethra may interfere with complete emptying of bladder and increase risk of infection related to stasis of urine
   b. A history of toxic shock syndrome; if diaphragm is left in place for a long period of time this may increase risk of infection

Practice to Pass

What patient education is indicated to reduce the potential of toxic shock syndrome for a client using a diaphragm?

F. Cervical cap

1. The **cervical cap** is a small thimble-shaped device made of soft rubber that fits over cervix, is held in place by suction, and acts as a barrier between sperm and cervix (see Figure 3-2)

Figure 3–2

A cervical cap

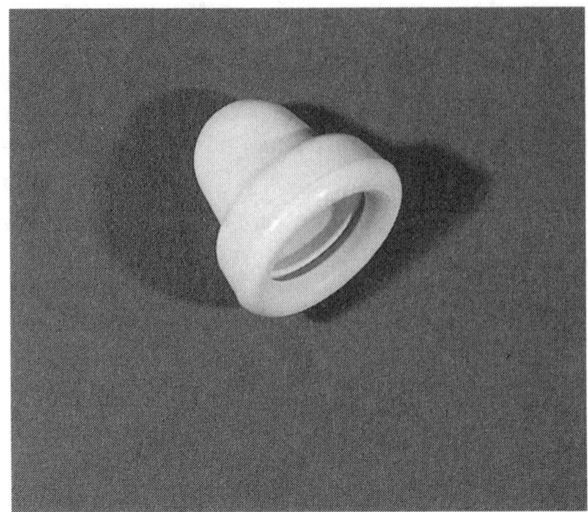

2. Effectiveness is influenced by childbearing history of woman; effectiveness for nulliparous women is 91% with perfect use and 80% with typical use; in parous women effectiveness is 74% with perfect use and 60% with typical use
3. Client education
   a. Teach client to apply spermicide inside cap
   b. Instruct client to insert cap at least 20 minutes but not longer than 4 hours prior to intercourse
   c. Advise client that cervical cap may be left in place up to 48 hours
   d. Counsel client that reapplication of spermicide with repeated intercourse is not needed
   e. Teach client not to use cap during menstruation, if any abnormal vaginal discharge is present, or if any signs or symptoms of infection or inflammation are present
   f. Instruct client to contact health care provider if warning signs develop as listed in Table 3-2
4. Advantages of cervical cap are similar to those of diaphragm
5. Disadvantages
   a. Cervical cap may be more difficult to fit because of limited sizes
   b. Cervical cap must be fit by a qualified health care provider and should be replaced annually
   c. Clients will need to be rechecked for fit following pregnancy or a 15-pound weight gain or loss; effectiveness is reduced for parous women
   d. If device dislodges or slips during sexual intercourse, risk for contraceptive failure or acquiring STIs is increased
   e. Some clients may have difficulty inserting and removing cervical cap

G. Contraceptive sponge

1. The **contraceptive sponge** is a small, round polyurethane sponge containing nonoxynol-9 spermicide
2. Effectiveness in nulliparous women is 91% with perfect use and 80% with typical use; in parous women effectiveness is 80% with perfect use and 60% with typical use
3. Client education
   a. Moisten sponge with water before insertion into vagina to activate spermicide
   b. Place concave side of sponge next to cervix for a better fit

c. Leave sponge in place for at least six hours after intercourse
d. Remove by pulling polyester loop on nonconcave side of sponge downward and out of vagina
e. Advise that sponge provides protection up to 24 hours and for repeated acts of intercourse
f. Leaving sponge in place for more than 24 to 30 hours should be avoided because of increased risk of toxic shock syndrome
g. Contact health care provider if warning signs develop as listed in Table 3-2

4. Advantages
   a. Same as for diaphragm
   b. Low cost
5. Disadvantages
   a. Some clients perceive sponge as bulky or awkward when in place
   b. Some clients perceive presence of sponge as uncomfortable during intercourse
   c. Effectiveness is reduced for parous women

H. *Intrauterine device (IUD)*

1. Specific method of action of IUD is unknown; contraception is achieved by triggering a spermicidal-type reaction with local inflammation of endometrium, thereby preventing fertilization
2. Types of IUDs available in United States (see Figure 3-3)
   a. Levonorgestrel-releasing intrauterine system (LNG-IUS) (Mirena) releases hormone gradually from a reservoir, and is recommended for women who are allergic to copper; may be left in place for up to five years; must be avoided by women with an allergy to levonorgestrel
   b. Copper T380A (ParaGard) can be left in place for 10 years; but must be avoided by women with an allergy to copper
   c. Effectiveness with perfect use is 98.5 to 99.4%; typical use effectiveness ranges from 98 to 99.2%
   d. Preferred candidates for use include parous women in a stable monogamous relationship (low risk for STI) with no history of pelvic inflammatory disease (PID) and normal uterine anatomy; nulliparous women at low risk for STI or women with a history of PID who are in a stable monogamous relationship and have had a pregnancy since the PID episode may also be considered on an individual basis
3. Client education
   a. Teach that cramping or intermittent bleeding may occur for two to six weeks after insertion
   b. Advise that the first few menses after placement may be irregular

Figure 3–3

Two types of IUDs.
A. Levonorgestrel-releasing,
B. Copper T380A.

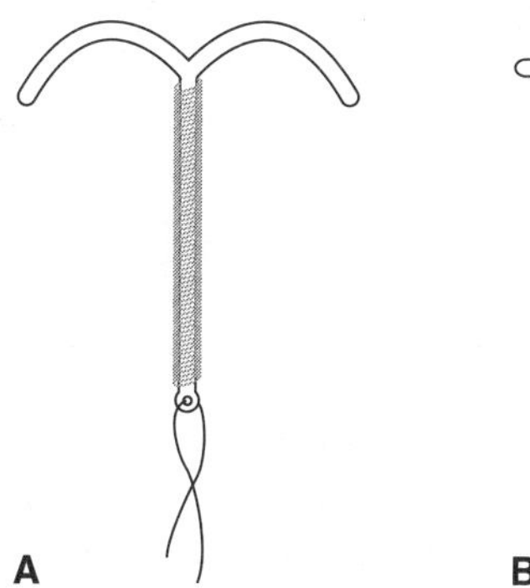

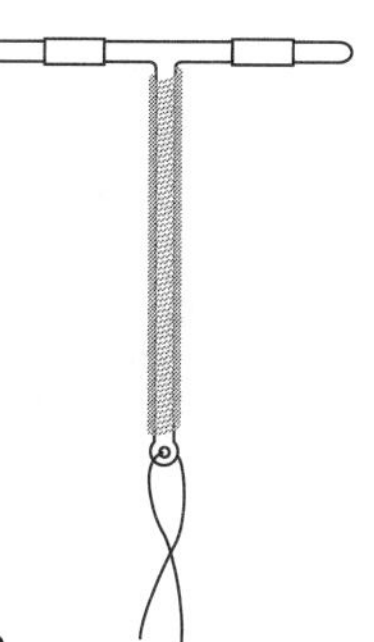

c. Instruct that follow-up examination is suggested in four to eight weeks
d. Instruct woman to check for presence of the string protruding through cervix by inserting a finger into vagina once a week for first month and then after each menstrual period
e. Counsel woman to contact health care provider if she is exposed to a STI or if any warning signs abbreviated as PAINS develop as shown in Table 3-2

4. Advantages
   a. IUDS are highly effective and provide continuous contraceptive protection
   b. They do not interact with medications
   c. They provide a good contraceptive option for women who cannot use hormone contraceptives, are breastfeeding, or are smokers over 35 years of age
5. Disadvantages
   a. IUD must be inserted by a qualified health care professional
   b. Some women experience discomfort, bleeding, and cramping, both during and between menses

   c. Client is at increased risk of pelvic infection for first three weeks following insertion
   d. Uterus may perforate during insertion
   e. IUD may be expelled spontaneously
   f. IUDs do not protect clients from acquiring STIs
   g. Adolescents rarely meet criteria for IUD candidates

VI. HORMONAL METHODS OF FAMILY PLANNING AND CONTRACEPTION

A. ***Oral contraceptives* (birth control pills):** act by inhibiting release of an ovum, blocking cyclical release of gonadotropin-releasing hormone, and changing cervical mucus

1. Types of oral contraceptives
   a. Standard combined oral contraceptives (COCs) contain both estrogen and progestin and are available in 21-day and 28-day packages; effectiveness is 99.1% with perfect use and 95% with typical use
   b. Newer extended use COCs (containing estrogen and progestin) include Seasonale and Seasonique as a 91-day package; women using either of these have 4 withdrawal periods per year instead of 12; effectiveness is similar to standard COCs
      1) With Seasonale the client takes 84 "active" estrogen/progestin pills followed by 7 "blank" pills
      2) With Seasonique the client takes 84 "active" pills followed by 7 pills with a reduced estrogen dose intended to promote less bleeding
   c. Progestin-only pill, also known as mini-pill, does not contain estrogen, contains less progestin than combination pills, and may be used by lactating women, women with mild hypertension, and those who experienced side effects from oral contraceptives containing estrogen; effectiveness is 95.5% with perfect use and 95% with typical use
2. Client education
   a. When starting oral contraceptives, instruct client to begin pills on first Sunday after onset of menstrual period and take one pill at same time each day
   b. If a 28-day or 91-day pack is prescribed or client is taking progestin-only pills, advise client not to skip days between packages
   c. Clients using a 21-day pack should wait seven days before starting the next cycle of pills
   d. Advise client regarding menstrual periods
      1) If using 21-day or 28-day packages, expect monthly menses
      2) If using 91-day packages, expect a menstrual period every three months (four times yearly)

3) Women using 91-day dosing regimens may experience more unplanned bleeding and spotting between expected menstrual periods during first few cycles of use than women on 28-day regimens

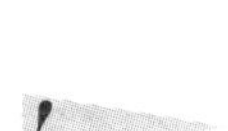

e. Instruct client what to do if progestin-only oral contraceptives are missed
   1) If client misses one pill at any time during cycle, missed pill should be taken immediately and next pill taken at regular time
   2) Any time a pill is missed, client should get back onto a regular schedule for taking pill and use an additional method of contraception through end of that cycle

f. Instruct client what to do if COCs are missed
   1) If one pill is missed at any time during cycle, client should take missed pill immediately, next pill at regular time, and no back-up method is needed
   2) If two pills are missed during first two weeks, client is advised to take two pills for next two days and resume taking pills on regular schedule
   3) If two pills are missed during third week, client is advised to take one pill daily until Sunday, then begin a new pack on Sunday without missing any days
   4) If three or more pills are missed at any time, client is advised to take one pill daily until Sunday, then begin a new pack on Sunday without missing any days
   5) If two or more pills are missed at any time, a back-up method should be used for one week or emergency contraception considered, if unprotected intercourse occurs

g. Observe for side effects of oral contraceptives, which can be estrogen-related (such as thromboembolic disease, headache, fluid retention, and nausea) or progestin-related (including acne, increased HDL cholesterol level, depression, and hirsutism)

h. Contact health care provider immediately if warning signs develop, which are known as ACHES and are shown in Table 3-2

3. Advantages
   a. Use of method is not directly related to act of sexual intercourse
   b. Menstrual periods are usually more regular and predictable
   c. Amount of menstrual flow and premenstrual symptoms are decreased
   d. Incidence or degree of iron-deficiency anemia may be reduced
   e. Oral contraceptives are safe throughout reproductive years for women who do not smoke
   f. Use of extended COCs (91-day pack) reduces side effects such as bloating, headache, breast tenderness, cramping, and swelling over time
   g. Noncontraceptive benefits include a decreased risk of ectopic pregnancy, fibrocystic breast disease, and ovarian and endometrial cancers; improvement of acne; and some protection against development of functional ovarian cysts

4. Disadvantages
   a. Risk of ectopic pregnancy is increased if client conceives while taking progestin-only pill
   b. Progestin-only pills are more likely to cause irregular bleeding or amenorrhea
   c. Oral contraceptives offer no protection against STIs
   d. Clients need to remember to take a pill at same time each day
   e. Clients with preexisting medical problems may not be candidates for this method
   f. Oral contraceptives may decrease effectiveness of insulin and oral anticoagulants such as warfarin (Coumadin)
   g. Effectiveness of oral contraceptives may be decreased when taken with other drugs such as phenytoin (Dilantin), carbamazepine (Tegretol), primidone (Mysoline), topirimate (Topamax), griseofulvin (Grisactin), rifampin (Rifadin), ampicillin (Omnipen), and tetracycline (Achromycin)

Practice to Pass

A client calls the clinic reporting that she uses a 28-day dosing regimen and "forgot to take her birth control pills for the last 2 days." How would the nurse advise this client?

5. Contraindications
    a. COCs should not be taken by women with a history of thromboembolic or cardiovascular disorders, breast cancer, or estrogen-dependent neoplasms
    b. COCs should not be used if woman is currently pregnant, lactating of less than six weeks' duration, smokes more than 20 cigarettes per day and is over 35 years old, has headaches with focal neurological symptoms, is experiencing prolonged immobility or surgery on legs, or has hypertension with blood pressure greater than 160/100 or diabetes mellitus of 20 or more years duration with vascular disease

B. Long-acting progestin injections

1. The injectable contraceptive hormone contains medroxyprogesterone acetate (**Depo-Provera**) or (DMPA) 150 mg, a long-acting progestin that blocks luteinizing hormone surge, prevents pregnancy by suppressing ovulation, and thickens cervical mucus to prevent penetration of sperm; has 97.7% effectiveness with both perfect and typical use
2. Client education
    a. Inform client of potential side effects such as menstrual irregularities, headache, weight gain, breast tenderness, and depression
    b. Teach importance of following three-month injection regimen to maintain contraceptive effects; subsequent dose must be given 80 to 90 days after previous dose for continuous contraceptive protection
    c. Instruct client to contact health care provider if she experiences any warning signs of ACHES as identified in Table 3-2
3. Advantages
    a. Contraception is not related to sexual intercourse
    b. Safe for lactating women
    c. Does not contain estrogen
    d. Requires administration only every three months
4. Disadvantages
    a. Injection must be repeated within 80 to 90 days to maintain effectiveness
    b. Clients with cardiovascular disorders or breast cancer are not candidates for contraceptive hormone injection
    c. Return of fertility may be delayed up to one year after stopping method
    d. DMPA may be used for up to two years, then provider should reevaluate contraceptive options due to decreased calcium absorption while using DMPA; client should consider calcium supplementation during use

C. Transdermal contraceptive patch

1. Releases small amounts of estrogen and progestin to suppress ovulation
2. Client education
    a. Inform client of possible side effects such as breakthrough bleeding, breast tenderness, headache, and skin reactions
    b. Instruct client to remove patch once a week on same day and apply a new patch to abdomen, buttocks, upper outer arm or trunk (excluding breasts) for three weeks; avoid placing patch on areas with a great deal of movement
    c. Advise client that no patch is used during week four and menstrual period typically occurs
3. Advantages
    a. Patch requires only weekly application
    b. Patch stays on even when showering and swimming
4. Disadvantages
    a. Offers no protection against STIs
    b. Not recommended for obese women (weight >198 pounds) or women with skin disorders that may result in reactions at application site

c. Clients with preexisting medical diseases may not be candidates for this method
d. Medication precautions are similar to those for a client taking oral contraceptives
5. Contraindications are same as for a client using oral contraceptives

D. Vaginal contraceptive ring

1. Releases small amounts of estrogen and progestin to suppress ovulation
2. Client education
   a. Inform client of possible side effects such as vaginal infection, irritation, increased discharge, headache, or upper respiratory infection
   b. Instruct client to insert vaginal ring and leave in place for three weeks
   c. Advise client that no ring is used during week four and menstrual period typically occurs
   d. Instruct client that removing vaginal ring during intercourse is not recommended, however, it may be removed for up to three hours without need for a back-up method
3. Advantages
   a. Requires application only once every four weeks
   b. Requires no special fitting
   c. Can safely be left in place during exercise or intercourse and generally without discomfort to woman or partner
4. Disadvantages
   a. Offers no protection against STIs
   b. Clients with marked vaginal prolapse should be cautioned to check for expulsion of vaginal ring
   c. Medication precautions are similar to those taking oral contraceptives
5. Contraindications are same as for a client using oral contraceptives

E. *Emergency contraception*

1. Measures that may be utilized when woman is concerned about becoming pregnant because of unprotected intercourse or when a contraceptive method fails
2. Emergency or postcoital contraception should be considered an emergency method and not be used on a frequent or regular basis
3. ! Methods of emergency contraception should be initiated as soon as possible after unprotected intercourse or contraceptive failure; average reduction in pregnancy rate is 75 to 85%, with higher effectiveness if emergency contraception is initiated within 12 hours of unprotected intercourse; however, this method may be effective even up to 5 days (120 hours) following act of intercourse
   a. Oral contraceptives (Plan B, Preven), often called morning after pills (MAPs): initiate within 72 hours of unprotected intercourse or contraceptive failure
      1) ! Procedure used with combined oral contraceptive pills consists of one dose containing at least 100 mcg ethinyl estradiol and either 100 mg of norgestrel or 50 mg levonorgestrel and repeating the same dose 12 hours later
      2) Procedure for use with progestin-only oral contraceptive pills consists of one dose containing 0.75 mg levonorgestrel or 1.5 mg norgestrel and repeating the same dose in 12 hours
      3) ! An antiemetic, such as metoclopramide (Reglan), can be given one hour prior to administration of the oral contraceptives to control nausea; contraindicated in clients with epilepsy; adverse effects may include depression with suicidal thoughts
   b. Insertion of an IUD
      1) A device containing copper (ParaGard) can be inserted within five days of unprotected intercourse or contraceptive failure
      2) This method of emergency contraception is only recommended for women wanting long-term protection and meeting criteria for an IUD

- **c.** Mifepristone (RU 486)
  - **1)** A progesterone antagonist that prevents implantation of a fertilized ovum
  - **2)** A 600-mg dose within 72 hours of unprotected intercourse or contraceptive failure is usually effective in preventing pregnancy

4. Client education
- **a.** Administration of oral contraceptives or insertion of an IUD may not be effective if the client is already pregnant
- **b.** The next menses can be expected about five days after last dose of oral contraceptives; if no bleeding occurs within 21 days, client should be evaluated for pregnancy
- **c.** Nausea and vomiting are common side effects of oral contraceptives unless an antiemetic has been given
- **d.** If postcoital contraception is sought repeatedly, explore reason(s) for unprotected intercourse or contraceptive failure
- **e.** Counsel client regarding safer and more reliable methods of contraception for regular use

5. Advantages
- **a.** Offers an opportunity to prevent an unwanted pregnancy after forced sexual intercourse, mistake, or method failure
- **b.** Reduces anxiety about pregnancy prior to next menses
- **c.** Provides an opportunity to teach and counsel about reliable contraceptive methods for long-term pregnancy protection

6. Disadvantages
- **a.** Timing of next menses can be affected
- **b.** Amount of next menstrual flow increases in many women
- **c.** Provides no protection against STIs

F. ***Subdermal implant*** **(Implanon)**

1. A single rod filled with synthetic progestin etonogestrel (Implanon) that is surgically inserted on inner side of a woman's upper arm to prevent pregnancy for three years by thickening cervical mucus, altering endometrium, and suppressing ovulation; is considered to be a birth control implant

2. Client education
- **a.** Inform client of potential side effects such as menstrual irregularities, headache, weight gain, breast tenderness, and depression
- **b.** Instruct client to contact health care provider if she experiences any warning signs of ACHES as identified in Table 3-2

3. Advantages
- **a.** Contraception is not related to sexual intercourse
- **b.** Safe for lactating women
- **c.** Does not contain estrogen
- **d.** Requires administration only every three years

4. Disadvantages
- **a.** The implant must be replaced every three years
- **b.** Clients with cardiovascular disorders or breast cancer are not candidates
- **c.** Return of fertility may be delayed after stopping method
- **d.** Scarring, infection, or related complications are possible at time of placement

VII. SURGICAL METHODS OF CONTRACEPTION

A. Surgical contraceptive methods: result in voluntary sterilization of male or female

B. Surgical consent: obtained after risks and benefits of specific method are explained

C. Vasectomy

1. During a **vasectomy**, vas deferens is resected through small incisions made in each side of scrotum resulting in blockage of passage of sperm
2. Client education
   a. Procedure takes about 15 to 20 minutes and can be performed in a clinic setting under local anesthesia
   b. Refrain from driving immediately after procedure and be discharged to someone who can drive and remain with client for 24 hours after procedure
   c. Remain at rest with minimal activity for 48 hours optimally
   d. Avoid tub baths for 48 hours
   e. Wear a scrotal support to increase comfort
   f. Use ice packs intermittently to minimize discomfort and swelling
   g. Use sitz baths after 48 hours
   h. Avoid strenuous activity for one week
   i. Contact health care provider if warning signs develop as listed in Table 3-2
   j. Sterility is not achieved until semen is free of sperm, about four to six weeks or 6 to 36 ejaculations; until then, use another contraceptive method
   k. Two or three semen samples should be analyzed to verify sterility prior to resuming unprotected intercourse
   l. Semen should be rechecked at 6 and 12 months to verify stertility has been maintained
3. Advantages
   a. Procedure is 99.85% effective
   b. Recovery time is short
   c. Simpler, safer, and more effective than female sterilization
   d. Complications are rare
   e. Sexual function is not affected
   f. Cost-effective and convenient
4. Disadvantages
   a. Although reversal of a vasectomy is possible in some cases, this method is considered permanent
   b. Potential complications include adverse reaction to anesthesia, infection, bleeding, sperm granuloma or spontaneous re-anastomosis of vas deferens
   c. Fertility, in rare instances, may occur spontaneously due to recanalization of vas deferens
   d. Female partner has no ability to influence control of fertility

D. Tubal ligation

1. During a **tubal ligation**, fallopian tubes are accessed through two small incisions into abdomen and visualized using a laparoscope, then cut, tied, cauterized, or banded to block passage of sperm and prevent ovum from being fertilized
2. Effectiveness ranges from 99.2 to 96.3% depending on method used; younger women have been reported to experience higher failure rates
3. Client education
   a. Procedure takes approximately 30 minutes and is performed under general or local anesthesia
   b. Client may be asked to restrict food and fluid intake for several hours before procedure, especially if general anesthesia is planned
   c. Pain may be experienced for several days after procedure
   d. Avoid tub baths for 48 hours
   e. Avoid driving, lifting, and strenuous activity for one week
   f. Contact health care provider if warning signs develop as listed in Table 3-2

Practice to Pass

A client tells the nurse "I am so tired of using contraception. I think I'm ready for something permanent." What additional information should the nurse obtain before responding to the question?

4. Advantages
   a. Permanent and effective in preventing pregnancy
   b. May be performed at any time; immediately after childbirth is optimal because uterus is enlarged and fallopian tubes are easy to identify
   c. Sexual function and spontaneity are not affected
5. Disadvantages
   a. Procedure requires outpatient surgery
   b. Potential complications include adverse reaction to anesthesia, infection, and bleeding
   c. If pregnancy occurs after tubal ligation, risk of ectopic pregnancy increases
   d. Reversal of procedure may not be possible or successful
   e. Possible changes in menstrual pattern: "post-tubal ligation syndrome"
   f. Male partner has no ability to influence control of fertility

Case Study

A client comes to the reproductive health clinic seeking contraception. She says she is interested in birth control pills but has never used them and needs more information before making a decision regarding their use.

1. What factors in the client's history would be contraindications to the use of oral contraceptives?
2. What advantages of birth control pills should be shared with the client?
3. What are the disadvantages of birth control pills that should be considered prior to use?
4. How should the nurse teach the client to use birth control pills?
5. What warning signs should the nurse teach the client to report immediately to the health care provider?

For suggested responses, see page 302.

POSTTEST

POSTTEST

1 Which intervention would be most effective in teaching a client with low literacy skills how to insert a diaphragm?

1. Assess the client's understanding of how a diaphragm works.
2. Give the client a printed handout explaining use of the diaphragm.
3. Provide the client with an opportunity to practice inserting and removing the diaphragm.
4. Use an audiotape to explain use of the diaphragm.

2 Which statement demonstrates that a male client understands how to correctly apply a condom? Select all that apply.

1. "I need to put it on before the penis is erect."
2. "I should unroll the condom, then place it on the penis."
3. "After putting on the condom, I need to leave some space at the tip to collect the sperm."
4. "I can use oil-based lubricants if needed."
5. "I can use a water-based lubricant if needed."

3 A client with a history of toxic shock syndrome comes to the reproductive clinic seeking contraception. Based on this information, which method should the nurse avoid recommending for this client?

1. Cervical cap
2. Female condom
3. Spermicide
4. Implanted progestin rod (Implanon)

4 The rationale for the nurse to ensure that a client gives informed consent for contraception prior to use is based on which fact about contraceptive methods?

1. Are usually invasive procedures
2. Require a surgical procedure
3. May not be reliable
4. Have potentially dangerous side effects

5 The nurse should instruct the client who has had an intrauterine device (IUD) inserted to do which of the following as part of follow-up self-care?

1. Have the IUD replaced every three years.
2. Check for the string periodically.
3. Use another method of contraception for two weeks after insertion.
4. Use a vinegar douche weekly for four weeks to decrease the risk of infection.

6 Following a teaching session on how to use the diaphragm as a contraceptive method, the nurse evaluates the client's understanding. Which statement made by the client demonstrates the need for additional teaching?

1. "If I choose a diaphragm, I won't need to use any spermicide."
2. "I will need to inspect the diaphragm after I take it out and clean it."
3. "When I want to get pregnant, I can just stop using my diaphragm."
4. "I need to leave the diaphragm in for at least six hours after having intercourse."

7 A client taking oral contraceptive pills calls the clinic and reports the presence of chest pain and shortness of breath. The nurse should instruct the client to do which of the following?

1. Go to the nearest emergency room to be evaluated.
2. Wait for the physician to return a telephone call to the client.
3. Stop taking the pills and use a nonhormonal contraceptive method.
4. Eat smaller meals more frequently to prevent gastric distention.

8 A client has decided to use a cervical cap for contraception. In providing instruction to the client on the correct use of this method, the nurse should tell the client to do which of the following?

1. Apply a spermicide to the inside of the cap.
2. Insert the cap no longer than four hours prior to intercourse.
3. Remove the cap within six hours of sexual activity.
4. Reapply spermicide with repeated acts of intercourse.

9 The nurse is teaching a client how to correctly use progestin-only oral contraceptives. The nurse should include which information in the teaching plan?

1. Take one pill at the same time each day.
2. Take the pills with calcium-rich foods to promote absorption.
3. Skip five days between the end of one pill cycle and the beginning of the next.
4. An additional method of contraception is not needed through the end of the cycle if a pill is missed.

10 A client comes to the family planning clinic for contraceptive advice. She states she has never used contraception before and does not know what options are available to her. The nurse determines that the priority nursing diagnosis for this client would be which of the following?

1. Anxiety related to fear of pregnancy
2. Ineffective Coping related to unprotected intercourse
3. Deficient Knowledge related to lack of information about contraceptives
4. Fear related to potential complications of contraception

➤ *See pages 65–67 for Answers and Rationales.*

ANSWERS & RATIONALES

Pretest

1 **Answer: 1, 2, 3** **Rationale:** A client interested in contraception should be informed about all options available to her before choosing one. Among these options are male condoms with spermicide, DMPA, and oral contraceptives. Screening for birth defects and semen analysis are not services helpful for birth control. **Cognitive Level:** Applying **Client Need:** Health Promotion and Maintenance **Integrated Process:** Teaching and Learning **Content Area:** Maternal-Newborn **Strategy:** Focus on the critical words *birth control* and *family planning* to focus on the option that deals with contraception. Eliminate options that relate to screening and increasing fertility, because these do not relate to contraception. **Reference:** Ladewig, P., London, M., & Davidson, M. (2010). *Contemporary maternal-newborn nursing care* (7th ed.). Upper Saddle River, NJ: Pearson Education, p. 83.

2 **Answer: 3** **Rationale:** Contraceptive counseling involves assessing the client's needs, desires, and risk factors. This will result in a contraceptive method that best suits the needs and health of the client. The client's partner does not need to be present to discuss contraceptive options. The information should be given without prejudgment on the nurse's part. The nurse would not be doing his or her job properly without giving the client all the information about possible side effects. **Cognitive Level:** Applying **Client Need:** Health Promotion and Maintenance **Integrated Process:** Communication and Documentation **Content Area:** Maternal-Newborn **Strategy:** Avoid options that give advice or use extreme words such as *only*. From there, use knowledge of counseling, effective communication, and family planning to choose the correct answer. **Reference:** Ladewig, P., London, M., & Davidson, M. (2010). *Contemporary maternal-newborn nursing care* (7th ed.). Upper Saddle River, NJ: Pearson Education, p. 84.

3 **Answer: 2** **Rationale:** Condoms, used with or without a spermicide, are mechanical methods of contraception. While abstinence is a natural method, since the woman is sexually active it will increase compliance if she only needs to be abstinent during fertile periods. Therefore, using the basal body temperature method permits her to be sexually active at certain times. **Cognitive Level:** Analyzing **Client Need:** Health Promotion and Maintenance **Integrated Process:** Nursing Process: Diagnosis **Content Area:** Maternal-Newborn **Strategy:** Critical words are *natural method of family planning*. Use knowledge of contraceptive methods to identify correct answer. **Reference:** Ladewig, P., London, M., & Davidson, M. (2010). *Contemporary maternal-newborn nursing care* (7th ed.). Upper Saddle River: Pearson Education, p. 83.

4 **Answer: 3** **Rationale:** Oil-based lubricants can break down latex condoms. The condom should be unrolled onto the penis, starting at the tip of the penis. Holding the rim keeps the condom from slipping off and leaking semen into the vagina. Small amounts of semen are released before ejaculation and can result in pregnancy. **Cognitive Level:** Analyzing **Client Need:** Health Promotion and Maintenance **Integrated Process:** Teaching and Learning **Content Area:** Maternal-Newborn **Strategy:** Note the critical words *understands* and *how to use condom*. Note that the question is worded to elicit a positive statement as the correct answer. The correct answer is a true statement about a point of client education. **Reference:** Ladewig, P., London, M., & Davidson, M. (2010). *Contemporary maternal-newborn nursing care* (7th ed.). Upper Saddle River, NJ: Pearson Education, p. 86.

5 **Answer: 3** **Rationale:** Female condoms can be applied up to eight hours before intercourse, are not made of latex, and do not require that the client be measured for proper fit. Both partners are protected from STIs during intercourse. **Cognitive Level:** Analyzing **Client Need:** Health Promotion and Maintenance **Integrated Process:** Teaching and Learning **Content Area:** Maternal-Newborn **Strategy:** The critical words are *female condoms* and *understood*. Since the question is worded in a positive manner, you are looking for a correct statement about the use of female condoms. **Reference:** Ladewig, P., London, M., & Davidson, M. (2010). *Contemporary maternal-newborn nursing care* (7th ed.). Upper Saddle River, NJ: Pearson Education, p. 86.

6 **Answer: 2, 3, 5** **Rationale:** Oil-based lubricants and cleaning agents other than soap and water can damage the

POSTTEST

ANSWERS & RATIONALES

rubber of the diaphragm. The chemical barrier (spermicidal cream or jelly) supplements the mechanical barrier (diaphragm) to increase the effectiveness of this contraceptive method. It takes at least six hours for the spermicidal cream or jelly at the rim to destroy sperm deposited in the vagina. Use during the menses increases the risk of toxic shock syndrome and should be avoided. **Cognitive Level:** Analyzing **Client Need:** Health Promotion and Maintenance **Integrated Process:** Nursing Process: Planning **Content Area:** Maternal-Newborn **Strategy:** This question is worded in a positive manner. Therefore, the correct options are also true statements about points of client education. **Reference:** Ladewig, P., London, M., & Davidson, M. (2010). *Contemporary maternal-newborn nursing care* (7th ed.). Upper Saddle River, NJ: Pearson Education, p. 86.

7 **Answer: 2 Rationale:** Oral contraceptives place the client at decreased risk for iron-deficiency anemia, ovarian cancer, and fibrocystic breast disease. Oral contraceptives can decrease the effectiveness of insulin. **Cognitive Level:** Analyzing **Client Need:** Health Promotion and Maintenance **Integrated Process:** Nursing Process: Planning **Content Area:** Maternal-Newborn **Strategy:** Note the critical words *assessment data* and *method other than oral contraceptives*. The focus of this question is to identify a disadvantage or reason not to use oral contraceptives. The incorrect options are all benefits of oral contraceptive use. **Reference:** Ladewig, P., London, M., & Davidson, M. (2010). *Contemporary maternal-newborn nursing care* (7th ed.). Upper Saddle River, NJ: Pearson Education, p. 85.

8 **Answer: 2 Rationale:** IUDs do not cause incomplete emptying of the bladder or increased production of cervical or vaginal mucus. IUDs do have the potential to increase the risk for pelvic inflammatory disease and possibly increase episodes of dysmenorrhea. **Cognitive Level:** Applying **Client Need:** Health Promotion and Maintenance **Integrated Process:** Nursing Process: Implementation **Content Area:** Maternal-Newborn **Strategy:** Critical words are *intrauterine device* and *side effects*. Specific knowledge of the side effects of IUDs is needed to choose increased risk for pelvic inflammatory disease. Eliminate options that are not related to the use of an IUD. **Reference:** Ladewig, P., London, M., & Davidson, M. (2010). *Contemporary maternal-newborn nursing care* (7th ed.). Upper Saddle River, NJ: Pearson Education, p. 89.

9 **Answer: 4 Rationale:** The procedure will not affect the client's sexual function. It is usually performed in a clinic under local anesthesia, and is not effective for four to six weeks. The client should rest with minimal activity for 48 hours following the procedure. **Cognitive Level:** Applying **Client Need:** Reduction of Risk Potential **Integrated Process:** Teaching and Learning **Content Area:** Maternal-Newborn **Strategy:** Critical words are *vasectomy* and *understands*, which indicate the correct option is also a correctly worded response from the client after the teaching. **Reference:** Ladewig, P., London, M., & Davidson, M. (2010). *Contemporary maternal-newborn nursing care* (7th ed.). Upper Saddle River, NJ: Pearson Education, p. 92.

10 **Answer: 3 Rationale:** The pregnancy rate following tubal ligation is 1 to 4 per 1000 women. Reversal of the procedure, not effectiveness, is affected by the method used for the procedure. The effectiveness of the method is not related to client behavior. **Cognitive Level:** Applying **Client Need:** Health Promotion and Maintenance **Integrated Process:** Communication and Documentation **Content Area:** Maternal-Newborn **Strategy:** The critical words in the question are *tubal ligation* and *effectiveness of the method*. Use specific knowledge of tubal ligation and its effectiveness to select the correct option. **Reference:** Ladewig, P., London, M., & Davidson, M. (2010). *Contemporary maternal-newborn nursing care* (7th ed.). Upper Saddle River, NJ: Pearson Education, p. 92.

Posttest

1 **Answer: 3 Rationale:** Assessing the client's knowledge should be performed before the teaching session, not during instructions on insertion. Printed materials may not be appropriate to the client's reading ability. An audiotape does not allow the client to see the insertion technique, while visual cues are provided by demonstration of the procedure. Practice sessions provide the nurse with an opportunity to give positive and corrective feedback integrating visual, auditory, and tactile senses. **Cognitive Level:** Applying **Client Need:** Health Promotion and Maintenance **Integrated Process:** Teaching and Learning **Content Area:** Maternal-Newborn **Strategy:** The critical words in this question are *low literacy*. The correct answer is the teaching strategy that relies the least on the use of words that the client may not be able to read or understand. **Reference:** Ladewig, P., London, M., & Davidson, M. (2010). *Contemporary maternal-newborn nursing care* (7th ed.). Upper Saddle River, NJ: Pearson Education, p. 88.

2 **Answer: 3, 5 Rationale:** Leaving space at the end of the condom to collect the semen can prevent breakage or spillage after ejaculation. The male condom is placed when the penis is erect, then rolled down. Water-based lubricants can be used to provide additional comfort, if needed. Oil-based lubricants are contraindicated. **Cognitive Level:** Analyzing **Client Need:** Health Promotion and Maintenance **Integrated Process:** Teaching and Learning **Content Area:** Maternal-Newborn **Strategy:** The wording of the question is positive, indicating that the correct options are true statements about points of client education. Use nursing knowledge to select these options. **Reference:** Ladewig, P., London, M., & Davidson, M. (2010). *Contemporary maternal-newborn nursing care* (7th ed.). Upper Saddle River, NJ: Pearson Education, p. 87.

3 **Answer: 1** **Rationale:** The cervical cap increases the risk of toxic shock syndrome because it may be left in place for up to 48 hours. The female condom, spermicide, and an implanted progestin rod pose no additional risk to this client based on her history and could be considered for contraception. **Cognitive Level:** Analyzing **Client Need:** Health Promotion and Maintenance **Integrated Process:** Nursing Process: Assessment **Content Area:** **Strategy:** Critical words are *toxic shock syndrome* and *avoid*. The focus of this question is a method that increases the client's risk of a reproductive tract infection. The incorrect options can be eliminated because they do not pose this risk for the client. **Reference:** Ladewig, P., London, M., & Davidson, M. (2009). *Contemporary maternal-newborn nursing care* (7th ed.). Upper Saddle River, NJ: Pearson Education, pp. 86–88.

4 **Answer: 4** **Rationale:** Ethical and legal considerations dictate that clients are knowledgeable of the benefits and risks of the contraceptive method. This empowers the client in making an informed decision. Not all contraceptive methods are invasive or require a surgical procedure. Informed consent is not related to the effectiveness of a method. **Cognitive Level:** Understanding **Client Need:** Management of Care **Integrated Process:** Nursing Process: Evaluation **Content Area:** Maternal-Newborn **Strategy:** Critical words are *informed consent* and *ensure*. Use knowledge of informed consent to determine that client should be told potential risks and benefits of contraceptives. The correct answer would be the option that includes information needed by the client to make a decision. **Reference:** Ladewig, P., London, M., & Davidson, M. (2010). *Contemporary maternal-newborn nursing care* (7th ed.). Upper Saddle River, NJ: Pearson Education, p. 83.

5 **Answer: 2** **Rationale:** Specific information about the type of IUD inserted is not provided; Progestasert needs to be replaced annually, Mirena is effective for up to 5 years, and the Copper T380A can be left in place for 10 years. The string should be checked once a week for the first month, then after the menses thereafter. Contraceptive effectiveness begins when the IUD is inserted. Although douching is sometimes used to treat vaginal infections, it is not a recommended practice to prevent infection. **Cognitive Level:** Applying **Client Need:** Health Promotion and Maintenance **Integrated Process:** Teaching and Learning **Content Area:** Maternal-Newborn **Strategy:** Critical words are *instruct* and *IUD*. Because the question is worded in a positive way, the correct option is also a true statement about a point of client education. **Reference:** Ladewig, P., London, M., & Davidson, M. (2010). *Contemporary maternal-newborn nursing care* (7th ed.). Upper Saddle River, NJ: Pearson Education, p. 87.

6 **Answer: 1** **Rationale:** A spermicidal cream or jelly is applied to the rim and dome of the diaphragm before inserting the device to increase the contraceptive effectiveness of the device. The other statements, needing to inspect the diaphragm after it is removed, being able to stop using the diaphragm at will, and needing to leave the diaphragm in for at least six hours after use, reflect correct client knowledge. **Cognitive Level:** Analyzing **Client Need:** Health Promotion and Maintenance **Integrated Process:** Teaching and Learning **Content Area:** Maternal-Newborn **Strategy:** Critical words are *diaphragm* and *need for additional teaching*. Use knowledge of diaphragms to answer the question. **Reference:** Ladewig, P., London, M., & Davidson, M. (2010). *Contemporary maternal-newborn nursing care* (7th ed.). Upper Saddle River, NJ: Pearson Education, p. 87.

7 **Answer: 1** **Rationale:** Shortness of breath and chest pain can indicate a serious complication associated with the use of oral contraceptives and require immediate evaluation. Waiting for a return telephone call could delay evaluation and treatment, jeopardizing the client's health. Changing the contraceptive method or food intake pattern does not reduce the immediate health risk to the client. **Cognitive Level:** Analyzing **Client Need:** Physiological Adaptation **Integrated Process:** Nursing Process: Implementation **Content Area:** Maternal-Newborn **Strategy:** Critical words are *chest pain* and *shortness of breath*, which indicate the need for immediate help from health care providers. The other answers indicate delayed responses on the part of the client rather than emergency care for potential emergency needs. **Reference:** Ladewig, P., London, M., & Davidson, M. (2010). *Contemporary maternal-newborn nursing care* (7th ed.). Upper Saddle River, NJ: Pearson Education, p. 90.

8 **Answer: 1** **Rationale:** Spermicide should be applied to the inside of the cervical cap. The device has no time limit between insertion and sexual activity, and may be left in place up to 48 hours after sexual activity. Reapplication of spermicide with repeated acts of intercourse is not needed. **Cognitive Level:** Applying **Client Need:** Health Promotion and Maintenance **Integrated Process:** Teaching and Learning **Content Area:** Maternal-Newborn **Strategy:** Critical words are *correct use of this method* and *cervical cap*. The correct answer must be a true statement about a point of client education. Use knowledge of cervical cap as a contraceptive device to determine the correct answer. **Reference:** Ladewig, P., London, M., & Davidson, M. (2010). *Contemporary maternal-newborn nursing care* (7th ed.). Upper Saddle River, NJ: Pearson Education, p. 88.

9 **Answer: 1** **Rationale:** Every pill contains a low dose of hormone and should be taken daily; consistency in taking the pills ensures a constant serum level of the hormone to maximize effectiveness. The pills are absorbed with or without the presence of calcium. If a pill is missed, it should be taken immediately and an additional method of contraception utilized through the remainder of that cycle. There is a seven-day period between the end of one pill cycle and the beginning of

the next. **Cognitive Level:** Applying **Client Need:** Health Promotion and Maintenance **Integrated Process:** Teaching and Learning **Content Area:** Maternal-Newborn **Strategy:** Critical words are *correctly use* and *progestin-only oral contraceptive.* The correct answer would include a true statement about a point of client education. Use knowledge of oral contraceptives to answer the question correctly. **Reference:** Ladewig, P., London, M., & Davidson, M. (2010). *Contemporary maternal-newborn nursing care* (7th ed.). Upper Saddle River, NJ: Pearson Education, p. 89.

10 **Answer: 3** **Rationale:** This client has a need for information about the various contraceptive methods available to her and their risks and benefits. No information is provided to determine if the client fears pregnancy or is engaging in unprotected sexual intercourse. If the client does not know what contraceptive methods are available, it is unlikely she knows or fears potential complications from using a method of contraception. **Cognitive Level:** Analyzing **Client Need:** Health Promotion and Maintenance **Integrated Process:** Nursing Process: Diagnosis **Content Area:** Maternal-Newborn **Strategy:** The critical focus in this question is the client's need for information. The correct answer includes knowledge as a focus. Use knowledge of contraceptives and nursing diagnosis to answer the question. **Reference:** Ladewig, P., London, M., & Davidson, M. (2010). *Contemporary maternal-newborn nursing care* (7th ed.). Upper Saddle River, NJ: Pearson Education, p. 83.

References

Birth Control: Implanon. Retrieved October 11, 2011, from http://www.plannedparenthood.org/health-topics/birth-control/birth-control-implant-implanon-4243.htm

Davidson, M., London, M., & Ladewig, P. (2012). *Olds' maternal newborn nursing & women's health across the lifespan* (9th ed.). Upper Saddle River, NJ: Pearson Education.

Hatcher, R. A., Trussell, J., Nelson, A. L., Cates, W., Stewart, F. & Kowal, D. (2008). *Contraceptive technology* (19th ed.). Atlanta, GA: Ardent Media Inc.

Ladewig, P., London, M., & Davidson, M. (2010). *Contemporary maternal-newborn nursing care* (7th ed.). Upper Saddle River, NJ: Pearson Education.

NANDA Nursing Diagnosis (2009). Retrieved January 29, 2011, from http://www.scribd.com/doc/11885949/NANDA-2009

Orshan, S. A. (2008). *Maternity, newborn, and women's health nursing: Comprehensive care across the life span.* Philadelphia: Lippincott Williams & Wilkins.

Ricci, S. (2009). *Essentials of maternity, newborn, and women's health nursing* (2nd ed.). Philadelphia: Lippincott Williams & Wilkins.

Reproductive Health Technologies Project. Retrieved January 27, 2011, from http://www.rhtp.org/

4 Fetal Development

Chapter Outline

Conception
Stages of Growth and Development
Preembryonic Development
Embryonic Development
Fetal Development

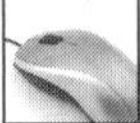

NCLEX-RN® Test Prep

Use the accompanying online resource, NursingReviewsandRationales, to test yourself with hundreds of NCLEX®-style practice questions.

Objectives

- Describe the process of conception.
- Differentiate among the preembryonic, embryonic, and fetal stages of development.
- Identify the function of extra-embryonic structures—the amniotic fluid, umbilical cord, and placenta.
- Describe fetal circulation.
- Summarize fetal development from conception to birth.

Review at a Glance

allele an alternate form of a gene

amnion inner fetal membranes

blastocyst inner mass of cells within morula that implants in uterus

chorion outer membrane of fetal membranes

decidua basalis part of decidua that unites with chorion to form placenta

decidua capsularis the part of decidua that surrounds chorionic sac

decidua vera decidua lining uterus other than placenta

ductus arteriosus a fetal cardiac connection between pulmonary artery and aorta to allow blood to bypass pulmonary circulation

ductus venosus a fetal circulatory adaptation to allow blood to bypass liver

ectoderm progenerators for neural and integument tissue

embryo an early stage in prenatal development between second and eighth week of gestation

endoderm progenerators for digestive and respiratory system

fertilization union of ovum and sperm

fetus period from eight weeks until end of intrauterine life

foramen ovale an opening in fetal heart between right and left atria allowing blood to bypass pulmonary circulation

gamete a haploid germ cell (i.e., sperm or ovum)

mesoderm intermediate layer of germ cells in embryo that gives rise to connective tissue, bone marrow, muscles, blood, lymphoid tissue, and epithelial tissue

morula an embryo in a 16-cell stage that resembles a mulberry

trophoblast outermost layer of developing blastocyst that comes into intimate relationship with uterine endometrium becoming the placenta

Wharton's jelly gelatinous connective tissue of umbilical cord

zygote fertilized ovum

PRETEST

1 A couple visits the genetic counseling clinic regarding a family history of cystic fibrosis, an autosomal recessive disorder. They ask the nurse, "What are the chances that we will have a child with cystic fibrosis if we are both carriers?" Which response by the nurse is best?

1. "It would be better not to have children because they will all have cystic fibrosis."
2. "The disorder occurs at random and there is no way to calculate the risk."
3. "There is a 50% chance that you will have a child with cystic fibrosis."
4. "There is a 25% chance that you will have a child with cystic fibrosis."

2 A nurse is counseling a couple about fertility awareness. The nurse determines they understand the ideal time for conception when the clients make which statement? Select all that apply.

1. "Ovulation occurs seven days after the beginning of the menstrual cycle."
2. "The ovum survives for 24 hours after ovulation."
3. "It is best to have intercourse 24 to 48 hours after ovulation."
4. "The ovum must be in contact with sperm for 48 hours in order for fertilization to occur."
5. "Sperm are most capable of fertilization 24 hours after intercourse."

3 After completing a health history in a prenatal clinic, the nurse concludes that which client has the greatest risk for potential birth anomalies?

1. A 23-year-old pregnant woman at seven months' gestation with a urinary tract infection
2. A 15-year-old primigravida with a sister who has Down syndrome
3. A 35-year-old multigravida at 16 weeks' gestation with a yeast infection
4. A 42-year-old multigravida at 5 months' gestation with a cold

4 A 30-year-old woman who is pregnant with twins tells the nurse that twins run in her family. She has a twin brother, her mother is a twin, and many relatives have twins. The nurse explains that which type of twinning most likely relates to her situation?

1. Identical
2. Monozygotic
3. Dizygotic
4. Monoamniotic

5 A client appears in the clinic for her first prenatal visit at 26 weeks of pregnancy. She states, "I didn't see any point in coming sooner since I felt fine." The nurse makes which statement to explain why prenatal care in the first trimester is important?

1. "We want to get to know our patients better. This gives us time to collect an accurate history and plan for potential problems."
2. "We need to monitor fetal lung maturity and fetal movement in case you go into labor early."
3. "Important cellular growth happens in the first trimester. Early assessment and education promotes a healthy pregnancy during this time."
4. "The most important thing is to see if you are even pregnant. Many women mistake a missed period for pregnancy."

PRETEST

6. A woman at seven months of pregnancy says that her 8-year-old daughter talks to the fetus and this calms the fetus when kicking her in the ribs. She asks the nurse if this is a possibility. What is the best response by the nurse?

    1. "This may very well be the case because the fetus begins to hear at 24 weeks."
    2. "We really don't know at what age the fetus begins to hear."
    3. "This is unlikely since the fetus doesn't hear until eight months' gestation."
    4. "You are both right and wrong. The fetus is able to hear, but it is silly to think your daughter's voice calms the fetus."

7. A client at eight months' gestation is diagnosed with oligohydramnios. She asks the nurse if this can harm the fetus. What is the nurse's best response?

    1. "Well, the reduced fluid around the fetus can allow for umbilical cord compression."
    2. "Yes, it means the fetus swallowed too much fluid."
    3. "No, this commonly occurs toward the end of pregnancy."
    4. "No, this is a sign that the lungs are maturing."

8. After delivery the nurse examines the umbilical cord. The nurse records the presence of a normal umbilical cord by documenting that the umbilical cord has which of the following?

    1. One artery and two veins
    2. Two arteries and one vein
    3. Two arteries and two veins
    4. One artery and one vein

9. During a prenatal class the nurse discusses weight gain in pregnancy. The nurse explains that the amniotic fluid in the third trimester weighs approximately how much?

    1. 1.5 kilograms
    2. 250 grams
    3. 500 grams
    4. 1 kilogram

10. A pregnant client asks the nurse when the fetal heart will begin beating. The nurse tells the client even though the fetal heart is not fully developed it begins to beat at gestational week _____.

    Fill in your answer below:

    ____

➤ *See pages 86–88 for Answers and Rationales.*

I. CONCEPTION

A. Genetic principles

1. Hereditary material
    a. Each human somatic cell contains 46 chromosomes or 23 pairs; there are 22 pairs of autosomes plus one pair of sex chromosomes; chromosomes are made of DNA, tightly coiled strands containing all genetic material; they can be arranged in a particular order known as karyotype
    b. Sex chromosomes
        1) Maternal ovum carries an X chromosome
        2) Male sperm carries either an X or Y chromosome
        3) A female results when an X chromosome is contributed by ovum and an X chromosome from sperm
        4) A male results when an X chromosome is contributed by ovum and a Y chromosome from sperm
    c. Genes are made of DNA; alone or in combination, they are smallest units of inheritance found on chromosomes; they perform a specific function in control of cellular activity
    d. Homozygous genes are a pair of genes carrying similar traits

e. Heterozygous genes are a pair of genes carrying dissimilar traits
f. Genome is the sum total of genes carried by all 46 chromosomes in a human
g. Human Genome Project: large coordinated effort to make a detailed map of human DNA and genes that guide development of a human being from a fertilized egg cell

2. Patterns of inheritance
   a. Mendelian inheritance (single gene inheritance)
      1) Autosomal dominant: a dominant gene is one gene of a heterozygous pair that is expressed
         a) A heterozygous genotype parent who carries a trait will manifest that trait; in other words: express the phenotype
         b) If a heterozygous parent has an infant with a homozygous parent without the trait there are four possible ways to combine the four genes: dominant/recessive, dominant/recessive, recessive/recessive, and recessive/recessive; there is a 50% chance of child expressing the trait and a 50% chance that the child will not express the trait
      2) Autosomal recessive genes are expressed only if homozygous
         a) When paired with a dominant gene it will not be expressed except in genotype
         b) Autosomal recessive diseases include phenylketonuria (PKU), Tay-Sachs, and cystic fibrosis
         c) As an example, if a parent carries a gene for PKU, the parent will not have PKU; if both parents have a gene for PKU, there are four possible ways to combine the genes: PKU/no PKU, no PKU/PKU, PKU/PKU, and no PKU/no PKU; there is a 25% chance of having a child with PKU, a 50% chance of the child being a carrier, and a 25% chance that the child will not carry or have PKU
      3) X-linked recessive genes are carried only on X chromosome; a female does not exhibit disease if she has an X chromosome without the trait; a male will exhibit trait because recessive gene is unopposed by the Y chromosome; i.e., if a man has an X chromosome with a recessive trait for colorblindness, he will be colorblind because Y chromosome has no comparable dominant gene to counteract this gene
      4) X-linked dominant: the gene is carried dominantly on X chromosome; it manifests itself in both males and females with the trait; for example, vitamin D–resistant rickets is X-linked dominant—both males and females are affected

Practice to Pass

A client reveals that she has PKU. She asks what the chances are for passing on the disease if the father does not have PKU. Knowing that this is an autosomal recessive trait, how would the nurse respond?

   b. Non-Mendelian inheritance is multifactorial; an interaction between the genetic material and the environment results in a trait, such as cleft palate
      1) Monosomy: one of an **allele**, an alternate form of a gene, is absent; an example is Turner's syndrome (XO); one of the sex chromosomes is missing so client has 45 chromosomes rather than 46
      2) Trisomy: an allele has an extra chromosome so client has 47 chromosomes rather than 46; examples include Klinefelter's syndrome (XXY) and Down syndrome (trisomy 21)
      3) Teratogens are nongenetic factors in environment that can produce mutations (changes in DNA that alter genes) in fetus; they include viruses and chemicals; greatest risk is during weeks two through eight of gestation

Practice to Pass

Following an amniocentesis a client learns she is carrying a fetus with Down syndrome, trisomy 21. Explain this to the client.

B. Role of the nurse related to genetics

1. Background information
   a. It is estimated that at least 50% of spontaneous abortions are caused by chromosomal abnormalities

Practice to Pass

A client learns that her fetus has anencephaly, a lethal congenital anomaly. What is the nurse's role in this situation?

b. Genetic counseling and testing takes place in many contexts and settings, such as birthing unit, prenatal clinic, well-child clinic, and family planning clinic
2. Genetic case finding and referral
3. Client education and counseling
4. Informed consent
5. Confidentiality
6. Communicating risks and dealing with uncertainty
7. Recognizing social, religious, and cultural differences
8. Autonomous, client-based decision making
9. Policy development

C. Sperm and ovum

1. A sexual reproductive cell, a **gamete**, is capable of uniting with a gamete of the opposite sex to form a new individual; gametes are also called germ cells
   a. Female gamete is the ovum
   b. Male gamete is the sperm
2. ! Gametogenesis occurs through cellular reproductive process of meiosis; through meiosis each gamete contains 23 chromosomes, the haploid state; this allows reshuffling of maternal and paternal genomes creating new combinations of genes
3. Oogenesis is a meiotic process by which female gametes are produced
   a. Primordial germ cells develop in ovary during fetal life; neonate is born with a lifetime supply of oogonia, which soon after birth begin to grow in size
   b. Oogonia that survive into female's sexual maturation become primary oocytes
   c. At sexual maturity, oocytes advance into first prophase of meiosis; when hormonal changes of puberty occur initiating menstrual cycle, one primary oocyte will continue through meiotic division in graffian follicle producing one primary oocyte and one nonfunctioning polar body; each contains the haploid state of 23 chromosomes
   d. Primary oocytes are released from ovary during ovulation (Figure 4-1); the second meiotic division begins as oocyte moves down fallopian tube; second division is completed with fertilization by a sperm resulting in a mature ovum and another polar body, each containing the haploid state
   e. At completion of meiotic division one oocyte results in three nonfunctioning polar bodies and one mature ovum
4. Spermatogenesis is a meiotic process by which male gametes are produced
   a. During puberty, germinal epithelium in seminiferous tubules of testes are stimulated to produce testosterone in testes
   b. As diploid spermatogonium enters first meiotic division, it is called a primary spermatocyte
   c. Each primary spermatocyte results in four mature spermatozoa, or sperm; the primary spermatocytes replicate to form two secondary spermatocytes containing haploid number of chromosomes; during second meiotic division, they divide to form four spermatids, each with a haploid number of chromosomes
   d. Spermatids continue to mature through process of spermatogenesis to become mature male gamete, spermatozoon or sperm

Practice to Pass

A client learning about fertility awareness asks, "When is the optimal time to have intercourse in relation to ovulation?" How will the nurse explain this?

! **D. *Fertilization*: occurs when sperm and ovum unite at conception (Figure 4-1)**

1. Usually within 12 hours of ovulation if coitus (intercourse) occurs; no more than 24 hours prior to ovulation
2. During intercourse 200 to 400 million sperm are ejaculated into vagina; they swim up into fallopian tubes to meet descending ovum, if present; only a few hundred sperm actually survive to ampulla (outer third) of fallopian tube where fertilization occurs

Figure 4-1

Ovulation, fertilization, and implantation

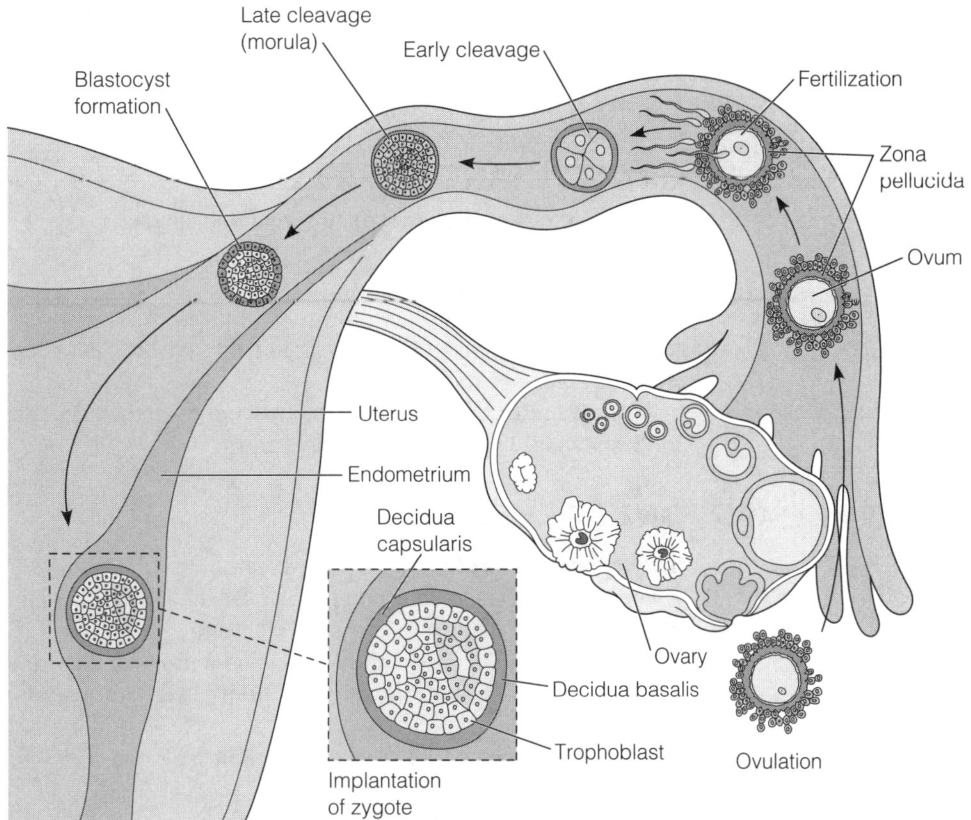

Practice to Pass

A nurse is a guest speaker at a support group for parents of twins. The topic for discussion is the biological difference between monozygotic and dizygotic twins. What information should the nurse include in the presentation?

3. Sperm survive in female reproductive tract for 24 to 48 hours but are most capable of fertilization for 24 hours
4. The ovum is enclosed in a glycoprotein matrix called zona pellucida, which is surrounded by corona radiata
   a. Zona pellucida binds sperm and prevents additional sperm from penetrating ovum
   b. Zona pellucida also initiates acrosomal reaction after sperm binding has occurred, mediating entry of sperm nucleus into ovum; release of lytic enzymes causes a small perforation in head of sperm; enzymes escape to digest a path through corona radiata and zona pellucida
   c. Capacitation occurs when protective coating around sperm is removed, facilitated by enzymes in fallopian tube
5. Fertilization occurs when sperm and ovum fuse, resulting in a **zygote** containing diploid number of chromosomes, or 46
6. Through cell division by mitosis, zygote increases in size 200 billion times before birth

! **E. Multiple pregnancies**

1. Dizygotic: fraternal or nonidentical twins result from release of two separate ova and fertilization by two separate sperm
   a. Incidence is 7 to 11 per 1000 births and accounts for ⅔ of twin births; incidence increases with maternal age
   b. They usually have separate placentas and membranes
2. Monozygotic: identical twins develop from a single fertilized ovum that splits into two separate zygotes
   a. They may share placentas and one or more fetal membranes
   b. If division occurs within three days of fertilization, zygotes will develop separate membranes

c. Twins who share one amnion are called "monamnionic"; these twins are at risk for intrauterine accidents such as knots in umbilical cords or "twin to twin transfusion syndrome"
d. Splitting of zygote in later stages may result in conjoined twins

II. STAGES OF GROWTH AND DEVELOPMENT

A. Human development before birth follows three stages
1. Preembryonic
2. Embryonic
3. Fetal

B. Intrauterine development from conception through birth is called gestation

C. Length of human gestation
1. 40 weeks after first day of last menstrual period, or 280 days
2. 38 weeks after fertilization, or 266 days

III. PREEMBRYONIC DEVELOPMENT

A. The first two weeks after fertilization: a time of cellular multiplication and implantation

B. Implantation: morula travels through fallopian tube for approximately three days while it undergoes rapid mitotic division called cleavage
1. When cells reach uterus they are called a **morula**; they float in uterus for several days prior to implantation and are nourished by nutrients within endometrial lining of uterus
2. Solid inner mass of cells is called **blastocyst**
3. Outer layer is called **trophoblast**
4. Adhesion occurs when blastocyst aligns with and adheres to uterine lining (endometrium)
5. Increased vascular permeability at implantation site facilitates a union between zygote and uterine tissues
6. Zygote implants in upper posterior uterine wall approximately seven to nine days after fertilization; some women may experience spotting at this time and mistake it for menses
7. Trophoblasts grow into endometrial lining and form fingerlike projections called villi

C. Endometrial lining: is rich in stored nutrients and provides nourishment until placenta is a functional unit of nutrient exchange

D. Decidua: layers of uterine tissue that grow around blastocyst
1. **Decidua capsularis**: portion that covers implanted blastocyst
2. **Decidua basalis**: portion directly under blastocyst
3. **Decidua vera**: portion that lines remainder of uterine cavity

IV. EMBRYONIC DEVELOPMENT

A. Development of an *embryo* occurs two to eight weeks following fertilization: characterized by rapid cell division and differentiation

B. Major functions of embryonic period
1. Cell multiplication and growth
2. Cell differentiation into organs
   a. Organogenesis: critical periods of development occur as organ systems develop; this is a time when embryo is particularly susceptible to teratogens and development of birth anomalies
   b. Morphogenesis: development of shape
   c. By end of eighth week, every organ system and external structure is present

C. **Primary germ layers**: develop into all tissues, organs, and body systems
1. **Ectoderm**: forms trophoblast that develops into placenta, integument, neural tissue, and glands
2. **Mesoderm**: forms muscles, bones, connective tissue, circulatory system, and genitourinary system
3. **Endoderm**: develops into digestive, respiratory, and parts of genitourinary systems

! D. **Fetal membranes**
1. **Amnion**: innermost lining of membrane that produces amniotic fluid
2. **Chorion**: outermost lining of membrane that forms from trophoblasts; chorionic villi develop into placenta
3. Membranes in multiple gestation
   a. Dizygotic twins: both zygotes implant separately and usually have separate placenta and membranes; occasionally zygotes implant so close together that placenta and membranes fuse
   b. Monozygotic twins
      1) If zygote separates at two-cell stage, two zygotes implant separately and have separate placentas and membranes
      2) Later splitting results in a common placenta; chorion develops in early blastocyst stage so twins have a common placenta and chorion, but separate amnions
      3) Twin to twin transfusion syndrome occurs when twins have a common placenta and membranes resulting in unequal circulation; one twin receives little circulation while the other most of the circulation; outcome is usually poor for both twins
4. ! Amniotic fluid is produced by amnion and derived from maternal blood
   a. Functions
      1) Cushions embryo, umbilical cord, and fetus
      2) Controls temperature
      3) Promotes symmetrical growth of embryo and fetus
      4) Prevents fetal adherence to amnion
      5) Allows freedom of movement within amniotic cavity
   b. Amount
      1) 30 mL at 10 weeks
      2) 350 mL at 20 weeks
      3) 700 to 1000 mL by 37 weeks
      4) Oligohydramnios is a condition of diminished amniotic fluid often related to renal system malfunction, intrauterine growth restriction, and postmaturity; it can contribute to skin and skeletal abnormalities, pulmonary hypoplasia, and cord compression
      5) Hydramnios or polyhydramnios is a condition of excess amniotic fluid often related to gastrointestinal malfunction
      6) Fetus swallows and urinates into fluid after 23 to 25 weeks
   c. Contains fetal cells and many chemicals that can be used to diagnose fetal well-being
      1) Alkaline in pH
      2) DNA for genetic analysis
      3) Surfactant for lung maturity analysis

E. **Yolk sac**: develops in blastocyst and forms early red blood cells during embryonic stage; it is then integrated into umbilical cord

F. **Body stalk**: connects embryo to yolk sac; as circulation develops in stalk, it becomes the umbilical cord connecting embryo to placenta

! **G. Placenta**

1. Purpose is to connect fetus to uterine wall so nutritive, respiratory, and excretory exchange can occur between mother and fetus
2. Development begins in third week of gestation and begins early function by fourth week
3. Uterine circulation prior to implantation
   a. Uterine arteries encircle uterus in a wreath called the arcuate arteries
   b. Radial arteries come off of these and divide into basal and spiral arteries
   c. Spiral arteries are responsive to hormonal changes and grow during luteal phase of menstrual cycle
   d. By time of implantation, spiral arteries are elongated and extend into endometrium
   e. Endometrium is rich in glycogen and protein to nourish blastocyst
4. Ectoderm develops into decidua basalis found directly below implanted morula
5. Small arteries work their way through entire decidua and open into intervillous spaces of developing placenta
6. Large venous sinuses develop
7. Uterine circulation after implantation (Figure 4-2)
   ! a. Maternal and fetal circulation remains independent of one another separated by a thin membrane
   b. Development of chorionic villi: trophoblastic cells form intervillous spaces within decidua for collection of maternal blood; as villi grow into these spaces, fetal blood enters villi via arteries and returns to fetus through fetal veins
   c. Trophoblasts: by end of four weeks, trophoblastic tissue has a radial appearance and contains a number of secondary and tertiary villi; villi are anchored in mesoderm and attached peripherally to maternal decidua

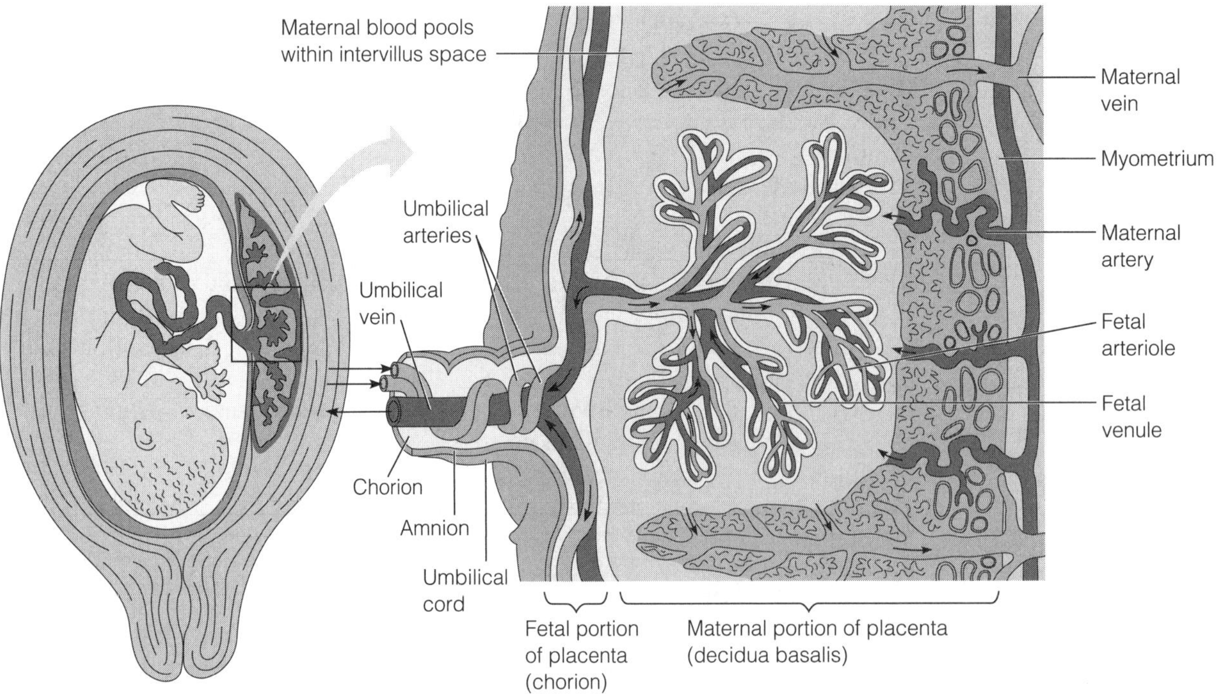

Figure 4-2

Vascular arrangement of the placenta

d. Prior to 12 weeks, there is little maternal blood in what will become intervillous spaces
e. Capillaries develop, giving rise to a vascular system between embryo and decidua that allows metabolic exchange but does not allow mixing of maternal and fetal blood
f. Maternal blood flows from uterine arteries into maternal sinuses surrounding villi and then back into uterine veins of mother
g. Maternal blood enters intervillous spaces through numerous spiral arteries
h. Blood enters deep into intervillous lakes and is drained away by endometrial veins following metabolic exchange
! **i.** Umbilical cord: two arteries and one vein
  1) Umbilical vessels are surrounded by **Wharton's jelly**, a gelatinous connective tissue that serves as a protective layer around umbilical vessels
  2) Fetal circulation enters placenta through arterial villi, then into capillary villi, finally returning to fetus through venous villi and umbilical vein following metabolic exchange
  3) At birth, umbilical cord is 2 centimeters in diameter and 50 to 60 centimeters in length

8. Placental structure
a. By beginning of fourth week, a fetal placental portion, made from trophoblasts, becomes a unit of metabolic transfer tissue
b. A maternal placental portion is made from decidua basalis
c. Trophoblasts and decidua intermingle in a junctional zone where trophoblasts are directly exposed to maternal blood flow
! **d.** Metabolic transfer occurs across trophoblastic cell membrane
e. Septums divide placenta into sections called cotyledons
f. Placenta enlarges as fetus grows
g. Umbilical cord has one vein that carries blood from placenta to fetus and two arteries that carry blood from fetus back to placenta, is surrounded by gelatinous connective tissue of umbilical cord, Wharton's jelly

! **9.** Metabolic functions of placenta
a. Placenta begins to function as a means of metabolic exchange by fourth week and is fully functional by eight weeks
b. Gases: exchange of oxygen and carbon dioxide
c. Nutrients and electrolytes: amino acids, free fatty acids, carbohydrates, and vitamins
d. Excretory products transfer from fetus to mother
! **e.** Production of hormones
  1) Progesterone to maintain pregnancy
  2) Estriol to stimulate uterine growth and mammary glands
! **3)** Human chorionic gonadotropin (hCG) functions similar to luteinizing hormone
  4) Human placental lactogen (hPL) functions similar to growth hormone; causes decreased insulin sensitivity resulting in a diabetogenic effect in mother and stimulates maternal breast development
f. Immunologic
! **1)** Transfer of maternal antibodies: immunoglobulin G (IgG)
  2) Poorly understood immunologic suppression occurs through actions of progesterone and hCG to protect fetus from rejection
g. Mechanisms of metabolic transport of placenta
! **1)** Simple diffusion moves substances including oxygen, carbon dioxide, carbon monoxide, water, electrolytes, and some drugs, from an area of higher concentration to an area of lower concentration

2) Facilitated diffusion requires a carrier to move molecules from an area of greater concentration to lesser concentration, such as glucose
3) Active transport moves substances, including amino acids, calcium, iron, vitamins, and glucose against a gradient
4) Pinocytosis transfers large molecules, including albumin and IgG by engulfment
5) Hydrostatic and osmotic pressures regulate water balance

V. FETAL DEVELOPMENT

A. **Fetal period**: extends from end of eighth week until birth; the *fetus* undergoes rapid growth and organ maturation during this time.

B. **Table 4-1 summarizes organ system development from 2 to 40 weeks' gestation**

C. **Table 4-2 lists important developmental highlights of interest to parents**

D. **Growth and appearance**

1. Greatest increase in length occurs during third, fourth, and fifth months of pregnancy
   a. At three months the head is ½ of the length; at full gestation it is ¼ of the length
   b. Growth in length: 12 weeks—11.5 centimeters, 20 weeks—25 centimeters, 40 weeks—53 centimeters
2. Growth-weight: greatest weight gain occurs in eighth and ninth month of pregnancy
   a. By 20 weeks = 1 pound
   b. 24 weeks = 1.7 pounds
   c. 32 weeks = 4.5 pounds or approximately 2000 grams
   d. 36 weeks = 5.5–6 pounds or approximately 2500–2750 grams
   e. 40 weeks = 7 pounds or approximately 3200 grams
3. After 8 weeks, the fetus takes on a human appearance
   a. Eyes and ears are positioned on face
   b. Limbs are relatively proportionate to rest of body although lower limbs are a bit short

E. **Integumentary growth**

1. Epidermis production begins at 3 weeks; by 11th week, it has three layers, and four layers exist by end of 4th month; by 24 weeks integument is fully present but immature
2. Lanugo forms at 13 weeks and begins to disappear at 36 weeks
3. Vernix caseosa appears at five months' gestation when an earlier skin layer is shed and mixes with secretions from sebaceous glands; it protects fetus from amniotic fluid skin maceration
4. At 24 weeks, skin is red, wrinkled, and lacks underlying connective tissue
5. Brown fat is deposited after 28 weeks' gestation in neck, subscapula, axillae, mediastinum, and perineal tissues
6. Subcutaneous fat is deposited during last two months
7. Innervation develops in third month; it is greatest around lips, sucking pad, and perioral zone

F. **Cardiac**

1. Heart begins beating 22 days after fertilization
2. Septation of heart is completed by fifth week
3. Fetal heart rate at 20 weeks' gestation averages 155 beats/minute; at term it averages 140 beats/minute
4. Primitive RBCs appear at three to four weeks' gestation
5. Fetal hemoglobin compensates for low fetal oxygen content
   a. Fetal hemoglobin has 20–30% greater oxygen-carrying capacity than maternal hemoglobin
   b. After 30 to 32 weeks' gestation, fetal hemoglobin production slows and formation of adult hemoglobin begins

Table 4-1 Summary of Organ System Development

Age: 2–3 weeks
Length: 2 mm = CRL (Crown-to-Rump Length)
Nervous system: Groove forms along middle back as cells thicken; neural tube forms from closure of neural groove.
Cardiovascular system: Beginning of blood circulation; tubular heart begins to form during third week.
Gastrointestinal system: Liver begins to function.
Genitourinary system: Formation of kidneys beginning.
Respiratory system: Nasal pits forming.
Endocrine system: Thyroid tissue appears.
Eyes: Optic cup and lens pit have formed; pigment in eyes.
Ear: Auditory pit is now enclosed structure.

Age: 4 weeks
Length: 4–6 mm = CRL
Weight: 0.4 grams
Nervous system: Anterior portion of neural tube closes to form brain; closure of posterior end forms spinal cord.
Musculoskeletal system: Noticeable limb buds.
Cardiovascular system: Tubular heart beats at 28 days and primitive red blood cells circulate through fetus and chorionic villi.
Gastrointestinal system: Mouth: formation of oral cavity; primitive jaws present; esophagotracheal septum begins division of esophagus and trachea. Digestive tract: stomach forms; esophagus and intestine become tubular; ducts of pancreas and liver forming.

Age: 5 weeks
Length: 8 mm = CRL
Weight: Only 0.5% of total body weight is fat (to 20 weeks)
Nervous System: Brain has differentiated and cranial nerves are present.
Musculoskeletal system: Developing muscles have innervation.
Cardiovascular system: Atrial division has occurred.

Age: 6 weeks
Length: 12 mm = CRL
Musculoskeletal system: Bone rudiments present; primitive skeletal shape forming; muscle mass begins to develop; ossification of skull and jaws begins.
Cardiovascular system: Chambers present in heart; groups of blood cells can be identified.
Gastrointestinal system: Oral and nasal cavities and upper lip formed; liver begins to form red blood cells.
Respiratory system: Trachea, bronchi, and lung buds present.
Ear: Formation of external, middle, and inner ear continues.
Sexual development: Embryonic sex glands appear.

Age: 7 weeks
Length: 18 mm = CRL
Cardiovascular system: Fetal heartbeats can be detected.
Gastrointestinal system: Mouth: tongue separates; palate folds. Digestive tract: stomach attains final form.
Genitourinary system: Separation of bladder and urethra from rectum.
Respiratory system: Diaphragm separates abdominal and thoracic cavities.
Eyes: Optic nerve formed; eyelids appear, thickening of lens.
Sexual development: Differentiation of sex glands into ovaries and testes begins.

Age: 8 weeks
Length: 2.5–3 cm = CRL
Weight: 2 grams
Musculoskeletal system: Digits formed; further differentiation of cells in primitive skeleton; cartilaginous bones show first signs of ossification; development of muscles in trunk, limbs, and head; some movement of fetus now possible.
Cardiovascular system: Development of heart essentially complete; fetal circulation follows two circuits—four extraembryonic and two intraembryonic.
Gastrointestinal system: Mouth: completion of lip fusion. Digestive tract: rotation in midgut; anal membrane has perforated.
Ear: External, middle, and inner ear assuming final forms.
Sexual development: Male and female external genitals appear similar until end of ninth week.

Age: 10 weeks
Length: 5–6 cm = C-H (Crown-to-Heel)
Weight: 14 grams
Nervous system: Neurons appear at caudal end of spinal cord; basic divisions of brain present.
Musculoskeletal system: Fingers and toes begin nail growth.
Cardiovascular system: Heartbeat can be heard with Doppler at 10–12 weeks.
Gastrointestinal system: Mouth: separation of lips from jaw; fusion of palate folds. Digestive tract: developing intestines enclosed in abdomen.
Genitourinary system: Bladder sac formed.
Endocrine system: Islets of Langerhans differentiated.
Eyes: Eyelids fused closed; development of lacrimal duct.
Sexual development: Males: production of testosterone and physical characteristics between 8 and 12 weeks.

Age: 12 weeks
Length: 8 cm = CRL; 11.5 cm = C-H
Weight: 45 grams
Musculoskeletal system: Clear outlining of miniature bones (12–20 weeks); process of ossification is established throughout fetal body; appearance of involuntary muscles in viscera.
Gastrointestinal system: Mouth: completion of palate. Digestive tract: appearance of muscles in gut; bile secretion begins; liver is major producer of red blood cells.
Respiratory system: Lungs acquire definitive shape.
Skin: Pink and delicate.

(continued)

Table 4-1 Summary of Organ System Development (Continued)

Endocrine system: Hormonal secretion from thyroid; insulin present in pancreas.
Immunologic system: Appearance of lymphoid tissue in fetal thymus gland.

Age: 16 weeks
Length: 13.5 cm = CRL; 15 cm = C-H
Weight: 200 grams
Musculoskeletal system: Teeth beginning to form hard tissue that will become central incisors.
Gastrointestinal system: Mouth: differentiation of hard and soft palate. Digestive tract: development of gastric and intestinal glands; intestines begin to collect meconium.
Genitourinary system: Kidneys assume typical shape and organization.
Skin: Appearance of scalp hair; lanugo present on body; transparent skin with visible blood vessels; sweat glands developing.
Eye, ear, and nose: Formed.
Sexual development: Sex determination possible.

Age: 18 weeks
Musculoskeletal system: Teeth beginning to form hard tissue (enamel and dentine) that will become lateral incisors.
Cardiovascular system: Fetal heart tones audible with fetoscope at 16–20 weeks.

Age: 20 weeks
Length: 19 cm = CRL; 25 cm = C-H
Weight: 435 grams (6% of total body weight is fat)
Nervous system: Myelination of spinal cord begins.
Musculoskeletal system: Teeth beginning to form hard tissue that will become canine and first molar. Lower limbs are of final relative proportions.
Gastrointestinal system: Fetus actively sucks and swallows amniotic fluid; peristaltic movements begin.
Skin: Lanugo covers entire body; brown fat begins to form; vernix caseosa begins to form.
Immunologic system: Detectable levels of fetal antibodies (IgG type).
Blood formation: Iron is stored and bone marrow is increasingly important.

Age: 24 weeks
Length: 23 cm = CRL; 28 cm = C-H
Weight: 780 grams
Nervous system: Brain looks like mature brain.
Musculoskeletal system: Teeth are beginning to form hard tissue that will become the second molars.
Respiratory system: Respiratory movements may occur (24–40 weeks). Nostrils reopen. Alveoli appear in lungs and begin production of surfactant; gas exchange possible.
Skin: Reddish and wrinkled, vernix caseosa present.
Immunologic system: IgG levels reach maternal levels.
Eyes: Structurally complete.

Age: 28 weeks
Length: 27 cm = CRL; 35 cm = C-H
Weight: 1200–1250 grams
Nervous system: Begins regulation of some body functions.
Skin: Adipose tissue accumulates rapidly; nails appear; eyebrows and eyelashes present.
Eyes: Eyelids open (28–32 weeks).
Sexual development: Males: testes descend into inguinal canal and upper scrotum.

Age: 32 weeks
Length: 31 cm = CRL; 38–43 cm = C-H
Weight: 2000 grams
Nervous system: More reflexes present.

Age: 36 weeks
Length: 35 cm = CRL; 42–48 cm = C-H
Weight: 2500–2750 grams
Musculoskeletal system: Distal femoral ossification centers present.
Skin: Pale; body rounded, lanugo disappearing, hair fuzzy or woolly; few sole creases; sebaceous glands active and helping to produce vernix caseosa (36–40 weeks).
Ears: Ear lobes with little cartilage.
Sexual development: Males: scrotum small and few rugae present; descent of testes into upper scrotum to stay (36–40 weeks). Females: labia majora and minora equally prominent.

Age: 40 weeks
Length: 40 cm = CRL; 48–52 cm = C-H
Weight: 3200+ grams (16% of total body weight is fat)
Respiratory system: At 38 weeks, lecithin-sphingomyelin (L/S) ratio approaches 2:1 (indicates decreased risk of respiratory distress from inadequate surfactant production if born now).
Skin: Smooth and pink; vernix present in skinfolds; moderate to profuse silky hair; lanugo hair on shoulders and upper back; nails extend over tips or digits; creases cover sole.
Ears: Ear lobes firmer due to increased cartilage.
Sexual development: Males: rugous scrotum. Females: labia majora well developed and minora small or completely covered.

Note: Age refers to gestational age of fetus/conceptus; fertilization age.
Source: Sadler, T. W. (2010). *Langman's medical embryology* (11th ed.). Philadelphia, PA: Lippincott Williams & Wilkins.

Table 4-2 Fetal Development: What Parents Want to Know

4 weeks	The fetal heart begins to beat.
8 weeks	All body organs are formed.
10–12 weeks	Fetal heart tones can be heard by Doppler device.
16 weeks	Baby's sex can be seen. Although thin, the fetus looks like a baby.
20 weeks	Heartbeat can be heard with a fetoscope. Mother feels movement (quickening). Baby develops a regular schedule of sleeping, sucking, and kicking. Hands can grasp. Baby assumes a favorite position in utero. Vernix (lanolin-like covering) protects body, and lanugo (fine hair) keeps oil on skin. Head hair, eyebrows, and eyelashes present.
24 weeks	Weighs 1 lb 10 oz. Activity is increasing. Fetal respiratory movements begin.
28 weeks	Eyes begin to open and close. Baby can breathe at this time. Surfactant needed for breathing at birth is formed. Baby is two-thirds its final size.
32 weeks	Baby has fingernails and toenails. Subcutaneous fat is being laid down. Baby appears less red and wrinkled.
38–40 weeks	Baby fills total uterus. Baby gets antibodies from mother.

Source: Davidson, Michele; London, Marcia L.; Ladewig, Patricia W., *Olds' maternal-newborn nursing & women's health across the lifespan*, 9th Ed., ©2012. Reprinted and Electronically reproduced by permission of Pearson Education, Inc., Upper Saddle River, New Jersey.

Practice to Pass

Some infants have a heart defect called *patent ductus arteriosus*. In this condition, the ductus arteriosus does not close after birth. What are the consequences to the neonate of maintaining this circulatory pattern after birth?

6. Anatomical structure of fetal circulation (Figure 4-3)
   a. Lungs and liver are nonfunctional so circulation bypasses these organs through special fetal circulatory structures
   b. As blood returns from placenta through single umbilical vein, a majority of blood supply bypasses liver through **ductus venosus** and goes directly to inferior vena cava
   c. As blood enters right atrium from inferior vena cava, most of it is directed across right atrium into left atrium through an opening called **foramen ovale**; this enables oxygen-rich blood from placenta to bypass lungs and be circulated to body
   d. Blood that enters right atrium from superior vena cava is mostly deoxygenated and passes through tricuspid valve into right ventricle and pulmonary artery; blood in pulmonary artery mostly passes through **ductus arteriosus** into descending aorta; from there, it flows into two fetal arteries back to placenta where it becomes oxygenated
   e. Umbilical cord has three vessels, two arteries that move fetal blood to placenta and one vein that takes blood from placenta and returns it to fetus; infants born with only two vessels often have other fetal anomalies
7. Clotting ability begins at 11 to 12 weeks
   a. Fibrinogen production in liver begins at 5 weeks and reaches adult levels by 30 weeks' gestation
   b. By 13 weeks, platelet levels are about same as adults
   c. Vitamin K levels are 50% of adult because sterile fetal gut is unable to produce the vitamin; after birth, gastrointestinal bacteria produce vitamin K
8. Formation of WBCs begins in liver at 5 to 7 weeks' gestation, spleen at 8 weeks, thymus at 10 weeks, and lymph nodes at 12 weeks; at birth, the number of WBCs is same or greater than adults

G. Respiratory

1. Respiratory movements occur at end of first trimester
2. Respiratory movement is stimulated by tactile stimuli and asphyxia

Figure 4-3
Fetal circulation

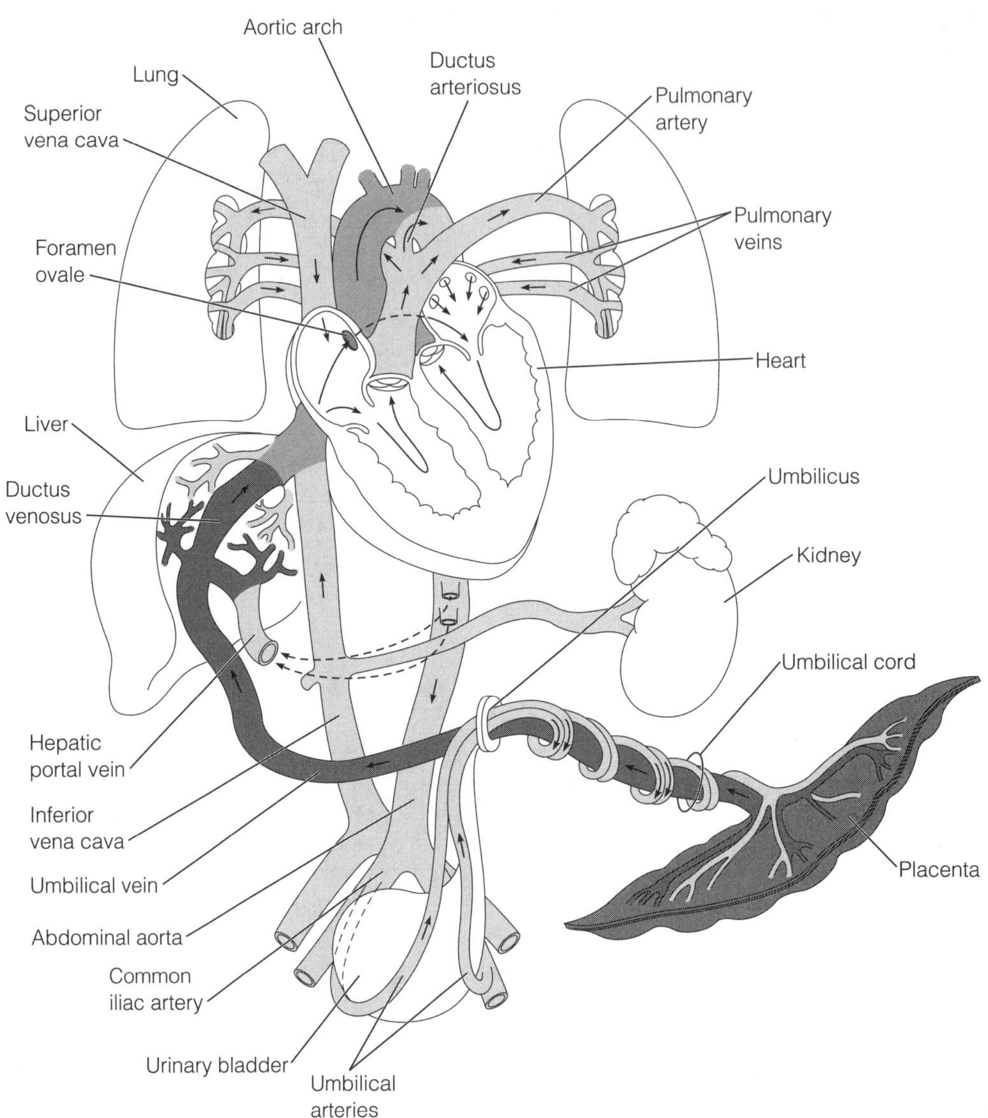

High oxygenation
Moderate oxygenation
Low oxygenation
Very low oxygenation

3. Respiratory inhibition occurs during the third and fourth month to prevent a collection of debris in alveoli
4. Fluid is secreted into lungs by alveolar epithelium
5. At 22 weeks, alveolar-capillary membrane comes into juxtaposition, allowing life outside womb to be possible, although survival is unlikely
6. At 24 weeks' gestation, terminal air sacs appear at end of terminal bronchioles
7. Mean fetal pO_2 after oxygenation is only 30 mm Hg; increased oxygen-carrying capacity of fetal hemoglobin prevents hypoxia
8. Surfactant secretion is detectable between 25 to 30 weeks' gestation and is mature by 36 weeks
9. Lungs mature at 36 weeks

H. Gastrointestinal (GI)

1. Anatomic development begins at four weeks
2. At 12 weeks, intestinal loops in umbilical cord withdraw into abdominal cavity
3. At beginning of fifth month, fetus swallows amniotic fluid
4. During last two to three months of pregnancy, GI development approaches that of term newborn
5. Liver is primarily hematopoetic; enzyme systems are immature at birth
6. Peristalsis is mature by third trimester
7. Meconium forms in intestine beginning at 16 weeks from unabsorbed residue of amniotic fluid and excretory products of GI mucosa and glands

I. Musculoskeletal

1. Primary ossification begins in long bones and skull by 12 weeks
2. Minimal reflexive muscle movement is noted by 12 weeks
3. Fetal movement is clearly detected by mother by 20 weeks
4. Bones are mostly unossified and cartilaginous until last four weeks of gestation; rapid ossification occurs when half of calcium and phosphate absorbed by fetus occurs during last month of pregnancy

J. Neurologic

1. Neural folds appear 22 to 23 days after conception and fuse at 28 days to form neural tube
   a. Tube closure begins at 22 days and progresses in a cephalocaudal direction
   b. Failure of closure results in neural tube defect
   c. Neural tube becomes central nervous system, brain, and spinal cord
2. Some reflex activity is present by 12 weeks
3. Neuronal proliferation maximizes at 12 to 18 weeks' gestation
4. Brain development
   a. Begins with lower levels such as basal ganglia, thalamus, midbrain, and brain stem
   b. Higher levels, cerebrum and cerebellum, form later
   c. Most neurons of cerebrum are formed from 10 to 18 weeks
   d. At birth, brain is 27% of adult weight
5. Neural organization begins at about six months and continues into adulthood
6. Myelinization occurs in third trimester and continues into adulthood; it progresses from peripheral to central nervous system and motor to sensory
7. Some body regulation control occurs at 25 to 28 weeks

Practice to Pass

A client wants to know the difference between an embryo and a fetus. How will the nurse respond to her inquiries?

K. Urinary

1. Nephron development begins at 8 weeks and filtration at 10 weeks
2. The absolute number of nephrons reaches adult levels by 34 to 35 weeks but are functionally immature
3. ! By fifth month, fetus urinates into amniotic fluid although urine contains little waste; in second half of pregnancy, urine makes up a major portion of amniotic fluid
4. ! Ability to concentrate urine is 20 to 30% that of adults

L. Sexual

1. Testosterone production begins by male fetal genital ridge at seven weeks' gestation; later, fetal testes produce it; it is responsible for male organ development
2. ! Without testosterone, fetus appears female
3. By 16 weeks, external genitalia are developed enough for identification by ultrasound

Case Study

A nurse working in a women's health clinic conducts prenatal classes. At each class, the nurse addresses a different topic related to prenatal development. The nurse includes information to support safe progression through pregnancy and assist parents to picture stages of fetal development.

1. The nurse explains the stage of preembryonic development. How would you describe the significant events of this time period?
2. The nurse explains organogenesis and critical periods of development in relationship to teratogens. Can you explain the connection between these concepts?
3. A class participant asks about genetic transmission of birth defects. What is the nurse's response?
4. The nurse includes information about the age of viability. When is this achieved and what developmental landmarks must be present for life outside of the womb?
5. The nurse describes the appearance of the fetus at the end of each trimester. How does the fetus appear at each stage?

For suggested responses, see pages 302–303.

POSTTEST

POSTTEST

1 Two married clients have one child with Tay-Sachs disease, but neither of the clients has the disease. They are in the clinic for genetic counseling prior to conceiving another child. The nurse formulates which nursing diagnosis that most likely applies to this couple?

1. Decisional Conflict related to knowledge deficit
2. Posttrauma Syndrome related to care of a disabled child
3. Powerlessness related to transmission of genetic disease
4. Ineffective Health Maintenance related to ineffective family coping

2. Following an ultrasound at six weeks' gestation, the pregnant client comments, "The embryo doesn't look human. When will it begin to look like a baby?" Which of the following is the best response by the nurse?

1. "In one more week the embryo will take on a human appearance."
2. "The embryo looks like a baby already. Let me show you again."
3. "The embryo becomes a fetus and looks more human after about eight weeks' gestation."
4. "You are right, the embryo doesn't look human. Is this important to you?"

3. A woman decides to use natural family planning as a means of contraception and states, "The ovum is fertile for 48 hours after ovulation, the same as sperm." What is the nurse's best response?

1. "Correct; avoid intercourse during this time."
2. "Sperm are fertile for 48 hours, while the ovum is fertile for 24 hours."
3. "Actually, the ovum is fertile for 36 hours and sperm for 24 hours."
4. "Let me explain again, the ovum may be fertile up to 72 hours."

4. A nurse discusses teratogens with a client during preconceptual counseling. The client demonstrates understanding by making which statement?

1. "I should stop taking all my medications while I am pregnant."
2. "The fetus is at greatest risk for developing anomalies during the first 16 weeks of pregnancy."
3. "After 12 weeks the placenta protects the fetus from teratogens."
4. "Exposure to teratogens poses the greatest risk during the first eight weeks."

5. Following an amniocentesis the parents discover that their fetus has Down syndrome. What should the nurse do at this time?

1. Provide information about Down syndrome in an empathetic and respectful manner.
2. Discuss the possibility of intrauterine surgery.
3. Refer the parents for karyotyping.
4. Refer the parents to their local public health agency.

6. A pregnant client asks about the functions of the placenta. What items of information should the nurse include in the teaching plan? Select all that apply.

1. The placenta filters fetal urine.
2. Fetal and maternal blood mix in the placenta to exchange nutrients.
3. The placenta filters alcohol from the mother's blood.
4. Substances are exchanged by the placenta without mixing maternal and fetal blood.
5. Fetal respiration, nutrition, and excretion are carried out by the placenta.

7. At 36 weeks' gestation, a primigravida enters the birthing unit in labor and is concerned about delivering early. The nurse reassures the client by making which statement?

1. "Luckily, there is no need to worry; you are at term."
2. "Most likely everything is going to be fine. Your baby has a strong heart rate."
3. "Many babies born at this age have lungs that are just about mature."
4. "This is nothing to be excessively concerned about. We deliver babies at this age very often."

8 A nurse evaluates understanding of fetal development in a prenatal class. The nurse concludes that more teaching is required when one of the group members make which statement?

1. "Smoking will help me have an easy labor because the baby will be small."
2. "I should not smoke at all during pregnancy."
3. "Infants born to mothers who smoke may suffer lung problems."
4. "Chemicals from smoking pass through the placenta to the fetus."

9 A client is pregnant with twins, a boy and a girl, and asks if they will be identical. What is the nurse's best response?

1. "They are not identical because the ultrasound showed one was bigger than the other."
2. "I'll discuss this with the doctor and give you a call later."
3. "We won't know until the babies are delivered."
4. "The twins are not identical. Identical twins are virtually always the same sex."

10 A pregnant client asks the nurse when the fetal heart will begin beating. The nurse tells the client even though the fetal heart is not fully developed it begins to beat at about _____ days of gestation.

Fill in your answer below:
______ days

➤ *See pages 88–89 for Answers and Rationales.*

POSTTEST

ANSWERS & RATIONALES

Pretest

1 **Answer: 4** **Rationale:** A carrier for cystic fibrosis is an individual who does not have the illness but is heterozygous for the abnormal gene. It is not until two carriers mate and produce children that the abnormal gene will be manifested in the offspring. The risk can be calculated. The affected offspring must carry two of the abnormal genes to be affected. There is a 25% chance of this occurring, a 50% chance that the offspring will be a carrier without the disease, and a 25% chance of not having the gene at all. **Cognitive Level:** Analyzing **Client Need:** Physiological Adaptation **Integrated Process:** Communication and Documentation **Content Area:** Maternal-Newborn **Strategy:** Critical words are *autosomal recessive*, *cystic fibrosis*, and *both are carriers.* Knowledge of genetic transmission of autosomal recessive illnesses such as cystic fibrosis is needed to answer the question. **Reference:** Ladewig, P., London, M., & Davidson, M. (2010). *Contemporary maternal-newborn nursing care* (7th ed.). Upper Saddle River, NJ: Pearson Education, p. 151.

2 **Answer: 2, 5** **Rationale:** The ovum survives 24 hours after ovulation. Sperm are most capable of fertilization 24 hours after introduction into the female's reproductive tract. Ovulation usually occurs 14 days prior to the first day of the menstrual period. If sperm are introduced 24 hours after ovulation the ovum cannot be fertilized. The ovum does not need to be in contact with the sperm for 48 hours for fertilization to occur. **Cognitive Level:** Applying **Client Need:** Health Promotion and Maintenance **Integrated Process:** Teaching and Learning **Content Area:** Maternal-Newborn **Strategy:** Critical words are *understand* and *ideal time*. Because the question is worded positively, the correct answer is a true statement about a point of client education. Knowledge of ovulation and conception are necessary to answer the question. **Reference:** Ladewig, P., London, M., & Davidson, M. (2010). *Contemporary maternal-newborn nursing care* (7th ed.). Upper Saddle River, NJ: Pearson Education, p. 83.

3 **Answer: 4** **Rationale:** The risk of Down syndrome increases markedly after the age of 40. The 42-year-old woman is at greatest risk, the 23-year-old is at lesser risk, and the 15-year-old is at least risk related to age. Infection is more likely to result in a birth anomaly if it occurs in the first trimester. **Cognitive Level:** Analyzing **Client Need:** Physiological Adaptation **Integrated Process:** Nursing Process: Diagnosis **Content Area:** Maternal-Newborn **Strategy:** Critical words are *greatest risk* and *birth anomalies*. Recall that the incidence of birth anomalies, particularly genetically determined disorders, increases with the age of the mother. The correct answer is the oldest woman. **Reference:** Ladewig, P., London, M.,

ANSWERS & RATIONALES

& Davidson, M. (2010). *Contemporary maternal-newborn nursing care* (7th ed.). Upper Saddle River, NJ: Pearson Education, p. 151.

4 **Answer: 3** **Rationale:** Dizygotic twins, also known as fraternal or nonidentical, do run in families. The pregnancy results from the fertilization of two different ova by two different sperm. The zygotes develop separately and carry their own distinct genetic code and develop their own placentas and amniotic sacs. Monozygotic, also known as identical, result from a single fertilized ovum. They share the same genetic code and often share placentas and amniotic sacs. This type of twinning occurs at random. **Cognitive Level:** Applying **Client Need:** Health Promotion and Maintenance **Integrated Process:** Teaching and Learning **Content Area:** Maternal-Newborn **Strategy:** Critical words are *pregnant with twins* and *twins run in the family*. The focus of this question is dizygotic twins. Eliminate the incorrect answers because they describe monozygotic twins. **Reference:** Ladewig, P., London, M., & Davidson, M. (2010). *Contemporary maternal-newborn nursing care* (7th ed.). Upper Saddle River, NJ: Pearson Education, p. 493.

5 **Answer: 3** **Rationale:** The primary reason for early prenatal care relates to the critical periods of development that occur in the first trimester and to promote safety during this particularly vulnerable time of pregnancy. While it is important to establish a relationship with clients and verify pregnancy, monitoring client and fetal safety during the first trimester is of highest importance. Fetal movements are usually felt in the second trimester, and viability is not possible until 24 weeks, when fetal lung maturity would arise as a concern. **Cognitive Level:** Applying **Client Need:** Health Promotion and Maintenance **Integrated Process:** Communication and Documentation **Content Area:** Maternal-Newborn **Strategy:** Critical words are *26 weeks of pregnancy* and *prenatal care in first trimester*. The focus of this question is importance of prenatal care to health promotion and maintenance. The incorrect answers focus on health problems. **Reference:** Ladewig, P., London, M., & Davidson, M. (2010). *Contemporary maternal-newborn nursing care* (7th ed.). Upper Saddle River, NJ: Pearson Education, p. 66.

6 **Answer: 1** **Rationale:** The ears ossify at 20 weeks' gestation and the fetus has the ability to hear at 24 weeks. Telling the client that it's uncertain when the fetus begins to hear or that the fetus does not hear until eight months' gestation is factually incorrect. Telling the client that she is "silly" to think the fetus can be calmed by a sibling's voice creates distance between client and nurse from possibly offensive language. **Cognitive Level:** Applying **Client Need:** Health Promotion and Maintenance **Integrated Process:** Communication and Documentation **Content Area:** Maternal-Newborn **Strategy:** Critical words are *seven months' pregnant*, *talks to fetus*, and *calms the fetus*. Knowledge of the fetal development is necessary to answer the question. Because the question is worded positively, the correct answer is a true statement that would be included in client education. **Reference:** Ladewig, P., London, M., & Davidson, M. (2010). *Contemporary maternal-newborn nursing care* (7th ed.). Upper Saddle River, NJ: Pearson Education, p. 66.

7 **Answer: 1** **Rationale:** Oligohydramnios is an insufficient amount of amniotic fluid, which impairs the normal functions of the fluid, resulting in potential complications such as fetal skin and skeletal abnormalities, pulmonary hypoplasia, and umbilical cord compression. It does not indicate that the fetus has swallowed too much amniotic fluid. It is an abnormal condition occurring when amniotic fluid volume is less than expected for a given stage of pregnancy. Oligohydramnios is not a sign of maturing lungs. **Cognitive Level:** Applying **Client Need:** Physiological Adaptation **Integrated Process:** Communication and Documentation **Content Area:** Maternal-Newborn **Strategy:** The critical words are *oligohydramnios* and *harm the fetus*. Because the stem of the question is positively worded, the correct answer is a true statement about a point of client education. Knowledge of potential complications of oligohydramnios is necessary to answer the question. **Reference:** Ladewig,P., London, M., & Davidson, M. (2009). *Contemporary maternal-newborn nursing care* (7th ed.). Upper Saddle River, NJ: Pearson Education, p. 499.

8 **Answer: 2** **Rationale:** There are two umbilical arteries that carry blood from the fetal common iliac artery to the placenta. These two arteries are twisted around a large umbilical vein that carries blood from the placenta to the fetal heart. About 1% of umbilical cords contain only two vessels. This condition is more likely to be associated with congenital malformations. Having an umbilical cord with one artery and two veins or two arteries and two veins does not occur. **Cognitive Level:** Applying **Client Need:** Health Promotion and Maintenance **Integrated Process:** Nursing Process: Assessment **Content Area:** Maternal-Newborn **Strategy:** Critical words are *expects* and *umbilical cord*. Normal assessment findings are expected in this question, thus a three-vessel cord. Immediately eliminate two options because of this. Recall that there are two arteries and one vein to select correctly. **Reference:** Ladewig, P., London, M., & Davidson, M. (2010). *Contemporary maternal-newborn nursing care* (7th ed.). Upper Saddle River, NJ: Pearson Education, p. 59.

9 **Answer: 4** **Rationale:** At term the amniotic fluid volume ranges from 700 to 1000 milliliters (mL). Each mL weighs about 1 gram, so the amniotic fluid contributes about 700 to 1000 grams to the weight of pregnancy. This is the same as 0.7 to 1 kilogram, since 1000 gram equals a kilogram. **Cognitive Level:** Applying **Client Need:** Health Promotion and Maintenance **Integrated Process:** Teaching and Learning **Content Area:** Maternal-Newborn **Strategy:** Critical words are *amniotic fluid* and *third trimester weighs*. Recall that amniotic fluid makes a significant contribution to pregnancy weight gain and use ability to do weight and volume conversions to increase the

likelihood of selecting the correct option. **Reference:** Ladewig, P., London, M., & Davidson, M. (2010). *Contemporary maternal-newborn nursing care* (7th ed.). Upper Saddle River, NJ: Pearson Education, p. 57.

10 **Answer: 4** **Rationale:** By the end of 28 days (4 gestational weeks) the tubular heart is beating at a regular rhythm and circulating primitive red blood cells through the main blood vessels. **Cognitive Level:** Applying **Client Need:** Health Promotion and Maintenance **Integrated Process:** Nursing Process: Implementation **Content Area:** Maternal-Newborn **Strategy:** Recall that the fetal heart begins beating early, often before the woman knows she's pregnant. This should help to select an early stage of fetal development. **Reference:** Ladewig, P., London, M., & Davidson, M. (2010). *Contemporary maternal-newborn nursing care* (7th ed.). Upper Saddle River, NJ: Pearson Education, p. 66.

Posttest

1 **Answer: 1** **Rationale:** Families with genetic disease are faced with difficult decisions regarding pregnancy. One of the purposes of genetic counseling is to provide the best information available so families can make knowledgeable decisions. The fact that the family is seeking professional help is evidence that they feel some power regarding the situation. There is no evidence one way or another regarding their coping abilities with a disabled child. There is no evidence to support posttrauma syndrome. **Cognitive Level:** Analyzing **Client Need:** Psychosocial Integrity **Integrated Process:** Nursing Process: Diagnosis **Content Area:** Maternal-Newborn **Strategy:** The focus of this question is genetic counseling, which is intended to provide information to facilitate decision making. Eliminate options not focused on this purpose. **Reference:** Ladewig, P., London, M., & Davidson, M. (2010). *Contemporary maternal-newborn nursing care* (7th ed.). Upper Saddle River, NJ: Pearson Education, p. 151.

2 **Answer: 3** **Rationale:** The embryonic phase of development is a time of organogenesis. By the end of eight weeks' gestation, all of the tissue and organ foundations have developed. Once this occurs, the embryo appears human and enters the fetal phase. The fetal phase is one of organ maturation. Agreeing with the client and asking about an additional question does not answer the client's original question. **Cognitive Level:** Applying **Client Need:** Health Promotion and Maintenance **Integrated Process:** Teaching and Learning **Content Area:** Maternal-Newborn **Strategy:** Critical words are *ultrasound at six weeks* and *when will it look like a baby.* The question is worded positively, so the correct response will also be a true statement. Knowledge of fetal development is necessary to answer the question. **Reference:** Ladewig, P., London, M., & Davidson, M. (2010). *Contemporary maternal-newborn nursing care* (7th ed.). Upper Saddle River, NJ: Pearson Education, p. 292.

3 **Answer: 2** **Rationale:** Ova are capable of being fertilized for 24 hours after ovulation. Sperm live for 48 to 72 hours after coitus but are most capable of fertilization in the first 24 hours. **Cognitive Level:** Applying **Client Need:** Health Promotion and Maintenance **Integrated Process:** Teaching and Learning **Content Area:** Maternal-Newborn **Strategy:** The wording of the question indicates that the correct answer is an incorrect statement by the client. It is necessary to understand fertilization in order to correct the client's misunderstanding. **Reference:** Ladewig, P., London, M., & Davidson, M. (2010). *Contemporary maternal-newborn nursing care* (7th ed.). Upper Saddle River, NJ: Pearson Education, p. 183.

4 **Answer: 4** **Rationale:** Organogenesis and cell differentiation occur during the first eight weeks of pregnancy, making the embryo particularly sensitive to teratogens during this time. Although medications may have teratogenic effects, each medication's risk versus benefit needs to be evaluated by the health care provider. **Cognitive Level:** Analyzing **Client Need:** Health Promotion and Maintenance **Integrated Process:** Teaching and Learning **Content Area:** Maternal-Newborn **Strategy:** Critical words are *teratogens* and *demonstrated understanding*. Specific knowledge of teratogenic effects on the fetus is needed to answer the question. **Reference:** Ladewig, P., London, M., & Davidson, M. (2010). *Contemporary maternal-newborn nursing care* (7th ed.). Upper Saddle River, NJ: Pearson Education, p. 72.

5 **Answer: 1** **Rationale:** The nurse is in an ideal position to provide information, educate families, and review what has been discussed in genetic counseling sessions. The nurse provides information about Down syndrome. Karyotyping is not indicated because they have a diagnosis. Intrauterine surgery cannot cure a chromosomal anomaly. Referral to public health may be indicated after the parents make a decision regarding the pregnancy. **Cognitive Level:** Applying **Client Need:** Reduction of Risk Potential **Integrated Process:** Caring **Content Area:** Maternal-Newborn **Strategy:** The focus of this question is the role of the nurse as educator. The correct option will provide information to the client about a new diagnosis. **Reference:** Ladewig,P., London, M., & Davidson, M. (2010). *Contemporary maternal-newborn nursing care* (7th ed.). Upper Saddle River, NJ: Pearson Education, p. 226.

6 **Answer: 4, 5** **Rationale:** Fetal gas exchange occurs in the intervillous spaces of the placenta through simple diffusion of oxygen, carbon dioxide, and carbon monoxide. Substance exchange between the maternal and fetal blood occurs without mixing of the blood. Fetal waste products are excreted via the placenta, but urine is excreted by the fetus into the amniotic fluid. While the placenta is capable of filtering some substances, most substances consumed by the mother are exchanged with the fetus, including alcohol. **Cognitive Level:** Analyzing **Client Need:** Health Promotion and Maintenance **Integrated Process:** Teaching and Learning

Content Area: Maternal-Newborn **Strategy:** Critical words are *functions of the placenta.* Knowledge of the basic functions of the placenta is needed. The wording of the question indicates that the correct option is also a true statement. **Reference:** Ladewig, P., London, M., & Davidson, M. (2010). *Contemporary maternal-newborn nursing care* (7th ed.). Upper Saddle River, NJ: Pearson Education, p. 72.

7 **Answer: 3** **Rationale:** Surfactant with a lecithin:sphingomyelin ratio of 2:1 is required for mature lung function. This occurs at about 36 weeks' gestation. An infant born prior to 38 weeks' gestation is considered preterm. A reassuring fetal heart rate is not indicative of lung maturity. Stating there is nothing to be excessively concerned about ignores the client's concern and is not reassuring. **Cognitive Level:** Applying **Client Need:** Physiological Adaptation **Integrated Process:** Communication and Documentation **Content Area:** Maternal-Newborn **Strategy:** Critical words are *36 weeks' gestation* and *concerns about delivering early.* Knowledge of normal development of fetus and lung maturity is needed to answer the question correctly. Use of therapeutic communication techniques also aids in eliminating incorrect options. **Reference:** Ladewig, P., London, M., & Davidson, M. (2010). *Contemporary maternal-newborn nursing care* (7th ed.). Upper Saddle River, NJ: Pearson Education, p. 183.

8 **Answer: 1** **Rationale:** Smoking causes vasoconstriction that can interfere with placental circulation. The infant may suffer negative effects including intrauterine growth restriction. Any chemical the mother is exposed to during pregnancy has the potential to pass through the placenta to the fetus. **Cognitive Level:** Analyzing **Client Need:** Health Promotion and Maintenance **Integrated Process:** Teaching and Learning **Content Area:** Maternal-Newborn **Strategy:** Critical words are *more teaching is required*, indicating you are looking for a high-risk behavior and response that would be incorrect. **Reference:** Ladewig, P., London, M., & Davidson, M. (2010). *Contemporary maternal-newborn nursing care* (7th ed.). Upper Saddle River, NJ: Pearson Education, p. 72.

9 **Answer: 4** **Rationale:** Twins of opposite sex are always fraternal because it indicates two sperm were involved in fertilization, one carrying a Y chromosome and one carrying an X chromosome. Identical twins develop from one ovum and one sperm. Therefore, the genotype is the same, including sex. Identical twins may be different sizes because one twin may receive a greater amount of placental circulation than the other. It is unnecessary to discuss this with the health care provider; the question requires a simple factual answer. **Cognitive Level:** Applying **Client Need:** Health Promotion and Maintenance **Integrated Process:** Communication and Documentation **Content Area:** Maternal-Newborn **Strategy:** The core issue of this question is identical twins. The correct answer provides true information. **Reference:** Ladewig, P., London, M., & Davidson, M. (2010). *Contemporary maternal-newborn nursing care* (7th ed.). Upper Saddle River, NJ: Pearson Education, p. 59.

10 **Answer: 28** **Rationale:** By the end of 28 days (four gestational weeks) the tubular heart is beating at a regular rhythm and circulating primitive red blood cells through the main blood vessels. **Cognitive Level:** Applying **Client Need:** Health Promotion and Maintenance **Integrated Process:** Teaching and Learning **Content Area:** Maternal-Newborn **Strategy:** Recall that the fetal heart begins beating early, often before the woman knows she is pregnant. This should help to select an early stage of fetal development. **Reference:** Ladewig, P., London, M., & Davidson, M. (2010). *Contemporary maternal-newborn nursing care* (7th ed.). Upper Saddle River, NJ: Pearson Education, p. 66.

References

Davidson, M., London, M., & Ladewig, P. (2012). *Olds' maternal newborn nursing & women's health across the lifespan* (9th ed.). Upper Saddle River, NJ: Pearson Education.

Ladewig, P., London, M., & Davidson, M. (2009). *Contemporary maternal-newborn nursing care* (7th ed.). Upper Saddle River, NJ: Pearson Education.

NANDA Nursing Diagnosis (2009). Retrieved January 29, 2011, from http://www.scribd.com/doc/11885949/NANDA-2009

Orshan, S. A. (2008). *Maternity, newborn, and women's health nursing: Comprehensive care across the life span.* Philadelphia: Lippincott Williams & Wilkins.

Ricci, S. (2009). *Essentials of maternity, newborn, and women's health nursing* (2nd ed.). Philadelphia: Lippincott Williams & Wilkins.

Sadler, T. W. (2010). *Langman's medical embryology* (11th ed.). Philadelphia: Lippincott Williams & Wilkins.

5 The Normal Prenatal Experience

Chapter Outline

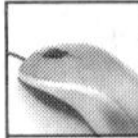

NCLEX-RN® Test Prep

Use the accompanying online resource, NursingReviewsandRationales, to test yourself with hundreds of NCLEX®-style practice questions.

Objectives

- Describe the nursing care provided to the maternity client during the first prenatal visit.
- Identify assessment needs of maternity clients during subsequent prenatal visits.
- Differentiate between presumptive, probable, and positive signs of pregnancy.
- Describe the physical changes that occur in each body system of the pregnant woman.
- Identify discomforts commonly experienced in pregnancy and related nursing interventions.
- Describe the content areas that nurses should include in an educational program for a pregnant client.

Review at a Glance

Chadwick's sign a bluish color of vaginal mucous membrane resulting from increased vascularity; can be seen beginning at about fourth month of pregnancy

chloasma increased pigmentation, commonly seen over nose and cheeks during pregnancy; sometimes called "mask of pregnancy"

colostrum a thin, bluish-white breast secretion that appears before onset of lactation; comprised mainly of serum and white blood corpuscles, fluid is high in protein and contains immune properties

estimated date of birth (EDB) sometimes called "due date" or "estimated date of confinement (EDC)"; this is the date in pregnancy when birth is expected

fetal heart tones sounds produced by fetal heart; can be counted to determine fetal heart rate

fundal height distance (in centimeters) from symphysis pubis to top edge of fundus; this measurement can be used to calculate gestational age

Goodell's sign a softening of cervix that begins in second month of pregnancy

gravida term used to indicate a pregnant woman; sometimes used to indicate number of times a woman has been pregnant

linea nigra a dark line of pigment extending from umbilicus to the pubis, sometimes seen in later part of pregnancy

McDonald's method procedure used to determine gestational age by measuring fundal height; is most accurate between 22 and 34 weeks; can also be used serially to monitor fetal growth; may be inaccurate in presence of maternal obesity, uterine fibroids, and polyhydramnios

Nägele's Rule a commonly used method for determining estimated date of birth; is calculated by determining first day of last menstrual period, subtracting three months from that date, and then adding seven days

para a woman who has delivered an infant who had reached age of viability

positive signs of pregnancy findings that confirm pregnancy such as auscultation of fetal heart tones, fetal movement, and visualization of fetus

presumptive signs of pregnancy findings reported by mother that suggest presence of a pregnancy, such as cessation of menses, morning sickness, and quickening

probable signs of pregnancy findings noted by health care provider that suggest a pregnancy is present, including Goodell's sign, McDonald's sign, enlargement of abdomen, and palpation of fetal outline

quickening first fetal movement felt by pregnant woman, usually between 16 and 18 weeks' gestation

striae gravidarum shiny red lines on skin of breasts, abdomen, thighs, and buttocks caused by stretching of skin

PRETEST

1 During the client's initial prenatal visit, which assessment data obtained by the nurse would indicate a need for further assessment?

1. History of diabetes for six years
2. Exercises three times a week
3. Occasional use of over-the-counter pain relievers
4. Maternal age 30 years

2 The nurse should instruct the low-risk client who is 16 weeks' pregnant to return to the prenatal clinic in ______ weeks.

Fill in your answer below:

____________ weeks

3 The client has completed an at-home pregnancy test with positive results. Which client statement indicates that the client understands the meaning of the test results?

1. "I understand that this means I have ovulated in the past 24 hours."
2. "I understand that this means I am not pregnant."
3. "I understand that this means I might be pregnant."
4. "I understand that this means I am pregnant."

4 A client comes to the clinic for her first prenatal visit and reports that July 10 was the first day of her last menstrual period. Using Näegele's rule, the nurse calculates the estimated date of birth for the client to be ______. (Use format month-day, i.e., July 10 = 07-10)

Fill in your answer below:

____

5 The pregnant client reports that she has a 3-year-old child at home who was born at term, had a miscarriage at 10 weeks' gestation, and delivered a set of twins at 28 weeks' gestation that died within 24 hours. How should the nurse record the client's status in the prenatal record?

1. Gravida 2, para 1
2. Gravida 3, para 3
3. Gravida 4, para 2
4. Gravida 5, para 4

6 The client, who is 36 weeks' gestation, calls her prenatal care provider because she is concerned about a thin, bluish-white fluid leaking from her breasts. What is an appropriate response by the nurse? Select all that apply.

1. "This probably indicates an infection in your breasts. You will need to come into the office."
2. "This usually happens when you are going into premature labor. You should go to the hospital."
3. "This normally occurs as your breasts prepare for breastfeeding. You should continue to wear a good-fitting bra."
4. "This is an indication that you may have some problems with breastfeeding. I will have the lactation consultant call you."
5. "The fluid is colostrum and normally leaks from the breast during the last trimester of pregnancy."

PRETEST

7 The client's prenatal education includes danger signs to report. Which of the following, if reported, would indicate that the client understood the teaching?

1. Dizziness and blurred vision
2. Occasional nausea and vomiting
3. No bowel movement for three days
4. Ankle edema

8 The client, a pregnant 20-year-old single woman, tells the nurse that she wants to keep her baby, but she isn't sure she can manage by herself. What is the best response by the nurse?

1. "It is hard to raise a child by yourself. Perhaps it would help to contact Child Protective Services."
2. "Try to not become concerned too early; lots of women manage by themselves."
3. "I can see you are concerned, let's talk about possible support systems."
4. "If you are having some concerns, maybe you should talk to an adoption agency."

9 The nurse is planning a childbirth education class for women in their first trimester of pregnancy. Which of the following topics will be most appropriate?

1. Breathing techniques for pain relief in labor
2. Choosing a prenatal care provider
3. Postpartum self-care
4. Care of the newborn infant

10 The client, who was an appropriate weight for height at the time she became pregnant, is 20 weeks' pregnant and has gained a total of 12 pounds. She is concerned about weight gain. What is the best reply by the nurse?

1. "I will tell the doctor that you are worried. He will tell you what to do."
2. "Your weight gain is about average for this point in your pregnancy. What concerns you about it?"
3. "You really have gained at lot. I will consult the nutritionist for you."
4. "A lot of your weight gain is probably fluid. Why don't you decrease your salt intake and see if that will help."

➤ *See pages 105–106 for Answers and Rationales.*

I. NURSING CARE OF THE PRENATAL CLIENT

A. First prenatal visit: should begin by finding out why the woman is seeking care and should include a complete health history and physical examination

1. Collect a history on pre-pregnant health including weight; nutrition; exercise pattern; over-the-counter, prescription, and illicit drug use; allergies; potential teratogens; history of surgery or present disease states, especially those with known implications for pregnancy (such as viral infections, diabetes, hypertension, cardiovascular disease, renal problems, and thyroid or bleeding disorders); gynecologic history including date and results of last Pap smear; previous infections; age at menarche, and menstrual, contraceptive, and obstetric histories
2. Physical assessment

a. **Fetal heart tones** (FHT), also referred to as fetal heart rate (FHR) per minute, can be assessed by fetoscope (beginning at about 16 weeks) or by ultrasonic Doppler device (beginning at about 10 weeks); FHTs are useful in determining gestational age and fetal well-being; FHR normally ranges from 110 to 160

b. **Fundal height**, the measurement from symphysis pubis to top of uterine fundus (in centimeters), can be used to assess approximate gestational age and fetal growth, plus or minus 2 weeks gestation; most accurate between 20 and 37 weeks (see Figure 5-1)

Figure 5-1

Fundal height during pregnancy at various weeks of gestation

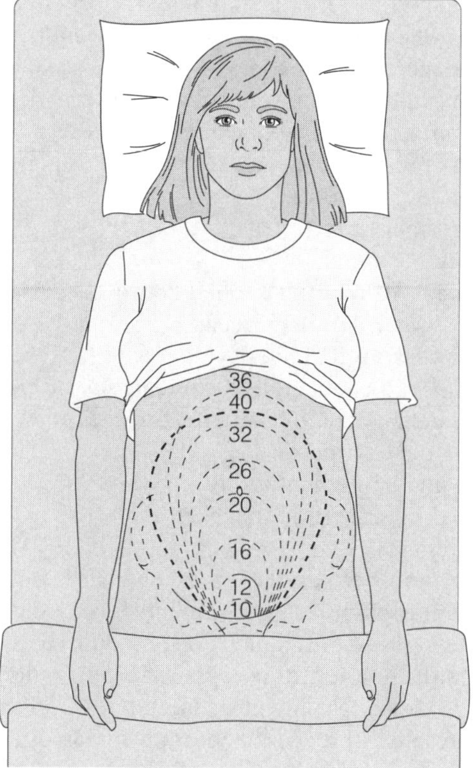

c. Complete maternal physical examination should be done including vital signs; height and weight; thyroid function; heart and breath sounds; and reproductive organs including pelvic musculature, size of uterus, and adequacy of pelvis for delivery

d. Laboratory assessment should include complete blood count with hematocrit and hemoglobin and white blood cell differential analysis; blood group and typing; Rh typing; rubella titer; blood glucose level; urinalysis and culture; serum syphilis test; screening for other sexually transmitted infections such as gonorrhea and chlamydia; Pap smear; and offer of HIV and illicit drug screen; other tests may be indicated for certain clients

e. Priority nursing diagnoses: Effective Therapeutic Regimen Management; Risk for Ineffective Health Maintenance; Deficient Knowledge

f. Planning and implementation
   1) Prepare for exam by telling woman what to expect
   2) Provide information about the prenatal care program, setting, and personnel
   3) Provide information about physiologic changes to be expected in pregnancy, over-the-counter medications that are considered safe during pregnancy as per health care provider, and danger signs to report
   4) Encourage paternal and sibling attendance at prenatal visits as able

g. Evaluation: client verbalizes knowledge of procedures for physical exam, future prenatal care, and expected changes related to normal and abnormal aspects of pregnancy

Practice to Pass

The client has just had her pregnancy confirmed by ultrasound. When she begins to cry, how should the nurse respond?

3. Psychosocial assessment
   a. Assess client for emotions such as excitement, anxiety, and/or ambivalence about pregnancy
   b. Explore available support systems

c. Assess stability and functional level of client's immediate and extended family
d. Assess whether economic support is adequate for housing, daily needs, transportation, and medical expenses

e. Discuss cultural preferences including practices to be used or avoided during pregnancy, preference of caregiver gender, and preferred support person(s)
f. Discuss pros and cons of decisions regarding circumcision and of breastfeeding versus bottle-feeding

B. Follow-up prenatal visits

1. Frequency
   a. Every 4 weeks during the first 28 weeks' gestation
   b. Every 2 weeks until 36 weeks
   c. Every week until delivery
   d. For high-risk clients follow-up visits should be scheduled more frequently
2. Priority nursing diagnoses: Ineffective Health Maintenance; Deficient Knowledge; Parental Role Conflict
3. Planning and implementation
   a. Visits should include teaching as well as assessment of maternal and fetal well-being
   b. Instruct mother about physical changes associated with pregnancy, such as **quickening** (first fetal movements felt) and colostrum production, as well as danger signs of pregnancy presented in Table 5-1
   c. Assess the mother for acceptance of pregnancy and adjustment to maternal role, changes from baseline measurement of vital signs, weight gain, nutritional status, and presence of glucose and/or protein in urine
   d. A quadruple (quad) screen, which tests blood levels of alpha-fetoprotein (AFP) to screen for fetal neural tube defects and to test for increased likelihood of Down syndrome and other indicators of fetal problems, should be assessed at 15 to 20 weeks; maternal blood glucose level should be assessed at 24 to 28 weeks to screen for gestational diabetes or sooner if indicated
   e. The fetus should be assessed at each visit for growth as measured by fundal height, movement, and heart rate
4. Evaluation: client reports extent to which she is engaged in positive health behaviors; maternal health indicators and uterine growth are comparable to normal parameters

Table 5-1 Danger Signs in Pregnancy

Danger Sign	Possible Cause
Gush of fluid from vagina	Rupture of membranes
Vaginal bleeding	Abruptio placentae, placenta previa, bloody show
Abdominal pain	Premature labor, abruptio placentae
Temperature > 101°F	Infection
Persistent vomiting	Hyperemesis gravidarum
Visual disturbances	Hypertension, preeclampsia
Edema of face or hands (or possibly including legs and feet)	Hypertension, preeclampsia
Severe headache	Hypertension, preeclampsia
Epigastric pain	Preeclampsia
Dysuria	Urinary tract infection
Decreased fetal movement	Compromised fetal well-being

C. Childbirth education

1. Childbirth classes provide information on pregnancy and childbirth to facilitate optimal decision making in families; topics should be timed to progress of pregnancy as outlined in Table 5-2
2. In addition, classes can be planned for special groups such as grandparents, siblings, adolescents, and clients who will deliver by cesarean section
3. Exercise is an important topic for childbirth education; encourage women to participate in regular exercise (at least three times per week) during pregnancy
   a. Benefits of exercise include maintaining muscle tone and bowel function, as well as fewer complications during labor and delivery
   b. Exercises especially helpful for childbirth include pelvic tilt, partial sit-ups, Kegel exercises, and exercises to stretch inner-thigh muscles
4. Classes on preparation for birth process provide information on selection of birthing method and relaxation techniques
   a. Commonly taught birthing methods include Lamaze, Kitzinger, Bradley, and Hypobirthing methods of prepared childbirth; see Table 5-3 for a comparison of these methods
   b. Relaxation techniques commonly taught for use during labor include touch, disassociation, and progressive relaxation

Practice to Pass

The client has come to the clinic for her first prenatal visit at 18 weeks' gestation. After the nurse explains the prenatal visit schedule, the client states, "I don't really see any need to come back until I go into labor." How should the nurse respond?

Table 5-2 Childbirth Education Topics by Trimester

Trimester	Educational Topic
First	Physical and psychosocial changes of pregnancy Self-care in pregnancy Protecting and nurturing the fetus Choosing a care provider and birth setting Prenatal exercise Relief of common early pregnancy discomforts
Second	Planning for breastfeeding Sexuality in pregnancy Relief of common later-pregnancy discomforts
Third	Preparation for childbirth Development of a birth plan Relaxation techniques Postpartum self-care Infant stimulation Infant care and safety

Table 5-3 Comparison of Common Birthing Methods

Method	Characteristics	Breathing Techniques
Lamaze	Uses education about fetal growth and changes associated with pregnancy, along with training in exercises that strengthen muscles used during labor and delivery to decrease fear and help woman cope with labor pain	Patterned, paced
Bradley	Relies on a partner to coach laboring woman; promotes relaxation through abdominal breathing and exercises	Primarily abdominal
Kitzinger	Prepares woman for birth through use of sensory memory and Stanislavsky acting method to teach relaxation	Chest breathing with abdominal relaxation
Hypnobirthing	Promotes relaxation and relief of fear to experience birth in a calm, stress-free environment	Deep and slow breathing with relaxation techniques

5. Classes geared toward knowledge that will be needed after delivery include sessions on postpartum self-care, newborn care, infant stimulation, and infant safety needs

D. Management of common discomforts of pregnancy (see Tables 5-4 and 5-5)

1. Discomforts occur as a result of physiologic or anatomic changes of pregnancy; they differ from trimester to trimester
2. While not dangerous, they constitute a significant problem for client and present an opportunity for nursing intervention

II. ESSENTIAL CONCEPTS OF PREGNANCY

A. *Estimated date of birth (EDB)* or "due date": can be determined by several methods

!

1. **Nägele's Rule** is used to determine EDB by taking first day of last menstrual period, subtracting 3 months and adding 7 days; this date is most accurate when woman remembers her last menstrual period, has menses every 28 days, and was not taking oral contraceptives at time of conception
2. First trimester ultrsound assessment; ultrasound later in pregnancy can assist in diagnosing gestational age but is much less accurate
3. **McDonald's method** uses uterine size to indicate gestational age by measuring (in centimeters) distance from symphysis pubis to top of uterine fundus
   a. This distance, **fundal height**, correlates well with number of weeks' gestation between 22 and 34 weeks, plus or minus 2 weeks
   b. Prediction of EDB (also known as EDC) using this method can be affected by maternal height, irregular fetal growth, multiple gestation, and abnormal amounts of amniotic fluid (confirmatory)
4. Quickening, feeling of fetal movement by mother, usually occurs between 16 and 18 weeks; because of wide range of times this is experienced, this method gives a less accurate EDB (confirmatory)
5. Auscultation of fetal heart rate can occur as early as 8 weeks' gestation using an ultrasonic Doppler device but is more commonly heard between 10 and 12 weeks; this variation can result in a less accurate date (confirmatory)

Practice to Pass

The client, who is a gravida 3, para 2, tells the nurse that she did not go to childbirth classes with her previous pregnancies and that she and the babies did fine. The client asks why she should go to classes with this pregnancy. How should the nurse respond?

Table 5-4 Management of Discomforts in Early Pregnancy

Discomfort	Management
Nausea and vomiting	Avoid strong odors Drink carbonated beverages Avoid drinking while eating Eat crackers or toast before getting out of bed Eat small, frequent meals Avoid spicy or greasy foods
Breast tenderness	Wear a well-fitting, supportive bra
Urinary frequency	Increase daytime fluid intake Decrease evening fluid intake Empty bladder as soon as urge is felt
Fatigue	Plan a rest period or nap during day Go to bed as early as possible
Ptyalism (excessive saliva)	Use gum, mints, hard candy, or mouthwash
Nasal stuffiness/bleeding	Use cool air vaporizer

Table 5-5 Management of Discomforts in Late Pregnancy

Discomfort	Management
Heartburn	Eat small, frequent meals Avoid spicy or greasy foods Refrain from lying down immediately after eating Use low-sodium antacids
Constipation	Increase fluid and fiber intake Exercise Develop regular bowel habits Use stool softeners as per health care provider
Hemorrhoids	Avoid constipation Apply topical anesthetics, ointments, or ice packs Use sitz baths or warm soaks Reinsert into rectum, if necessary
Backache	Practice good body mechanics Practice pelvic tilt exercise Avoid high heels, heavy lifting, overfatigue, and excessive bending or reaching
Leg cramps	Dorsiflex feet Apply heat to affected muscle Evaluate calcium to phosphorus ratio in diet
Varicose veins	Elevate legs Wear support hose Avoid crossing legs at the knee, restrictive clothing, and standing for long periods of time
Ankle edema	Practice frequent dorsiflexion of feet Avoid standing for long periods of time Elevate legs when sitting or resting
Faintness	Arise slowly Avoid prolonged standing Maintain hematocrit and hemoglobin
Flatulence	Avoid gas-forming foods Chew food thoroughly Establish regular bowel habits

Practice to Pass

The client, who states that she and her partner use condoms "most of the time," presents with amenorrhea for one month, fatigue, and breast tenderness. The client suspects that she is pregnant. How can this be confirmed?

6. Ultrasound examination may be used to assess EDB; first trimester ultrasound is so accurate that if ultrasound-derived EDB differs from LMP-derived EDB by more than one week, the ultrsound derived by EDB will prevail; beyond first trimester, dating by ultrsound becomes much less reliable

B. Gravida and para

1. *Gravida* and *para* are terms used to describe childbearing history
2. **Gravida** is number of times a woman has been pregnant
3. **Para** is number of infants delivered after 20 weeks' gestation, born dead or alive; multiple births count as one delivery regardless of number of infants delivered

4. TPAL is a more detailed description of para
   a. *T* is number of term infants born after 37 completed weeks
   b. *P* is number of premature infants born between 20 and 37 weeks
   c. *A* is number of pregnancies that end in spontaneous or therapeutic abortion prior to 20 weeks
   d. *L* is number of children currently alive

III. SIGNS AND SYMPTOMS OF PREGNANCY (SEE BOX 5-1)

A. ***Presumptive signs of pregnancy* (subjective)**: signs and symptoms that woman reports, which may or may not be associated with pregnancy
B. ***Probable signs of pregnancy* (objective)**: noted by examiner, which may or may not be associated with pregnancy
C. ***Positive signs of pregnancy* (diagnostic)**: noted by examiner and can only be caused by pregnancy

IV. PHYSIOLOGIC CHANGES OF PREGNANCY

A. Reproductive

1. Uterus: during pregnancy, uterus takes on an ovoid shape and increases in capacity from 10 mL to 5 liters; this increase is primarily caused by an increase in size of cells (hypertrophy) in response to estrogen, as well as distention caused by growing fetus; by end of pregnancy, uterus and its contents require up to $\frac{1}{6}$ of total maternal blood flow
2. Cervix: under influence of estrogen, cervix secretes mucus that forms a plug at opening of endocervical canal to limit ability of bacteria to enter uterus; increased blood flow to cervix results in **Goodell's sign** (softening of cervix) and **Chadwick's sign** (bluish color of cervix during pregnancy)
3. Vagina: under influence of estrogen, vaginal mucosa thickens and connective tissue relaxes; vaginal secretions thicken and increase in amount during pregnancy; pH is acidic, 3.6 to 6.0

Box 5-1

Signs and Symptoms of Pregnancy

Presumptive Signs
amenorrhea
nausea and vomiting
fatigue
urinary frequency
breast changes
quickening

Probable Signs
Hegar's sign (softening of isthmus of uterus where cervix meets uterine body)
McDonald's sign (an ease in flexing body of uterus against cervix)
enlargement of abdomen
pigmentation changes
abdominal striae
ballottement
positive pregnancy test
palpation of fetal outline

Positive Signs
fetal heartbeat
fetal movement palpable by the examiner
visualization of the fetus by ultrasound

! 4. Breasts: estrogen and progesterone cause breasts to increase in size and to increase in number of glands; **colostrum** (a thin bluish-white secretion high in protein and immune properties) is produced and may be expressed during last trimester; nipples darken

B. Cardiovascular

1. Cardiac output increases 30–40% over nonpregnant output with an increase in pulse of 10 to 15 beats/minute
2. Pulmonary and peripheral vascular resistance decreases 40–50%, lowering blood pressure throughout first and second trimesters; in third trimester, it begins to increase to pre-pregnant levels; postural hypotension may result as pregnant uterus presses on pelvic and femoral vessels limiting blood return to heart
3. ! Supine hypotensive syndrome or vena cava syndrome results when a pregnant woman lies flat on her back, which causes gravid uterus to compress vena cava, resulting in decreased blood flow to right atrium and a decrease in blood pressure
   a. Symptoms include pallor, dizziness, and clammy skin
   b. Problem can be prevented or treated by positioning woman on her left side with a pillow under her right hip
4. Blood volume increases 45% over pre-pregnant levels
   a. Red blood cells (RBCs) increase 18–30% depending on degree of iron supplementation
   b. Plasma volume increases 50%
   c. The greater increase in plasma over RBCs results in physiologic anemia with a decrease in hemoglobin (10–14 grams/dL) and hematocrit (32–42%); the drop in hematocrit is approximately 5–7%

Practice to Pass

The client, who is 28 weeks' gestation, complains of fatigue. She reports difficulty sleeping. She says that she slept on her back before becoming pregnant, but now she feels like she is going to faint in that position. How should the nurse respond?

C. Respiratory

1. Volume of air breathed increases 30–40% because of decreased airway resistance that occurs in response to progesterone
2. Intrathoracic volume remains unchanged, even though enlarged uterus presses up on diaphragm, because rib cage flares and chest circumference increases

D. Neurologic: no known changes

E. Musculoskeletal

1. Relaxation of pelvic joints results in classic "waddling" gait often seen in pregnancy
2. Physiological lordosis (Figure 5-2) develops as curvature of lumbar spine increases to compensate for weight of gravid uterus; this can result in low-back pain
3. Diastasis recti, separation of the rectus abdominis muscle, can result as the uterus enlarges

F. Gastrointestinal (GI)

1. Human chorionic gonadotropin (hCG) increases and can cause nausea and vomiting; this is usually worst during first trimester but can persist through pregnancy
2. Increased progesterone levels relax smooth muscles, resulting in decreased peristalsis as evidenced by bloating, reflux of gastric secretions, and constipation; GI sphincters lose tone and can contribute to reflux; GI problems worsen as gravid uterus presses on intestines
3. Constipation and increased pressure on blood vessels in rectum can result in hemorrhoids

G. Renal

1. In first trimester, gravid uterus presses on bladder, causing urinary frequency; this is relieved in second trimester because uterus moves upward into abdominal area; frequency returns in third trimester as presenting part presses on bladder
2. Glomerular filtration increases 50% during second trimester and remains elevated until delivery; kidneys may not be able to reabsorb all of glucose filtered, resulting in glycosuria

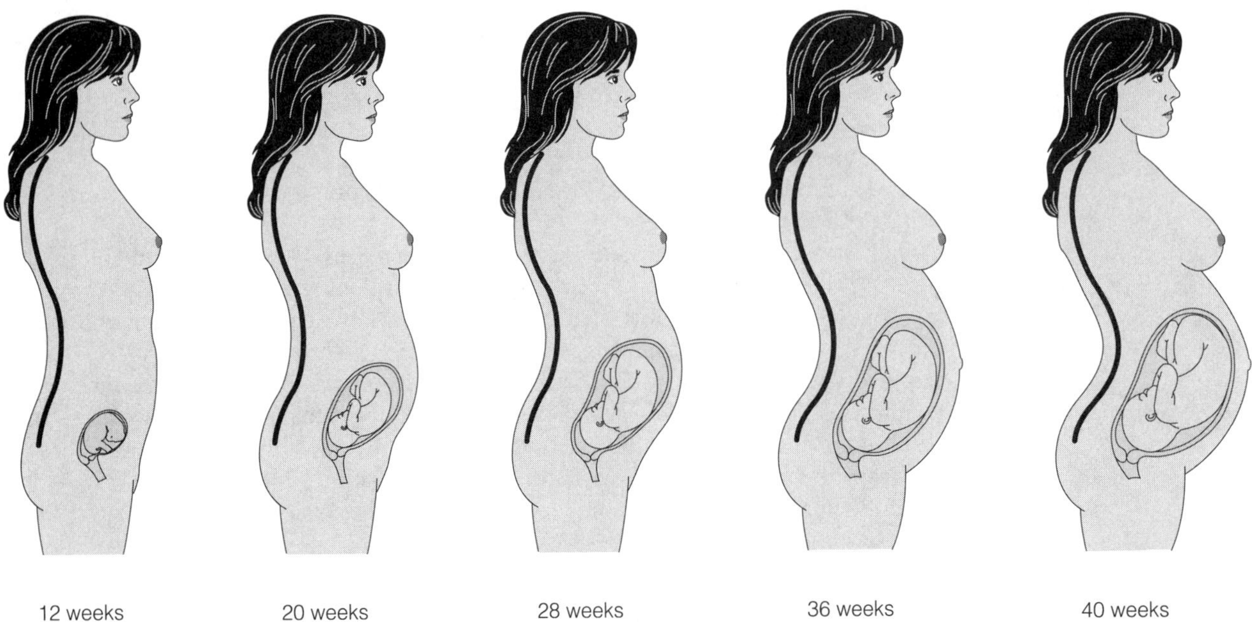

Figure 5-2

Postural changes during pregnancy that lead to physiological lordosis

Practice to Pass

The client, who is 24 weeks' gestation, is concerned about her weight. She has gained a total of 26 pounds over her pre-pregnant weight. She tells the nurse that she usually eats lunch at a fast-food restaurant and frequently snacks in the afternoon. How should the nurse respond?

H. Integumentary

1. In response to increased levels of estrogen, some areas of skin have an increase in pigmentation
   a. This is seen primarily in areas that already have increased pigmentation, such as areola, nipples, and vulva
   b. **Chloasma**, mask of pregnancy, is an increase in pigmentation on forehead and around eyes; it is seen most often in women of color and is aggravated by sun exposure
   c. **Linea nigra** is a darkly pigmented line that extends from umbilicus to pubic area
   d. **Striae gravidarum**, or stretch marks, appear as reddish streaks on trunk and thighs; they result from stretching of connective tissue caused by increased adrenal steroid levels; while these generally change to a shiny gray-white color after delivery, they do not disappear
2. Sweat and sebaceous gland activity increases during pregnancy

I. Endocrine

1. Metabolism
   a. Average weight gain is 3 to 5 pounds in first trimester and 12 to 15 pounds in each of second and third trimesters
   b. Water retention occurs during pregnancy caused by increased sex hormones and decreased serum protein
2. Hormones in pregnancy
   a. Human chorionic gonadotropin (hCG), which is secreted by trophoblast early in pregnancy, stimulates progesterone and estrogen production; it is thought to support pregnancy and cause nausea and vomiting in first trimester
   b. Human placental lactogen (hPL), also known as chorionic somatomammotropin, is an insulin antagonist; it promotes lipolysis, resulting in increased amounts of circulating free fatty acids available for maternal metabolic use

c. Estrogen and progesterone are produced by corpus luteum for first seven weeks of pregnancy and then by placenta
   1) Estrogen stimulates uterine development to support fetal growth and stimulates ductal system of breast for lactation
   2) Progesterone maintains endometrium, decreases uterine contractility, stimulates development of breast acini and lobules, and causes relaxation of smooth muscle

d. Relaxin, primarily made by corpus luteum, decreases uterine contractility, contributes to softening of cervix, and has long-term effects on collagen

e. Prostaglandins, lipids that are found throughout female reproductive system, contribute to decrease seen in placental vascular system, and probably contribute to onset of labor

V. NUTRITIONAL NEEDS

A. Requirements are affected by a variety of factors

1. Pre-pregnancy nutritional status: women who are underweight or overweight may need more or fewer calories for adequate fetal weight gain, respectively
2. Maternal age: teenage mothers may need increased caloric intake to allow for both maternal and fetal growth
3. Maternal parity: number of pregnancies and the interval between them can affect nutritional needs

Table 5-6 Nutritional Requirements during Pregnancy

Nutritional Element	Requirements	
	Pregnant	*Nonpregnant**
Protein	60 grams	46 grams
Vitamin A	800 mcgR	800 mcgR
Vitamin D	10 mcg	10 mcg
Vitamin E	10 mcg	8 mcg
Vitamin K	65 mcg	60 mcg
Vitamin C	70 mg	60 mg
Thiamine	1.5 mg	1.1 mg
Riboflavin	1.6 mg	1.3 mg
Niacin	17 mg NE	15 mg NE
Vitamin B_6	2.2 mg	1.6 mg
Folate	400 mcg	180 mcg
Vitamin B_{12}	2.2 mcg	2.0 mcg
Calcium	1200 mg	1200 mg
Phosphorus	1200 mg	1200 mg
Magnesium	320 mg	280 mg
Iron	30 mg	15 mg
Zinc	15 mg	12 mg
Iodine	175 mcg	150 mcg
Selenium	65 mcg	55 mcg

*Requirement for females aged 19–24.

Table 5-7 Maternal Weight Gain Distribution

Maternal Structure	Increase in Weight Gain
Fetus, placenta, and amniotic fluid	11 pounds
Uterus	2 pounds
Increased blood volume	4 pounds
Breast tissue	3 pounds
Maternal stores	5 to 10 pounds

B. Maternal nutrition

!

1. A normal pregnant woman requires an additional 300 calories per day
2. Other nutritional requirements are increased during pregnancy, as illustrated in Table 5-6
3. Appropriate pregnancy weight gain averages 25 to 35 pounds for women with a normal pre-pregnant weight (BMI 18.5–24.9), 15 to 25 pounds if overweight (BMI 25–29.9), 11 to 20 pounds if obese (BMI 30 or greater), and 28 to 40 pounds if underweight (BMI less than 18.5)
   a. 10 to 13 pounds in first 20 weeks
   b. About 1 pound per week after 20th week
4. Maternal weight gain is distributed to a variety of structures (see Table 5-7)

VI. PSYCHOSOCIAL CHANGES OF PREGNANCY

Practice to Pass

The pregnant client, who works full-time outside the home and is the mother of a 2-year-old and a 4-year-old, is 24 weeks' gestation. The woman seems very tired and reports little help at home from her husband. The client states, "If things continue like this, I just don't know what I'm going to do!" How should the nurse respond?

A. Role changes: occur as decisions are made concerning whether or not mother will continue or return to work, options for child care, and who will meet household responsibilities; roles of client, partner, and sibling(s) are all affected

B. Anxieties: related to birthing process, well-being of mother and infant, and finances

C. Family strengths in coping with psychosocial changes of pregnancy: communication skills, ability to resolve conflict and reach compromise, and willingness to seek and utilize support systems

D. Priority nursing diagnoses: Risk for Interrupted Family Processes, Risk for Impaired Parenting, Parental Role Conflict; Ineffective Role Performance

E. Planning and implementation

1. Discuss with client and partner the psychosocial processes that occur during pregnancy such as role changes, anxieties related to well-being of mother and infant, and additional financial responsibilities
2. Explore family coping mechanisms, communication skills, and support systems

Case Study

The client, who is a primigravida in her second trimester, has come in for a scheduled prenatal visit. When the nurse asks how things are going, the client replies, "Not very well. It seems like I'm just falling apart. I have heartburn after I eat, my ankles swell, I'm constipated all the time, and I think I may be getting hemorrhoids."

1. What questions should the nurse ask the client regarding the problems described?
2. What objective data should the nurse collect regarding the problems described?
3. What nursing diagnoses are appropriate for this client?
4. What teaching is needed in this situation?
5. How should the nurse followup with this client?

For suggested responses, see page 303.

POSTTEST

1 The nurse has given the client information on maternal serum alpha-fetoprotein (AFP) screening. Which statement by the mother indicates that she understood the information?

1. "If this test is negative, it means that my baby doesn't have any birth defects."
2. "It is best if this test is done before I reach 12 weeks' gestation."
3. "If the AFP level is high, it could indicate a problem with the baby's spinal cord."
4. "If my AFP level is below normal, I won't need any further testing."

2 The prenatal nurse considers that which of the following would be the best indicator of normal fetal growth?

1. Maternal weight gain seven pounds at 22 weeks' gestation
2. Fundal height 22 centimeters at 24 weeks' gestation
3. Maternal waist circumference 41 inches at 36 weeks' gestation
4. Maternal intake 1500 calories per day

3 The nurse is planning an educational program for a client who is in her third trimester of pregnancy. Which of the following childbirth education topics would be appropriate at this time? Select all that apply.

1. Childbirth health care provider selection
2. Morning sickness management
3. Nutritional needs during pregnancy
4. Pain relief during labor and delivery
5. Breathing techniques for labor

4 Following confirmation of pregnancy, the client has come into the clinic for her first prenatal visit. She reports having a 5-year-old child who was born at 40 weeks' gestation, a set of 3-year-old triplets who were born at 34 weeks' gestation, and a first trimester abortion when she was in college. On her medical record, the nurse would make which entry?

1. Gravida 4, para 1114
2. Gravida 3, para 1314
3. Gravida 4, para 4014
4. Gravida 3, para 3112

5 The client has come to the clinic because she suspects that she is pregnant. Which of the following would be the most definitive way to confirm the diagnosis?

1. Client's report of amenorrhea for three months
2. Positive Hegar's sign
3. Pigmentation changes of the breasts
4. Palpation of fetal movement by the care provider

6 The client, who is 34 weeks' gestation, says to the nurse, "I had hoped to use the Lamaze method when my baby is born, but my husband doesn't want to . . . so I guess I'll just have an epidural." What is the best response by the nurse?

1. "Oh, let's wait and see, your husband will probably change his mind when delivery time gets closer."
2. "Well, prepared childbirth is really overrated for some people, although it is wonderful for others."
3. "Have you and your husband discussed what he thinks his role would be in being your coach in childbirth?"
4. "Could you just ask your mother or someone else to be your support person?"

7 The client, who is a primigravida, has come to the clinic for a scheduled prenatal visit. She is concerned about facial chloasma that has developed since her last prenatal visit. What is the best response by the nurse?

1. "You should apply a facial skin bleach twice a day."
2. "Avoiding sun exposure may keep the pigmentation from getting any darker."
3. "This is a permanent condition caused by hormonal changes. You may be able to cover it with makeup."
4. "This is a condition associated with the development of skin cancer. I will make an appointment for you with a dermatologist."

POSTTEST

8 The client, who is 32 weeks' gestation, reports severe heartburn, especially at night. Following instruction by the nurse, which client statement indicates that she understands the best course of management?

1. "I should eat small, frequent meals."
2. "I should try to lie down and rest after eating."
3. "I should avoid using antacids because medication can hurt the baby."
4. "Heartburn is a common discomfort in pregnancy, there is really nothing to do about it."

9 The client, who is eight weeks' gestation, is experiencing frequent nausea and vomiting. Following instruction by the nurse, which client statement demonstrates that she understands the best course of management?

1. "I should plan to arise early so that I will have time to eat a full breakfast."
2. "I should avoid carbonated beverages as they can cause gas."
3. "I should eat crackers or toast before arising."
4. "I should avoid eating more frequently than every four hours."

10 Which statement would indicate to the nurse that a client demonstrates acceptance of pregnancy?

1. "A feeling of hopelessness keeps coming over me in waves since I found out I was pregnant."
2. "I still can't believe I let my husband talk me into having unprotected sex. This baby is really not what I need right now."
3. "I've thrown up every day for the last week, but I guess it will be worth it when I have that tiny baby in my arms."
4. "This pregnancy is causing so many changes in my life; I'm just not sure I'm going to be able to deal with it."

➤ *See pages 106–107 for Answers and Rationales.*

ANSWERS & RATIONALES

Pretest

1 **Answer: 1 Rationale:** Maternal diabetes places both the mother and infant at risk during pregnancy and would require further follow-up. Exercising three times a week, the occasional use of over-the-counter pain relievers, and a maternal age of 30 years present no further untoward risk. **Cognitive Level:** Analyzing **Client Need:** Physiological Adaptation **Integrated Process:** Nursing Process: Assessment **Content Area:** Maternal-Newborn **Strategy:** Critical words are *initial prenatal visit* and *indicate a need for further assessment,* thereby indicating you need to look for a potential problem. Only one option indicates a problem. **Reference:** Ladewig, P., London, M., & Davidson, M. (2010). *Contemporary maternal-newborn nursing care* (7th ed.). Upper Saddle River, NJ: Pearson Education, p. 199.

2 **Answer: 4 Rationale:** The risk for the mother and fetus increases as the pregnancy progresses. Therefore, clients are seen more frequently as pregnancy nears term. Visits every 4 weeks for low-risk clients are appropriate until 28 weeks of gestation. **Cognitive Level:** Applying **Client Need:** Health Promotion and Maintenance **Integrated Process:** Nursing Process: Planning **Content Area:** Maternal-Newborn **Strategy:** Correlate low risk in early pregnancy in the question with knowledge of the visit schedule to identify the correct answer. Knowledge of the regular plan for prenatal visits helps to answer this question. **Reference:** Ladewig, P., London, M., & Davidson, M. (2010). *Contemporary maternal-newborn nursing care* (7th ed.). Upper Saddle River, NJ: Pearson Education, p. 226.

3 **Answer: 3 Rationale:** A positive at-home pregnancy test indicates the presence of growing trophoblastic tissue and not necessarily a uterine pregnancy. It could even indicate a potential ectopic pregnancy. An at-home pregnancy test is not done to detect ovulation. **Cognitive Level:** Analyzing **Client Need:** Health Promotion and Maintenance **Integrated Process:** Nursing Process: Evaluation **Content Area:** Maternal-Newborn **Strategy:** Critical words are *understands the results.* Knowledge of over-the-counter pregnancy tests and the interpretation of the results will help to choose the correct answer. **Reference:** Ladewig, P., London, M., & Davidson, M. (2010). *Contemporary maternal-newborn nursing care* (7th ed.). Upper Saddle River, NJ: Pearson Education, p. 188.

4 **Answer: 04-17 Rationale:** Using Näegele's rule, the estimated date of birth is calculated by subtracting three months from the first day of the last menstrual period and then adding seven days to that date. **Cognitive Level:** Analyzing **Client Need:** Health Promotion and Maintenance **Integrated Process:** Nursing Process: Diagnosis **Content Area:** Maternal-Newborn **Strategy:** Recall Näegele's rule to calculate the answer to this question. **Reference:** Ladewig, P., London, M., & Davidson, M. (2010). *Contemporary maternal-newborn nursing care* (7th ed.). Upper Saddle River, NJ: Pearson Education, p. 206.

5 **Answer: 3 Rationale:** Counting the current pregnancy, the client has been pregnant a total of four times for gravida 4. Para is the number of pregnancies that have reached viability, in this case two. **Cognitive Level:** Applying **Client Need:** Health Promotion and Maintenance **Integrated Process:** Communication and Documentation **Content Area:** Maternal-Newborn **Strategy:** Recall the definitions of gravida and para to aid in answering the question. **Reference:** Ladewig, P., London, M., & Davidson, M. (2010). *Contemporary maternal-newborn nursing care* (7th ed.). Upper Saddle River, NJ: Pearson Education, p. 200.

6 **Answer: 3, 5 Rationale:** The fluid leaking from her breasts is colostrum. It normally leaks from the breasts during the last trimester. The client should wear a supportive bra. It does not indicate an infection in the breasts, or that the client is going into premature labor. It does not mean that the client will have a problem with breastfeeding. **Cognitive Level:** Analyzing **Client Need:** Health Promotion and Maintenance **Integrated Process:** Teaching and Learning **Content Area:** Maternal-Newborn **Strategy:** Knowledge of the normal changes to the breast during pregnancy and the teaching needs will help to answer this question. **Reference:** Ladewig, P., London, M., & Davidson, M. (2010). *Contemporary maternal-newborn nursing care* (7th ed.). Upper Saddle River, NJ: Pearson Education, p. 183.

7 **Answer: 1 Rationale:** Dizziness and blurred vision can be symptoms of preeclampsia, a complication that requires further assessment and medical management. Occasional nausea and vomiting, no bowel movement for three days, and ankle edema are not danger signs of pregnancy. **Cognitive Level:** Applying **Client Need:** Health Promotion and Maintenance **Integrated Process:** Teaching and Learning **Content Area:** Maternal-Newborn **Strategy:** Recognize that only one option indicates a high risk; the other options are not danger signs of pregnancy. Often neurological signs can indicate a true concern. **Reference:** Ladewig, P., London, M., & Davidson, M. (2010). *Contemporary maternal-newborn nursing care* (7th ed.). Upper Saddle River, NJ: Pearson Education, p. 188.

8 **Answer: 3 Rationale:** The client has expressed a realistic concern. The nurse needs to help her explore what support systems are available for her and her child. There is no indication that Child Protective Services should be contacted. Disregarding a client's concern represents a communication block, such as telling a

client not to become concerned. The client has indicated she wants to keep the baby, and so it is inappropriate to suggest talking with an adoption agency at this time. **Cognitive Level:** Applying **Client Need:** Psychosocial Integrity **Integrated Process:** Communication and Documentation **Content Area:** Maternal-Newborn **Strategy:** Eliminate two options initially that are not what the client indicated. Then choose the only option that indicates the nurse's support and opens the opportunity to explore the client's concerns. **Reference:** Ladewig, P., London, M., & Davidson, M. (2010). *Contemporary maternal-newborn nursing care* (7th ed.). Upper Saddle River, NJ: Pearson Education, p. 168.

9 **Answer: 2 Rationale:** Topics should be timed to present information that the woman needs at that specific stage of pregnancy. Clients in the first trimester need to select a prenatal care provider, among other concerns. Breathing techniques for pain relief in labor, postpartum self-care and care of a newborn infant can be covered later in the pregnancy. **Cognitive Level:** Applying **Client Need:** Health Promotion and Maintenance **Integrated Process:** Nursing Process: Planning **Content Area:** Maternal-Newborn **Strategy:** Critical words are *childbirth classes in first trimester* and *most appropriate.* Use the process of elimination and knowledge about the progression of pregnancy to make a selection. **Reference:** Ladewig, P., London, M., & Davidson, M. (2010). *Contemporary maternal-newborn nursing care* (7th ed.). Upper Saddle River, NJ: Pearson Education, p.171.

10 **Answer: 2 Rationale:** For women of normal pre-pregnant weight, the recommended pattern of weight gain during pregnancy is three to five pounds during the first trimester and one pound per week thereafter. It is unnecessary to have the health care provider speak to the client about average weight gain. Nutritional counseling would be an appropriate action if the client was experiencing a large weight gain, but this is not the case. Salt intake during normal pregnancy should be moderate but not restricted. **Cognitive Level:** Applying **Client Need:** Health Promotion and Maintenance **Integrated Process:** Communication and Documentation **Content Area:** Maternal-Newborn **Strategy:** Specific knowledge of the recommended weight gain during pregnancy will aid in answering this question. The correct answer provides a true statement about a point of client education and explores the client's concerns. **Reference:** Ladewig, P., London, M., & Davidson, M. (2010). *Contemporary maternal-newborn nursing care* (7th ed.). Upper Saddle River, NJ: Pearson Education, p. 257.

Posttest

1 **Answer: 3 Rationale:** If the maternal level of AFP is elevated, it could indicate that fetal AFP from a fetal neural tube defect has leaked into the maternal serum. The test is most sensitive between 16 to 18 weeks' gestation. It is not definitive enough to make a diagnosis and is best used as a screening tool and so it may be repeated. **Cognitive Level:** Applying **Client Need:** Reduction of Risk Potential **Integrated Process:** Teaching and Learning **Content Area:** Maternal-Newborn **Strategy:** Knowledge of the test and its indications would help to answer the question correctly. **Reference:** Ladewig, P., London, M., & Davidson, M. (2010). *Contemporary maternal-newborn nursing care* (7th ed.). Upper Saddle River, NJ: Pearson Education, p. 290.

2 **Answer: 2 Rationale:** In singleton births with fetal growth within normal limits, fundal height in centimeters plus or minus two should correlate with gestational age in weeks. A low weight gain for the gestational age, the client's waist circumference, and the amount of calories consumed per day do not address this assessment. **Cognitive Level:** Analyzing **Client Need:** Health Promotion and Maintenance **Integrated Process:** Nursing Process: Evaluation **Content Area:** Maternal-Newborn **Strategy:** Remember that from about 22–34 weeks' gestation, fundal height correlates well with weeks of gestation, plus or minus 2 cm. **Reference:** Ladewig, P., London, M., & Davidson, M. (2010). *Contemporary maternal-newborn nursing care* (7th ed.). Upper Saddle River, NJ: Pearson Education, p. 204.

3 **Answer: 4, 5 Rationale:** Childbirth education should be geared to the time in pregnancy. In the third trimester, the pregnant woman begins to focus on labor, delivery, and newborn care. Selecting a health care provider, morning sickness management, and nutritional needs during pregnancy should be covered early in pregnancy. **Cognitive Level:** Analyzing **Client Need:** Health Promotion and Maintenance **Integrated Process:** Teaching and Learning **Content Area:** Maternal-Newborn **Strategy:** Critical words are *third trimester* and *appropriate.* Knowledge of childbirth education and the related information that corresponds to the trimester aids in answering this question. This question is time-sensitive. **Reference:** Ladewig, P., London, M., & Davidson, M. (2010). *Contemporary maternal-newborn nursing care* (7th ed.). Upper Saddle River, NJ: Pearson Education, p. 171.

4 **Answer: 1 Rationale:** The first number, gravida, represents the total number of pregnancies including the current one. In this case that equals 4. Para is represented by using the TPAL system. T represents the number of term births, 1; P represents the number of preterm births, 1; A represents the number of therapeutic or spontaneous abortions, 1; and L represents the number of living children, 4. Multiple births do not affect the parity in the T, P, or A categories; they are counted in the L category. **Cognitive Level:** Analyzing **Client Need:** Health Promotion and Maintenance **Integrated Process:** Communication and Documentation **Content Area:** Maternal-Newborn **Strategy:** Specific knowledge of the TPAL system to document pregnancies, preterm births, abortions, and living children is needed to choose the

correct answer. **Reference:** Ladewig, P., London, M., & Davidson, M. (2010). *Contemporary maternal-newborn nursing care* (7th ed.). Upper Saddle River, NJ: Pearson Education, p. 200.

5 **Answer: 4** **Rationale:** Palpation of fetal movement is considered to be a positive sign of pregnancy that cannot have any other cause. Amenorrhea for three months is a presumptive sign, and positive Hegar's sign (softening of the cervix) and pigmentation changes of the breasts are probable signs of pregnancy. **Cognitive Level:** Analyzing **Client Need:** Health Promotion and Maintenance **Integrated Process:** Nursing Process: Assessment **Content Area:** Maternal-Newborn **Strategy:** A critical word in the stem of the question is *confirm*. Eliminate the answers that could have another etiology. Fetal movement by a trained examiner after about 20 weeks' gestation is a diagnostic (positive) sign of pregnancy. **Reference:** Ladewig, P., London, M., & Davidson, M. (2010). *Contemporary maternal-newborn nursing care* (7th ed.). Upper Saddle River, NJ: Pearson Education, p. 188.

6 **Answer: 3** **Rationale:** The husband can take on a variety of roles during labor and delivery including coach, teammate, and observer. Exploring both partners' expectations may help to clarify reasons for the husband's hesitancy, which could result in improved communication and family coping. A wait-and-see attitude does not help the client in planning for labor. Referring to prepared childbirth as overrated for some ignores the concern that the client has raised. Asking someone else to be the support person may not be of interest to the client, and discounts the importance of the husband's role during labor and delivery. **Cognitive Level:** Applying **Client Need:** Psychosocial Integrity **Integrated Process:** Communication and Documentation **Content Area:** Maternal-Newborn **Strategy:** The core issue of this question is expectations and communication. The correct answer includes the most therapeutic response to facilitate couple communication. Discussing if the husband will be the coach is the only therapeutic response that could open the communication between the husband and wife about the upcoming delivery expectations. **Reference:** Ladewig, P., London, M., & Davidson, M. (2010). *Contemporary maternal-newborn nursing care* (7th ed.). Upper Saddle River, NJ: Pearson Education, p. 168.

7 **Answer: 2** **Rationale:** Increased pigmentation during pregnancy is a response to increased estrogen levels. It can be worsened by the sun, is harmless, and generally fades after the pregnancy ends. Recommending that the client uses a facial bleach is inappropriate. Informing the client the condition is permanent is incorrect. Telling the client the increased pigmentation is indicative of skin cancer is both incorrect and inappropriate. **Cognitive Level:** Applying **Client Need:** Health Promotion and Maintenance **Integrated Process:** Teaching and Learning **Content Area:** Maternal-Newborn **Strategy:** Knowledge of the normal changes during pregnancy and the educational needs of the mother are essential to choose the correct answer. **Reference:** Ladewig, P., London, M., & Davidson, M. (2010). *Contemporary maternal-newborn nursing care* (7th ed.). Upper Saddle River, NJ: Pearson Education, p. 188.

8 **Answer: 1** **Rationale:** Heartburn is usually caused by gastric reflux. Remaining in an upright position after meals, eating smaller and more frequent meals, and use of low-sodium antacids all help to relieve the problem. **Cognitive Level:** Applying **Client Need:** Health Promotion and Maintenance **Integrated Process:** Teaching and Learning **Content Area:** Maternal-Newborn **Strategy:** Knowledge of the changes in the GI system as a result of pregnancy and the educational needs of the mother will aid in answering this question. Since the question is worded positively, the correct option will also be a true statement. **Reference:** Ladewig, P., London, M., & Davidson, M. (2010). *Contemporary maternal-newborn nursing care* (7th ed.). Upper Saddle River, NJ: Pearson Education, p. 183.

9 **Answer: 3** **Rationale:** Nausea and vomiting, probably related to hormonal changes, usually disappear by the 12th week of pregnancy. Small, frequent meals, carbonated beverages, and crackers or toast sometimes relieve the symptoms. **Cognitive Level:** Applying **Client Need:** Health Promotion and Maintenance **Integrated Process:** Teaching and Learning **Content Area:** Maternal-Newborn **Strategy:** Knowledge of the self-care measures for common discomforts of pregnancy will help to choose the correct answer. **Reference:** Ladewig, P., London, M., & Davidson, M. (2010). *Contemporary maternal-newborn nursing care* (7th ed.). Upper Saddle River, NJ: Pearson Education, p. 226.

10 **Answer: 3** **Rationale:** While some ambivalence is common during pregnancy, the client should also have some feelings of happiness, tolerance of physical discomforts, and a feeling that she can deal with the changes and problems related to the pregnancy. **Cognitive Level:** Analyzing **Client Need:** Psychosocial Integrity **Integrated Process:** Nursing Process: Assessment **Content Area:** Maternal-Newborn **Strategy:** Knowledge of the emotional responses to pregnancy and the common responses toward the pregnancy will help to choose the answer that identifies the acceptance of the pregnancy. **Reference:** Ladewig, P., London, M., & Davidson, M. (2010). *Contemporary maternal-newborn nursing care* (7th ed.). Upper Saddle River, NJ: Pearson Education, p. 191.

References

Davidson, M., London, M. & Ladewig, P. (2012). *Olds' maternal newborn nursing & women's health across the lifespan* (9th ed.). Upper Saddle River, NJ: Pearson Education.

Ladewig, P., London, M., & Davidson, M. (2009). *Contemporary maternal-newborn nursing care* (7th ed.). Upper Saddle River, NJ: Pearson Education.

NANDA Nursing Diagnosis (2009). Retrieved January 29, 2011, from http://www.scribd.com/doc/11885949/NANDA-2009

Orshan, S. A. (2008). *Maternity, newborn, and women's health nursing: Comprehensive care across the life span.* Philadelphia: Lippincott Williams & Wilkins.

Ricci, S. (2009). *Essentials of maternity, newborn, and women's health nursing* (2nd ed.). Philadelphia: Lippincott Williams & Wilkins.

Common Laboratory and Diagnostic Tests

6

Chapter Outline

Objectives

- ➤ Describe laboratory tests used to evaluate the status of the pregnant client.
- ➤ Describe diagnostic tests used to assess fetal well-being.

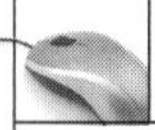

NCLEX-RN® Test Prep

Use the accompanying online resource, NursingReviewsandRationales, to test yourself with hundreds of NCLEX®-style practice questions.

Review at a Glance

alpha-fetoprotein (AFP) a fetal antigen leaked into amniotic fluid and absorbed into the maternal circulation; used as a screening tool for body wall defects, especially of neural tube; may be tested as part of quadruple screen

amniocentesis a procedure to collect amniotic fluid via a needle inserted through maternal abdominal wall; used to diagnose genetic problems and, later in pregnancy, to determine maturity

biophysical profile an assessment of fetal well-being that uses ultrasound to determine fetal breathing movements, body movements, muscle tone, heart rate reactivity, and amniotic fluid volume; based on assessment findings, scores range from 0 to 10

chorionic villus sampling (CVS) collection of a specimen from fetal side of placenta, obtained transcervically or transabdominally and used for fetal genetic testing

contraction stress test (CST) an assessment of ability of fetus to withstand stress of uterine contractions, which occur spontaneously or are artificially induced by oxytocin or nipple stimulation

Doppler blood flow analysis an assessment of fetal blood flow across placenta; non-invasive and useful for detection of intrauterine growth restriction

glucose tolerance test (GTT) a screening test for gestational diabetes at 24 to 28 weeks' gestation; 50-gram oral glucose is administered followed by venous plasma glucose assessment in one hour; results >140 mg/dL are abnormal and indicate need for further testing

karyotype schematic arrangement of chromosomes used to assess chromosome number and morphology

lecithin to sphingomyelin (L/S) ratio used to denote ratio of lecithin to sphingomyelin in amniotic fluid and assess fetal lung maturity; a ratio of 2:1 or > indicates probable lung maturity

nonstress test (NST) an assessment of fetal well-being that analyzes response of fetal heart rate to fetal movement

oral glucose tolerance test (OGTT) diagnostic test for gestational diabetes and indicated following an abnormal GTT; glucose levels are assessed at one, two, and three hours following a three-day high-carbohydrate diet, eight-hour fast, fasting glucose assessment, and administration of 100 grams of oral glucose

phosphatidylglycerol (PG) a phospholipid found in pulmonary surfactant; evidence of it in amniotic fluid is an indicator of fetal lung maturity

quadruple screen an elective prenatal test that assesses alpha-fetoprotein and several other agents detectible in the maternal circulation; measured at 14 to 20 weeks as a screening tool, has high false-positive rate

sexually transmitted infections (STIs) a group of infections that are spread by sexual contact including human papillomavirus (HPV), human immunodeficiency virus (HIV), group B streptococcus (GBS), syphilis, gonorrhea, and chlamydia; also called sexually transmitted or venereal diseases

TORCH infections a group of infections caused by viruses or protozoa that cause serious fetal problems when contracted by mother during pregnancy including toxoplasmosis (T), other infections such as hepatitis (O), rubella (R), cytomegalovirus (C), and herpes simplex virus (H)

ultrasound use of high-frequency sound waves to identify maternal and fetal tissues, bones, and fluids; can determine gestational, structural problems, and fetal well-being

PRETEST

1 A 42-year-old client who is six weeks pregnant has requested genetic testing. During the counseling session, the client asks the nurse about the advantages of chorionic villus sampling (CVS) over amniocentesis. What is the nurse's best response? Select all that apply.

1. "CVS can be done earlier in your pregnancy."
2. "CVS is a safer procedure for you and the baby."
3. "CVS provides more information than amniocentesis."
4. "You will need anesthesia for amniocentesis, but not for CVS."
5. "The results are available more quickly."

2 The pregnant client, who is one week past her due date, is to have a nonstress test (NST). After receiving an explanation of the test, which statement by the client would indicate a need for further teaching?

1. "I understand that you will start an IV containing medicine to cause me to have contractions."
2. "During the test I will need to push a button when I feel the baby move."
3. "I won't need to be admitted to the hospital for this test."
4. "The test should take 20–30 minutes."

3 The pregnant client, who is in her first trimester, is scheduled for an abdominal ultrasound. When explaining the reason for early pregnancy ultrasound, what information should the nurse share with the client?

1. "The test will help to determine if your baby is in a good position for delivery."
2. "The test will help to determine how many weeks you have been pregnant."
3. "The test will help to determine if your baby has intrauterine growth restriction."
4. "The test will help to determine if you have enough amniotic fluid."

4 The pregnant client is to be screened for gestational diabetes with an oral glucose tolerance test (GTT) using a 50-gram glucose load. The nurse explains that the client should schedule the test to be done at what point in the pregnancy?

1. 12 weeks' gestation
2. 16 weeks' gestation
3. 24 weeks' gestation
4. 36 weeks' gestation

5 The nurse is reviewing results from a client's initial prenatal visit and notes that the urine contained an increased number of white blood cells, nitrites, and greater than 10,000 bacteria/mL of urine. These findings lead the nurse to suspect which of the following?

1. Renal insufficiency
2. Contamination of the urine with amniotic fluid
3. Urinary tract infection
4. Nothing unusual, this is a normal finding in pregnancy

6 The client is considering having maternal alpha-fetoprotein (AFP) screening. She asks the nurse how a test on her blood can indicate a fetal birth defect. Which response by the nurse is best?

1. "We aren't sure why this test works, but it does."
2. "Neural tube defects are passed in genetic material so determining the amount of AFP in your DNA will show if it was passed to your baby."
3. "When babies have a neural tube defect, some of their AFP leaks out and is absorbed into your blood, which causes your level to rise. This test detects that rise."
4. "When a fetus has a neural tube defect, not enough AFP is produced so some of your AFP moves across the placenta into the baby's circulation. This makes your level decrease and that is reflected in your AFP level."

7 A female client's test for syphilis has come back positive. In talking with the woman about how the infection is spread, the nurse would discuss that syphilis can be contracted in which ways?

1. Shaking hands, kissing, and oral–genital sexual contact
2. Kissing, oral–genital or genital–genital sexual contact, and biting
3. Exposure to contaminated toilet seats and oral–genital sexual contact
4. Only oral–genital sexual contact

8 In explaining to a client during her initial prenatal exam the importance of testing pregnant women for gonorrhea, the nurse should tell the client that gonorrhea can cause which problem in the neonate?

1. Perineal discharge
2. Eye infections
3. Liver damage
4. Congenital anomalies

9 The nurse concludes that which client manifestation indicates a need for colposcopy and biopsy for human papilloma virus?

1. Rash on the palms of the hands and soles of the feet
2. Chancre sore noted on the vulva
3. A crusted ulcer inside the vagina
4. 2–3 mm soft, papillary swellings either singly or in clusters noted on the genitalia

10 A client has come in for her initial prenatal visit. When the testing to be done at this visit is explained, the client asks why it all has to be done today. What is the nurse's best response?

1. "Actually, we need to do it all on the first visit because sometimes the client does not come back."
2. "Insurance won't pay for testing unless it is done in the first trimester."
3. "It is best to find any current problems so that they can be treated as early as possible."
4. "It's great that you are concerned, but your doctor is keeping up with current practice about what is best for you and your baby."

➤ *See pages 126–127 for Answers and Rationales.*

I. LABORATORY AND DIAGNOSTIC TESTING DURING FIRST PRENATAL VISIT

Practice to Pass

During the initial interview with the nurse, a woman tells the nurse that her mother had "that problem with her blood that causes the baby to turn yellow." The client wants to know if she will also have that problem. How should the nurse respond?

A. **Complete blood count (CBC)**: a series of blood tests that provide information on hematologic system as well as other body systems; advantages include that it is inexpensive and easy to perform, and results are quickly available; for individual tests, their purpose, normal results, and changes in pregnancy, see Table 6-1

1. Test procedure: after explaining procedure to client, obtain 5 to 7 mL of blood in a lavender-top tube; mix well but avoid hemolysis
2. Interfering factors
   a. Changes in fluid balance
   b. Living at a high altitude
   c. Drugs including antibiotics, methyldopa, hydantoins, antineoplastic drugs, aspirin, and quinidine
   d. Abnormalities in RBC size
3. Significant results: preeclampsia is often associated with low platelet counts, falsely elevated hemoglobin and hematocrit levels, and RBC morphology abnormalities

Table 6-1 Complete Blood Count

Test	Purpose	Normal Results	Changes in Pregnancy
RBC Count	A count of number of circulating RBCs in 1 mm^3 of peripheral venous blood; can be used to evaluate client for anemia	4.2–5.4 million/mm^3	5–6.25 million/mm^3
Hemoglobin	A measure of total amount of hemoglobin in peripheral blood; indicates oxygen-carrying capacity of blood	12–16 grams/dL	>11grams/dL
Hematocrit	A percentage of total blood volume that is comprised of RBCs	37–47%	>33%
Mean Corpuscular Volume	A measure of average volume of a single RBC; used to classify types of anemia	80–95/cubic micrometer	none
Mean Corpuscular Hemoglobin	A measure of average amount of hemoglobin within a single RBC	27–31/picogram	none
Mean Corpuscular Hemoglobin Concentration	A measure of average concentration or percentage of hemoglobin within a single RBC	32–36 grams/dL packed RBCs	none
WBC Count	A measure of total white blood cells (WBCs) in mm^3 in peripheral venous blood; can indicate client's ability to fight infection and react against foreign bodies or tissues	5000–10,000/mm^3	5000–15,000/mm^3
Polymorphonuclear Cells	Sometimes called granulocytes, an increase in these cells can indicate an acute infection, parasitic infestation, or allergic response	55–70% of WBCs	60–85% of WBCs
Lymphocytes	Sometimes called agranulocytes, an increase can indicate chronic bacterial infection or acute viral infection	20–40% of WBCs	15–40% of WBCs
Platelet Count	A measure of number of platelets/mm^3 of blood; platelets are essential to blood clotting	150,000–400,000/mm^3	none until 3–5 days after delivery

B. Blood group and Rh typing

1. Purpose: to determine client's blood group and Rh status to identify a fetus at risk for developing erythroblastosis fetalis or hyperbilirubinemia in neonatal period
2. Test procedure: after explaining procedure to client, collect 7 to 10 mL of venous blood in a nonadditive tube; avoid hemolysis
3. Interfering factors: none
4. ! Significant results: mothers who are type O and/or Rh negative may require further fetal or infant testing
5. Mothers with Rh negative blood type should receive Rhogam Immunoglobulin when having any prenatal bleeding or abdominal trauma, at 28 weeks' gestation, and within 72 hours of birth if infant is Rh positive

C. *TORCH infections*: a group of infections caused by viruses and protozoa that cause serious fetal problems when contracted by mother during pregnancy; each letter represents a different infection including Toxoplasmosis, Other infections (usually hepatitis), Rubella, Cytomegalovirus, and Herpes simplex virus

1. Toxoplasmosis
   a. Cause: infection with protozoan parasite *toxoplasma gondii*
   b. Transmission: development of this infection in mother is associated with consumption of infested undercooked meat and poor handwashing after handling cat litter; fetal infection occurs if mother acquires toxoplasmosis after conception and passes it to fetus via placenta
   c. Diagnosis: because it is difficult to grow toxoplasmosis cultures, diagnosis is made by serologic testing; the indirect fluorescent antibody test is most commonly used; IgG titers greater than 1:256 suggest a recent infection, whereas IgM titers greater than 1:256 indicate an acute infection
   d. Maternal effects: flu-like symptoms in acute phase
   e. Fetal/neonatal effects: miscarriage is likely in early pregnancy; in neonates central nervous system lesions can result in hydrocephaly, microcephaly, chronic retinitis, and seizures
   f. Test procedure: after explaining procedure to client, collect 5 mL of venous blood in a nonadditive tube; indicate on lab slip if client is pregnant or has been exposed to cats
   g. Prevention: advise clients who have cats *not* to clean cat litter box while pregnant or trying to conceive
2. Other infections, usually hepatitis virus
   a. Cause: infection with hepatitis A (HAV) or B (HBV) virus; hepatitis B is most common infection in fetus
   b. Transmission: HAV is spread by droplets or hands and is associated with poor hand-washing after defecation; transmission to fetus is rare but can occur; hepatitis B can be transmitted to fetus via placenta, but transmission usually occurs when infant is exposed to blood and genital secretions during labor and delivery
   c. Diagnosis: radioimmunoassay and enzyme-linked immunosorbent assay methods are used to detect HAV antibodies; elevated IgM antibody in absence of IgG antibody indicates probable acute hepatitis; elevated IgG in absence of IgM indicates a convalescent or chronic stage of HAV; hepatitis B is detected through hepatitis B surface antigen (HbsAg)
   d. Maternal effects: fever, malaise, nausea, and abdominal discomfort; may be associated with liver failure
   e. Fetal/neonatal effects: preterm birth, hepatitis infection, and intrauterine fetal death
   f. ! Test procedure: after explaining procedure to client, collect 5 to 7 mL of venous blood in a nonadditive tube; handle blood as though it were capable of transmitting virus

g. Prevention: while not pregnant and using contraception, client should receive hepatitis B vaccination series

3. Rubella, sometimes called German measles or three-day measles
   a. Cause: infection with rubella virus
   b. Transmission: infection is spread by droplets
   c. Diagnosis: IgG antibodies to rubella are measured to determine client's rubella immunity status; a titer of 1:10 or greater indicates that woman is immune to rubella; a titer of 1:8 or less indicates minimal or no immunity
   d. Maternal effects: fever, rash, and mild lymphedema
   e. Fetal/neonatal effects: miscarriage, congenital anomalies, and death
   f. Test procedure: after explaining procedure to client, collect 3 to 5 mL of venous blood in a serum separator tube (SST), a vacuum tube
   g. Prevention: clients who do not have immunity to Rubella should receive a rubella vaccination during postpartum period to protect future pregnancies while not affecting a current pregnancy
4. Cytomegalovirus (CMV)
   a. Cause: exposure to cytomegalovirus
   b. Transmission: cytomegalovirus can be transmitted through respiratory droplets, semen, cervical and vaginal secretions, breast milk, placental tissue, urine, feces, and banked blood; most common mode of transmission is respiratory droplets; workers in daycare centers, institutions for developmentally delayed clients, and health care delivery settings are especially at risk
   c. Diagnosis: a viral culture is most definitive diagnostic tool; CMV antibodies indicate a recent infection; a fourfold increase in CMV titer in paired sera drawn 10 to 14 days apart usually indicates an acute infection
   d. Maternal effects: asymptomatic illness, cervical discharge, and mononucleosis-like syndrome
   e. Fetal/neonatal effects: fetal death or severe generalized disease with hemolytic anemia and jaundice, hydrocephaly or microcephaly, pneumonitis, hepatosplenomegaly, and deafness
   f. Test procedure: after explaining procedure to client, collect a swab specimen from urine, sputum, or mouth for a viral culture; culture requires three to seven days; if an antibody or antigen titer is desired, collect 5 to 7 mL venous blood in a red-top tube; in a client with suspected active CMV, collect a specimen as soon as possible and repeat in 10 to 14 days
   g. Prevention: advise clients to avoid exposure to children and adults who are ill with flu-like symptoms if at all possible
5. Herpes simplex virus (HSV)
   a. Cause: exposure to herpes simplex virus
   b. Transmission: HSV type 2 is a sexually transmitted infection transmitted by exposure to vesicular lesions on penis, scrotum, vulva, perineum, perianal region, vagina, or cervix; infant is usually infected during exposure to a lesion in birth canal; infant is most at risk during a primary infection in mother
   c. Diagnosis: viral culture is used for definitive diagnosis; serologic tests have a lower accuracy
   d. Maternal effects: blisters, rash, fever, malaise, nausea, and headache
   e. Fetal/neonatal effects: miscarriage, preterm labor, or stillbirth; transplacental infection is rare but can cause skin lesions, intrauterine growth restriction, mental retardation, and microcephaly
   f. Test procedure: after explaining test to client, client is placed in lithotomy position and cervix is visualized; a cotton-tipped swab is used to obtain a specimen from endocervical canal; swab specimens may also be obtained from visible lesions

Practice to Pass

The client tells you that she does not need to be tested for TORCH infections because she has not been ill. How will you respond?

g. Significant results: vaginal delivery is recommended if client has no visible lesions or prodromal symptoms
h. If visible lesions or prodromal symptoms are present, cesarean delivery is indicated

D. Urinalysis

1. Findings
   a. pH may be decreased with poor glucose metabolism and ketone acids in urine
   b. Specific gravity may be increased with dehydration caused by excessive vomiting as seen in hyperemesis gravidarum
   c. Color should be pale yellow to amber depending on foods ingested and urine concentration
   d. Glucose reabsorption is impaired in pregnancy resulting in spilling of glucose into urine at a blood glucose level of 160 mg/dL
   e. Protein may normally be found in urine during pregnancy at a level of trace to +1 using dipstick method; increased protein may indicate gestational hypertension or preeclampsia
   f. WBCs or nitrites can indicate a possible urinary tract infection, which can place client at risk for preterm labor
   g. Casts, which are formed from clumps of materials or cells in renal distal and collecting tubules, form when urine is acidic and concentrated; they can be associated with proteinuria and stasis in renal tubules
   h. Ketones may indicate diabetes, hyperglycemia, or breakdown of fats or proteins for calories
   i. Urine culture should be done to identify women with asyptomatic bacteriuria; greater than 10,000 bacteria/mL urine is indicative of a urinary tract infection
   j. Urine toxicology can be used to screen for illicit drug use
2. Test procedure: after explaining test, collect a fresh urine specimen in a urine container; if a culture is to be done, collect a midstream, clean-catch specimen

Practice to Pass

On her third prenatal visit, the client asks why a urine sample is needed at every visit. What should you tell her?

II. LABORATORY TESTING DURING FOLLOW-UP PRENATAL VISITS

A. Clean-catch urine specimen

1. Specimen is collected at each visit to assess for glucose, protein, nitrites, and leukocytes
2. Abnormal results can indicate diabetes, gestational hypertension or preeclampsia, or infection

B. Hemoglobin

1. Hemoglobin (normal 12–16 grams/dL) is assessed monthly to monitor for iron-deficiency anemia
2. If level is less than 12 grams/dL, client should have nutritional counseling; if level drops below 11 grams/dL, client should receive iron supplementation

C. Glucose tolerance test (GTT)

1. GTT is used to screen pregnant clients for gestational diabetes; is a standard part of prenatal care for all clients; is generally completed between 24 and 28 weeks' gestation, although it is indicated earlier for clients with a history of gestational diabetes or those who are overweight
2. Test procedure: after explaining test to client, a 50-gram oral glucose load is administered; the time of day or time since last meal is not a factor; venous plasma glucose is assessed one hour after glucose load
3. Findings: a level greater than 140 mg/dL is considered abnormal, and indicates a need for further testing

Table 6-2 Abnormal Oral Glucose Tolerance Test Results (per 100 grams of glucose)

Time	Abnormal Result
Fasting	greater than 95 mg/dL
1 hour	greater than 180 mg/dL
2 hour	greater than 155 mg/dL
3 hour	greater than 140 mg/dL

4. Follow-up: clients with abnormal GTT results should be assessed with a three-hour, 100-gram **oral glucose tolerance test (OGTT)** used to diagnose gestational diabetes
   a. Test procedure: client is told to eat a conventional unrestricted diet with at least 150 grams of carbohydrates per day for three days before test and then, on day of test, to fast for eight hours (overnight); a fasting serum glucose is obtained; following the fast, 100 grams of oral glucose is administered and glucose levels are measured at one, two, and three hours
   ! b. Findings: gestational diabetes is diagnosed if two or more results are abnormal (see Table 6-2); results are borderline if one value is abnormal; with borderline results, OGTT is repeated in one month

D. **Quadruple screen test**
1. Description
   a. **Quadruple screen**, also called quad screen, is an optional screening test of mother's serum at 15 to 21 weeks of gestation in which specific substances are tested for and quantified according to expected norms
   b. Measurements of **alpha-fetoprotein (AFP)**, which is a fetal protein, human chorionic gonadotropin (hCG), unconjugated estriol (UE), and inhibin-A (a placental hormone) are included in quad screen
   c. Quad screen tests have a high false-positive rate; clients need to understand this before choosing whether or not to have it done
2. Test procedure: after explaining procedure to client, collect 5 to 10 mL of venous blood in a serum separator tube; gestational age should be indicated on laboratory slip
3. ! Findings: elevated AFP level may indicate neural tube or body wall defects, multiple gestation, or a later gestational age than is currently estimated; low AFP level could indicate increased risk of trisomy 18 or trisomy 21 (Down syndrome); elevated hCG and inhibin-A levels and low UE level could also indicate increased risk of Down syndrome
4. Interfering factors include multiple pregnancy and incorrect estimation of gestational age
5. ! Follow-up: abnormal results may indicate a need for a repeated test, then an ultrasound or amniocentesis

III. DIAGNOSTIC TESTS FOR SEXUALLY TRANSMITTED INFECTIONS

A. **Overview**
1. **Sexually transmitted infections (STIs)**: sometimes called sexually transmitted diseases, STIs are caused by bacteria, viruses, protozoa, or ectoparasites
2. Infections include human papillomavirus (HPV), human immunodeficiency virus (HIV), group B streptococcus (GBS), syphilis, gonorrhea, and chlamydia
3. All sexual partners of clients with STIs should be contacted and treated, as indicated

B. Human papillomavirus (HPV)

1. Cause/transmission: sometimes called genital or venereal warts, HPV infection is caused by spread of human papillomavirus through sexual contact; neonates can acquire infection during birth
2. Diagnosis: by direct visualization of warts and confirmed by biopsy
3. Maternal effects: symptoms depend on viral strain causing infection but can include genital lesions, chronic vaginal discharge, pruritis, and cervical dysplasia; some strains are asymptomatic
4. Fetal/neonatal effects: juvenile laryngeal papillomata
5. Test procedure: after explaining test to client, colposcopy and direct visualization of warts, sometimes with biopsy, is completed; vinegar solution may be used to highlight early or flat cervical lesions
6. Prevention: vaccination with HPV vaccine as a series is recommended for boys age 9–26, and for females ages 9–45 who are not currently pregnant; it is acceptable for administration during breastfeeding
7. Treatment: topical agents are used to eradicate affected tissue; some of these agents are contraindicated in pregnancy

C. Human immunodeficiency virus (HIV)

1. Cause/transmission: transmission is primarily through exchange of body fluids including semen, blood, or vaginal secretions
   a. In women, now the fastest-growing population of people with HIV, infection is most commonly spread through heterosexual contact
   b. Neonatal transmission can occur transplacentally and is less likely if mother receives treatment during pregnancy; transmission can also occur by contact at time of delivery or through breast milk
2. Diagnosis: made with a reactive enzyme immunoassay (EIA) and a positive Western blot or immunofluorescence assay; the p24 antigen capture assay can be used as early as two to six weeks after infection and is used to diagnose neonatal HIV infection, to detect HIV before seroconversion, and to determine progression of AIDS; viral culture is best diagnostic tool for neonates; but is expensive and requires four to six weeks for results
3. Maternal effects: opportunistic diseases including *Pneumocystis carinii* pneumonia, candida esophagitis, and wasting syndrome; HSV and CMV infections are also common; fever, headache, night sweats, malaise, generalized lymphadenopathy, myalgias, nausea, diarrhea, weight loss, sore throat, and rash are associated with seroconversion
4. Fetal/neonatal effects: asymptomatic at birth followed by opportunistic infections, immunodeficiency, failure to thrive, parotitis, lymphadenopathy, hepatosplenomegaly, fever, chronic diarrhea, dermatitis, thrush, and death
5. Test procedure: after explaining test to client, an informed consent must be obtained; 5 to 10 mL of peripheral venous blood is collected in a nonadditive tube; clients may remain anonymous through use of number identification
6. HIV positive women are high-risk patients and warrant treatment with drug therapy according to Centers for Disease Control (CDC)'s most current recommendations

Practice to Pass

The client, who has come to the clinic for her first prenatal visit, asks you why she needs to be tested for HIV when only homosexual men are at risk for contracting the infection. How should you respond to the client?

D. Group B streptococcus (GBS)

1. Cause/transmission: considered normal vaginal flora, is found in 10–30% of healthy pregnant women; is transmitted vertically from birth canal of infected mother to fetus
2. Diagnosis: current recommendations are to screen all women at 35 to 37 weeks' gestation with a GBS culture
3. Maternal effects: preterm labor, chorioamnionitis, premature rupture of membranes, urinary tract infections and postpartum infections

4. Fetal/neonatal effects: neonatal meningitis, sepsis, and septic shock; early onset GBS has a significant infant mortality rate
5. Test procedure: after explaining need for test to client, collect GBS cultures from anorectal and vaginal areas, not cervix
6. Women who are GBS positive need treatment during labor according to CDC's most current recommendations; infants who are either not screened or not adequately treated during labor require special surveillance as newborns, including blood work, cultures, and extended assessments

E. Syphilis

1. Cause/transmission: syphilis is caused by *Treponema pallidum*, a motile spirochete transmitted through microscopic abrasions in subcutaneous tissue; it can be transmitted through kissing, biting, intercourse or oral–genital sex; transmission to fetus can occur via placenta at any time during pregnancy
2. Diagnosis: can be made by microscopic examination of primary and secondary lesion tissue; serology is used for diagnosis during latency and late infection; women should be screened at first prenatal visit and possibly again late in third trimester; screening is done with VDRL (Venereal Disease Research Laboratories) or RPR (rapid plasma reagin) test; both tests detect antibodies to *Treponema* organism; if VDRL or RPR is positive, diagnosis is confirmed with a flourescent treponemal antibody absorption test (FTA-ABS)
3. ! Maternal effects: during acute stage, a chancre develops on skin near infection; second stage is marked by lymphadenopathy and a rash located on palms of hands and soles of feet; the third or latent stage, which can last up to five years, is asymptomatic; disease can progress to a tertiary stage that involves central nervous system (CNS), cardiovascular, and ocular signs and symptoms; infection can cause miscarriage or premature labor
4. Fetal/neonatal effects: include CNS damage, hearing loss, or death
5. Test procedure: after explaining test to client, collect 7 mL of venous blood in a collection tube
6. Syphilis can be safely treated in pregnancy using penicillin-type antibiotics

F. Gonorrhea

1. Cause/transmission: caused by *Neisseria gonorrhoeae*, which are aerobic, gram-negative diplococci bacteria; transmitted by all types of sexual activity; neonates can acquire infection by exposure to bacteria in birth canal
2. Diagnosis: all pregnant women should be screened at initial prenatal visit and at-risk women should be screened again at 36 weeks' gestation; a Thayer-Martin culture of endocervix, rectum, or pharynx is completed for diagnosis
3. Maternal effects: sometimes asymptomatic but can cause purulent endocervical discharge, menstrual irregularities, pelvic or lower abdominal pain, and premature rupture of membranes
4. ! Fetal/neonatal effects: preterm birth, neonatal sepsis, intrauterine growth restriction and ophthalmia neonatorum, which can cause blindness
5. Test procedure: after explaining procedure to client, cervix is cleaned of mucus and a swab specimen is collected from endocervical canal; rectum or pharynx may also be cultured; results may be affected by douching within 24 hours prior to specimen collection; specimen contamination with fecal material, lubricants, disinfectants, or menstrual blood can also affect results
6. Treatment: clients infected with gonorrhea should be treated during pregnancy using most recent CDC guidelines; partner(s) also need treatment; retesting should be done following treatment
7. ! Prevention: all infants are treated prophylactically with erythromycin ophthalmic ointment to prevent conjunctivitis

G. Chlamydia

1. Cause/transmission: *Chlamydia trachomatis* bacteria is spread through sexual contact; CDC recommends screening of asymptomatic, high-risk women
2. Diagnosis: cultures for chlamydia are expensive, require special transport and storage, and take up to 10 days
3. Maternal effects: although usually asymptomatic, infection can cause bleeding, mucoid or purulent cervical discharge, pelvic inflammatory disease, or dysuria
4. Fetal/neonatal effects: conjunctivitis, pneumonia, and ophthalmia neonatorum
5. Test procedure: after explaining test to client, cervix is swabbed to remove mucus from cervical os, and a scraping of endocervical cells is collected; special culture media and proper handling of specimens are important
6. Treatment: clients infected with gonorrhea should be treated during pregnancy using most recent CDC guidelines; partner(s) also require treatment; retesting should be done following treatment
7. Prevention: all infants are treated prophylactically with erythromycin ophthalmic ointment to prevent conjunctivitis

IV. OTHER DIAGNOSTIC TESTS USEFUL DURING PREGNANCY

A. Ultrasound

1. Description: **ultrasound** uses sound waves having a frequency higher than 20,000 Hz to produce a three-dimensional view and pictorial image to identify maternal and fetal tissues, bones, and fluids
2. Transvaginal ultrasound
   - **a.** Purpose: used primarily during first trimester to evaluate pelvic anatomy, assess developing embryo/fetus for number and size, locate placenta, diagnose intrauterine pregnancy, screen for fetal and placental anomalies, and establish gestational age
   - **b.** Advantages: eliminates need for a full bladder and clearer images in obese clients as sound waves do not pass through thick abdominal layers
   - **c.** Disadvantages: some clients are embarrassed or uncomfortable with vaginal insertion of probe; vaginal ultrasound is contraindicated in clients with latex allergies as probe is covered with a latex condom
   - **d.** Test procedure: after explaining procedure to client, an informed consent is obtained because probe is inserted into body; client is placed in a supine position and vaginal probe is inserted; allowing client to insert probe may promote comfort and decrease embarrassment; fetal structures should be pointed out to mother during procedure
3. Abdominal ultrasound
   - **a.** Purpose: to obtain information on fetal viability; number, position, gestational age, growth pattern, and anomalies; amniotic fluid volume; placental location and maturity; and assessment of fetal well-being
   - **b.** Advantages: ultrasound provides a safe, non-invasive fetal assessment; in situations where there is a problem, it allows early diagnosis of many fetal problems, allowing the family choices regarding intrauterine surgery or other therapies, termination of pregnancy, or preparation for birth of an infant with a problem
   - **c.** Disadvantages: during early pregnancy, procedure is best done when client's bladder is full; this can result in discomfort
   - **d.** Test procedure: in early pregnancy, clients are instructed to come to test with a full bladder; test is explained and transmission gel is applied to abdomen; transducer is moved over abdomen to produce an image; after examination, client's abdomen should be cleaned of transmission gel and client is allowed to empty her bladder

4. Findings
   a. Viability is determined by assessment of fetal heart activity; this is possible at six to seven weeks' gestation; fetal death can be determined by absence of heart activity
   b. Gestational age can best be established during the first 12 weeks' gestation as fetal growth rate is fairly consistent during this time; body part to be assessed is based on development; measurement of gestational sac is done in pregnancies that are about eight weeks' gestation, and crown-rump measurement is done on fetuses that are 7–14 weeks' gestation; in a fetus greater than 12 weeks' gestation, biparietal diameter (BPD) and femur length are measured
   c. Fetal growth is assessed by serial measurements of BPD and femur length; this information can assist health care provider in distinguishing between intrauterine growth restriction and inaccurate dating of pregnancy
5. **Biophysical profile** is a method of assessing fetal well-being after at least 23–24 weeks' gestation by determining scores on five criteria including fetal breathing movements, body movements, muscle tone, heart rate activity, and amniotic fluid volume
   a. Total score ranges from 0 to 10; a score of 2 is given if findings for a criterion are normal; a score of 0 is given if findings for that criterion are abnormal
   b. A total score of 8 to 10 is considered normal, a score of 4 to 6 is interpreted as possibly abnormal and a score of less than 4 may indicate a need for delivery; scoring is described in greater detail in Table 6-3
6. **Doppler blood flow analysis** (umbilical velocimetry) is a non-invasive assessment of fetal blood flow across placenta; provides information concerning blood flow and resistance in placental circulation and is useful in detecting intrauterine growth restriction
   a. Can be done as early as 16 to 18 weeks
   b. Velocity waveforms from umbilical and uterine arteries are reported as systolic/diastolic (S/D) ratios; persistently elevated ratios of greater than 3 after 30 weeks' gestation are considered abnormal and have been associated with intrauterine growth restriction

Table 6-3 Biophysical Profile Scoring

Assessment Variable	Normal Findings = score of 2	Abnormal Findings = score of 0
Fetal breathing movements	At least one episode of breathing movement lasting at least 60 seconds in a 30-minute assessment period	Absence of a 60-second breathing episode during a 30-minute assessment period
Fetal body movements	At least three episodes of fetal movement in a 30-minute assessment period	Two or fewer episodes of fetal movement in a 30-minute assessment period
Fetal muscle tone	At least one episode of extension and return to flexion during assessment period	Slow extension with return to only partial flexion during assessment period
Fetal heart rate reactivity	Two or more movement-associated heart rate increases of at least 15 beats per minute above baseline and 15 seconds in duration in a 20-minute assessment period	Fewer than two movement-associated heart rate increases of at least 15 beats per minute above baseline and 15 seconds in duration in a 20-minute assessment period
Amniotic fluid volume	At least one pocket of amniotic fluid measuring 1 cm in two perpendicular planes	Either fluid is absent in most areas of uterine cavity or largest pocket measures 1 cm or less in vertical axis

Practice to Pass

The client has just had a reactive nonstress test and asks you if this means that her baby will be able to tolerate labor. How will you respond?

B. Stress and nonstress tests

1. **Nonstress test (NST)** is an assessment of fetal well-being that analyzes the response of the fetal heart to fetal movement; it is performed after at least 23–24 weeks' gestation
   a. Advantages: non-invasive, easily interpreted, and can be performed in an outpatient setting at a low cost; the NST is a good indicator of fetal well-being
   b. Disadvantages: a high number of false-positive results caused by fetal sleep cycles, medications, and fetal immaturity; NST is not a good predictor of poor fetal outcomes
   c. Test procedure: client is placed in a semi-Fowler's position and an ultrasound transducer and tocodynamometer are used to record contractions and fetal heart rate (FHR); in some settings, client is asked to press a hand-held button when fetal movement is felt to make a mark on fetal heart tracing; with this information, episodes of fetal movement can then be compared to changes in the FHR; acoustical stimulation can be implemented in absence of fetal movement

   !

   d. Findings: test is considered normal (reactive) if there are two or more accelerations of 15 beats per minute lasting for 15 seconds over a 20-minute period or 10 beats per minute lasting for 10 seconds if the pregnancy is less than 32 weeks' gestation, and the baseline is normal; if these criteria are not met within 40 minutes, test is considered nonreassuring (nonreactive) and further testing is indicated
2. Fetal acoustic stimulation test (FAST) and vibroacoustic stimulation test (VST) are used to stimulate fetus while an NST is performed; non-invasive sound and vibrations shorten the time for NST
3. **Contraction stress test (CST)** assesses ability of fetus to withstand stress of uterine contractions and is a means of evaluating placental capacity for oxygen/carbon dioxide exchange; since contractions reduce blood flow to fetus, CST can be used to predict a fetus that may not be able to tolerate stress of labor; this test is done on pregnancies beyond 23 to 24 weeks' gestation
   a. Indications: factors that place fetus at risk for asphyxia such as intrauterine growth restriction, diabetes, postdates, nonreactive NST, and biophysical profile score less than 6
   b. Contraindications: third-trimester bleeding and previous cesarean birth with classical uterine incision; advantages of CST should be weighed against danger of preterm labor in situations where this is a risk, such as premature rupture of membranes or incompetent cervix
   c. Test procedure: after procedure is explained to client and informed consent is obtained, electronic monitoring of contractions and fetal heart rate are begun; after a baseline fetal heart tracing is obtained, contractions (if not occurring spontaneously) are initiated with intravenous oxytocin or breast self-stimulation

   !

   d. Findings: when a pattern of at least three contractions of 40–60 seconds duration in a 10-minute time period is obtained, FHR pattern is assessed; test is reassuring (negative) if no late decelerations occur (see Figure 6-1); test is not reassuring (positive) if there are late decelerations with at least 50% of contractions; test is suspicious (equivocal) if there are intermittent late decelerations, significant variable decelerations, decelerations in the presence of hyperstimulation; further assessment is needed with these results

C. Amniocentesis

1. Description and purpose: **amniocentesis** assesses fetal well-being and maturity; it assists in prenatal diagnosis of genetic disorders or congenital anomalies, assessment of pulmonary maturity, and diagnosis of fetal hemolytic disease; a needle is inserted through maternal abdominal wall to collect a sample of amniotic fluid, which contains fetal cells (see Figure 6-2); test can be done after 14–16 weeks' gestation

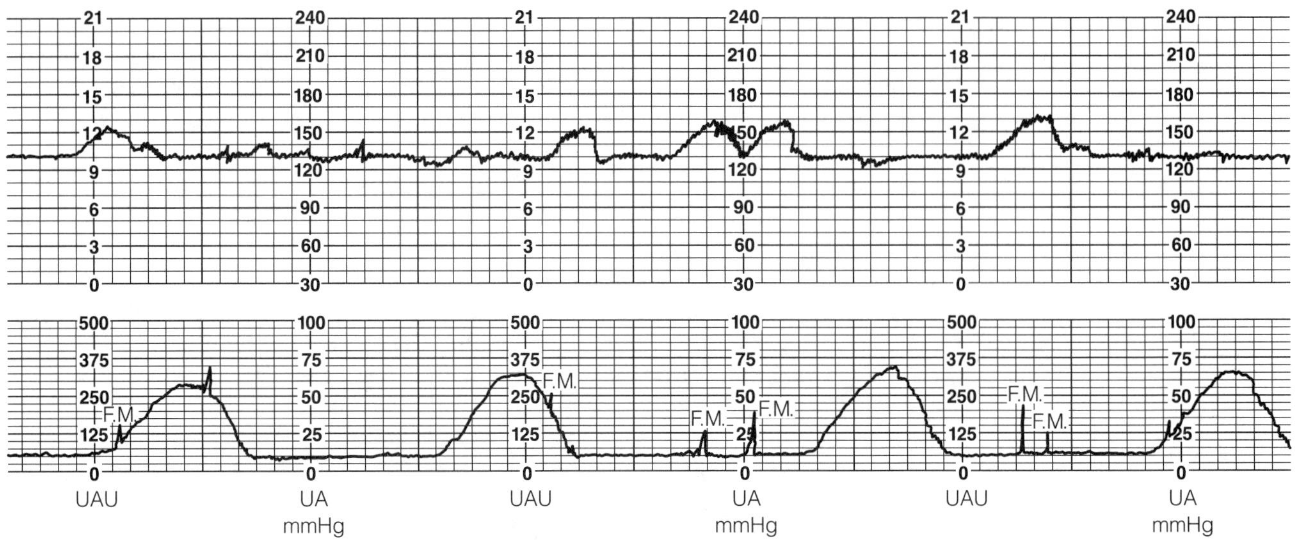

Figure 6-1

Contraction stress test

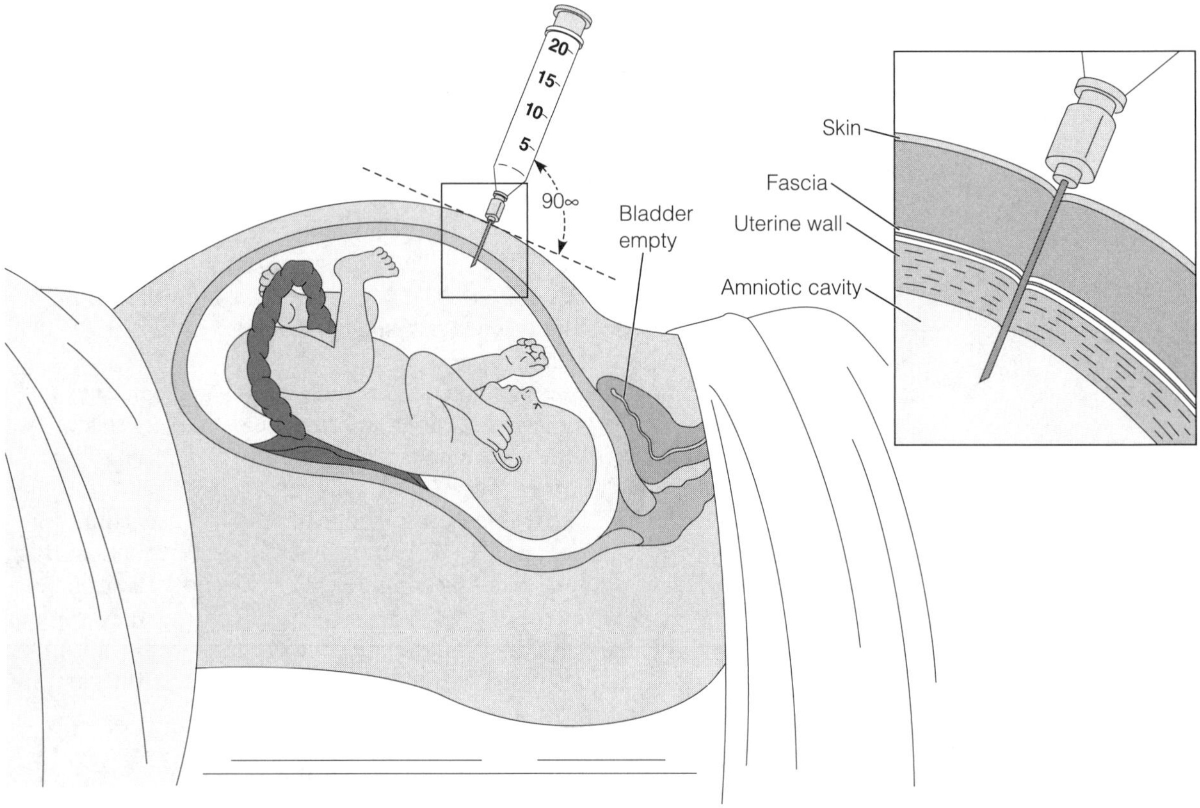

Figure 6-2

Amniocentesis

! 2. Complications occur in less than 1% of cases; possible maternal complications include hemorrhage, infection, labor, abruptio placentae, inadvertent damage to intestines or bladder, and amniotic fluid leakage or embolism; possible fetal complications include death, hemorrhage, infection, and direct injury from needle

! 3. Test procedure
   a. After explaining test to client, an informed consent is obtained
   b. If the client is greater than 20 weeks' gestation, she should empty her bladder
   c. With client in supine position, a sterile needle is inserted into uterus; ultrasound visualization is used to assist in guiding needle; 15–20 mL of fluid are withdrawn and placed in a light-resistant container
   d. FHR and maternal vital signs are monitored throughout procedure and for 30 minutes after; mothers who are Rh-negative should receive RhoGAM following procedure because of risk of isoimmunization from fetal blood

! 4. Follow-up: instruct client to contact health care provider if she experiences fluid loss, bleeding, fever, abdominal pain, or increased or decreased fetal activity; inform client that test results will be available in about two weeks

5. Findings
   a. **Lecithin to sphingomyelin (L/S) ratio** is used to assess fetal lung maturity; a ratio of 2:1 or greater indicates probable lung maturity; contamination with meconium or blood may alter results
   ! b. **Phosphatidylglycerol (PG)**, a phospholipid found in pulmonary surfactant; in amniotic fluid is an indicator of fetal lung maturity
   ! c. Genetic and chromosomal aberrations and gender of fetus can be determined from cells cultured for **karyotype** (schematic arrangement of chromosomes), which is used to assess chromosome number and morphology as well as enzymatic activity; determination of gender is important in assessment of sex-linked diseases
   d. Rh isoimmunization status and severity of hemolytic anemia can be assessed by measuring bilirubin pigment in amniotic fluid
   e. AFP levels, either increased or decreased, can indicate anatomic abnormalities; fetal blood contamination of amniotic fluid can alter AFP results

D. Chorionic villus sampling

1. Description: **chorionic villus sampling (CVS)** involves collecting a small specimen of tissue from fetal portion of placenta for fetal genetic studies; specimen can be obtained either transcervically or transabdominally; this test is done at approximately 10 weeks' gestation
2. Indications: women who are >35 years old (increased risk for Down syndrome), or who have had frequent spontaneous abortions, fetuses with chromosomal anomalies or other defects, or have a genetic defect themselves
3. Advantages: when compared to amniocentesis, include earlier diagnosis and rapid return of results; test can be performed at 10–12 weeks' gestation with results returned in one to two weeks
4. Test procedure
   a. Before procedure, instruct client to come for procedure with a full bladder
   b. After procedure is explained, informed consent is obtained
   c. Client is placed in lithotomy position and, using sterile technique, health care provider visualizes cervix; using ultrasound guidance, a suction cannula is used to collect specimen; if sample cannot be obtained transvaginally, transabdominal route is used
   d. Clients who are Rh-negative should be given RhoGAM following procedure
5. Complications: vaginal spotting or bleeding, miscarriage, rupture of membranes, and chorioamnionitis; limb anomalies have been reported when procedure is done before 10 weeks' gestation; complications are rare

6. Follow-up includes teaching client signs and symptoms of complications to report to physician, stating when results will be available, and assisting in arranging genetic counseling as needed

E. **Priority nursing diagnoses**: Deficient Knowledge; Health-Seeking Behaviors; Interrupted Family Processes; Ineffective Health Maintenance

F. **Planning and implementation**
1. Explain all planned testing including any special pretesting directions and obtain informed consents as needed
2. Answer all client questions including those regarding why tests are needed, what test entails, when results will be available and their significance
3. Protect client's privacy during testing
4. ! After specimens are collected, ensure accurate labeling, packaging, and storage until tests are completed; use standard precautions when handling specimens or diagnostic equipment that may result in exposure
5. Reassure client as to confidentiality of results and that she will be notified when results are available
6. After results are returned, place results in client's medical record
7. Contact client to arrange for follow-up testing, genetic counseling, and education as needed

G. **Evaluation:** follow up with client to see that appointments have been kept, results are understood, and sexual partners have been notified of infection or need for treatment, as indicated

Case Study

The client is a 38-year-old primigravida who has come to the clinic for confirmation of pregnancy and initial prenatal care. Her last menstrual period was six weeks ago. She is married, in good health, and this pregnancy was planned. She is concerned that her age may have an effect on the fetus.

1. What problem is this fetus at risk for because of maternal age?
2. In addition to regular prenatal screening, what additional testing should be offered to this client?
3. What advantages would chorionic villus sampling have over amniocentesis for this client?
4. The client shares with you that even if the baby has a defect, she would not consider terminating the pregnancy. She wonders if there would be any advantage to knowing before delivery if the baby has a problem. How will you respond?
5. The client is concerned that prenatal testing might injure the fetus. What will you tell her about possible complications from chorionic villus sampling and amniocentesis?

For suggested responses, see page 303.

POSTTEST

1. The results have been returned from a complete blood count for a pregnant client who came to the clinic for her initial prenatal visit. Which result would indicate a possible problem with oxygen-carrying capacity?

   1. Decreased white blood cell count
   2. Decreased red blood cell count
   3. Decreased polymorphonuclear cell count
   4. Decreased platelet count

2. A pregnant client who is 11 weeks' gestation has come to the office reporting flu-like symptoms. Laboratory studies indicate that she has contracted toxoplasmosis. From which of the following was the infection probably contracted? Select all that apply.

   1. Sexual contact with a heterosexual male
   2. Contact with toxoplasmosis-contaminated droplets in the air
   3. Exposure to infected saliva
   4. Poor handwashing after handling infected cat litter
   5. Eating raw or poorly cooked meat

3. The client's prenatal laboratory findings have been returned. Which of the following would indicate a need for further follow-up related to potential development of erythroblastosis fetalis?

   1. Blood type O
   2. Rh negative
   3. Blood type A
   4. Rh positive

4. During the first prenatal visit, the client denies having had rubella or the rubella vaccine. What would be an appropriate action by the nurse based on this information?

   1. Administer the rubella vaccine
   2. Take a blood sample to assess the rubella titer
   3. Have the client call her mother to ask if the client had German measles as a child
   4. State that since rubella has little effect on the fetus she shouldn't worry about exposure to the disease

5. The pregnant client, who had an abnormal screening glucose tolerance test (GTT) for gestational diabetes, has come to the clinic for a follow-up three-hour oral GTT. Which statement by the client indicates that she understands how the test is done?

   1. "I have eaten a low-protein diet for the past three days."
   2. "I ate a breakfast of toast and milk one hour ago."
   3. "I have eaten a high-carbohydrate diet for the past three days."
   4. "I just had black coffee for breakfast."

6. A pregnant client is scheduled to have an ultrasound. Which of the following might indicate a need to do the assessment transvaginally?

   1. Client is 5-feet 1-inch tall and weighs 230 pounds
   2. Client is 15 years old and easily embarrassed
   3. Client is 32 weeks' gestation
   4. Client is concerned about ultrasound waves hurting the baby

7. The client, who is 41 weeks' gestation, has just had a biophysical profile with a score of two. What nursing intervention would be most appropriate at this time?

   1. Tell the mother that this indicates fetal well-being.
   2. Reschedule the mother for a repeat of the test in one week.
   3. Recognize this as an equivocal test and schedule a repeat of it for the next day.
   4. Consult the physician as there is a probable need for immediate delivery.

8 The client has come to the clinic for her initial prenatal visit. Based on her menstrual history, the client is 9 weeks' gestation and is scheduled to have an ultrasound for estimation of gestational age of the fetus. Which fetal measurement would be the best indicator of gestational age at this time?

1. Biparietal diameter
2. Femur length
3. Abdominal circumference
4. Crown-rump measurement

9 The client, who is to have an amniocentesis for genetic testing, asks the nurse if there are any possible complications with this procedure. What is the nurse's best response?

1. "No, this procedure is completely safe."
2. "I don't know; you will need to speak with your health care provider about that."
3. "Yes, but if you are very still during the procedure they can be avoided."
4. "Yes, but they occur in less than 1% of the cases. Do you have any other questions about the procedure?"

10 A pregnant client at 40 weeks' gestation seems upset and says that the health care provider told her she needs to have a nonstress test. The client asks why she needs the test. What is the nurse's best response?

1. "This is a test to see if your stress level is affecting your baby's growth and well-being."
2. "This is a test to see if your baby will be able to withstand the stress of labor."
3. "This is a test to assess your baby's well-being now that you are due to deliver soon."
4. "This is a test to let us know if your baby needs to be delivered to avoid a bad outcome."

➤ *See pages 127–129 for Answers and Rationales.*

ANSWERS & RATIONALES

Pretest

1 **Answer: 1, 5** **Rationale:** CVS can be done at 10–12 weeks' gestation while amniocentesis cannot be done until 14 weeks' gestation. CVS has slightly more complications than amniocentesis and provides the same information on genetic makeup of the fetus as amniocentesis. Neither procedure requires anesthesia. Because CVS can be done earlier than amniocentesis, results are available more quickly. **Cognitive Level:** Analyzing **Client Need:** Reduction of Risk Potential **Integrated Process:** Teaching and Learning **Content Area:** Maternal-Newborn **Strategy:** Knowledge of genetic testing and the differences between CVS and amniocentesis are essential to choose the correct options. Use nursing knowledge and the process of elimination. **Reference:** Ladewig, P., London, M., & Davidson, M. (2010). *Contemporary maternal-newborn nursing care* (7th ed.). Upper Saddle River, NJ: Pearson Education, p. 305.

2 **Answer: 1** **Rationale:** A contraction stress test requires the client to have contractions, a nonstress test (NST) does not. Some testing sites ask the mother to push a button that marks the fetal heart rate strip when she feels the baby move. The NST can be done in an outpatient setting and requires 20–30 minutes of testing. **Cognitive Level:** Analyzing **Client Need:** Reduction of Risk Potential **Integrated Process:** Nursing Process: Evaluation **Content Area:** Maternal-Newborn **Strategy:** The critical words in the question are *need for further teaching.* This indicates that the correct option is a statement that is factually false. Recall what is involved with a nonstress test to answer the question correctly. **Reference:** Ladewig, P., London, M., & Davidson, M. (2010). *Contemporary maternal-newborn nursing care* (7th ed.). Upper Saddle River, NJ: Pearson Education, p. 298.

3 **Answer: 2** **Rationale:** Gestational age is best assessed in the first trimester when growth is fairly consistent among pregnancies. Position for delivery, intrauterine growth, and amniotic fluid volume are best assessed later in pregnancy. **Cognitive Level:** Applying **Client Need:** Reduction of Risk Potential **Integrated Process:** Teaching and Learning **Content Area:** Maternal-Newborn **Strategy:** The wording of the question indicates that the correct option is also a true statement. Recall the indications for an ultrasound to choose the correct option. **Reference:** Ladewig, P., London, M., & Davidson, M. (2010). *Contemporary maternal-newborn nursing care* (7th ed.). Upper Saddle River, NJ: Pearson Education, p. 292.

4 **Answer: 3 Rationale:** The oral GTT is done at about 24 weeks as this is when the fetal nutrient requirement rises, resulting in increased maternal intake and more sustained levels of blood glucose. **Cognitive Level:** Applying **Client Need:** Reduction of Risk Potential **Integrated Process:** Nursing Process: Planning **Content Area:** Maternal-Newborn **Strategy:** This question is time-dependent for a correct answer. Eliminate two options immediately as they occur too early in the pregnancy to provide valid information. Eliminate next the one that occurs too late in the pregnancy to provide intervention and reduce maternal-fetal risks. **Reference:** Ladewig, P., London, M., & Davidson, M. (2010). *Contemporary maternal-newborn nursing care* (7th ed.). Upper Saddle River, NJ: Pearson Education, p. 216.

5 **Answer: 3 Rationale:** The presence of nitrites, white blood cells, and bacteria are all indicative of a urinary tract infection. Renal insufficiency would show an increase in blood urea nitrogen and creatinine. Contamination of the urine with amniotic fluid is not realistic. Stating that the results are a normal finding in pregnancy is false because the urine should be sterile, not containing bacteria. **Cognitive Level:** Analyzing **Client Need:** **Integrated Process:** Nursing Process: Diagnosis **Content Area:** Maternal-Newborn **Strategy:** Knowledge of abnormal lab values and what they indicate is helpful to answer this question correctly. Associate the word *bacteria* in the stem of the question with the word *infection* in the correct option. **Reference:** Kee, J. L. (2010). *Laboratory and diagnostic tests with nursing implications* (8th ed.). Upper Saddle River, NJ: Pearson Education, p. 312.

6 **Answer: 3 Rationale:** When a fetal body wall defect is present, AFP leaks and is absorbed into the maternal circulation, causing the woman's serum AFP level to rise. AFP testing has nothing to do with DNA. The other explanations are inaccurate. **Cognitive Level:** Applying **Client Need:** Reduction of Risk Potential **Integrated Process:** Teaching and Learning **Content Area:** Maternal-Newborn **Strategy:** The wording of the question tells you the correct options will also be a correct statement. Knowledge of the AFP test and the indications will help to answer the question correctly. **Reference:** Ladewig, P., London, M., and Davidson, M. (2010). *Contemporary maternal-newborn nursing care* (7th ed.). Upper Saddle River, NJ: Pearson Education, p. 304.

7 **Answer: 2 Rationale:** Transmission occurs through entry of the spirochete into subcutaneous tissue through microscopic abrasions that can occur during sexual contact, kissing, and biting. It does not occur through contaminated toilet seats or shaking hands. **Cognitive Level:** Applying **Client Need:** Safety and Infection Control **Integrated Process:** Teaching and Learning **Content Area:** Maternal-Newborn **Strategy:** The wording of the question indicates that the correct option is also a true statement of fact. Knowledge of how syphilis is spread will help to answer the question correctly. **Reference:** Ladewig, P., London, M., & Davidson, M. (2010). *Contemporary maternal-newborn nursing care* (7th ed.). Upper Saddle River, NJ: Pearson Education, p. 204.

8 **Answer: 2 Rationale:** Gonorrhea contracted by the infant during the perinatal period can cause sepsis and intrauterine growth restriction. It does not cause liver damage or congenital anomalies. Most neonatal gonorrheal infections occur by the ascending route and result in ophthalmia neonatorum, an eye infection. Gonorrhea can cause perineal discharge for the mother. **Cognitive Level:** Applying **Client Need:** Physiological Adaptation **Integrated Process:** Teaching and Learning **Content Area:** Maternal-Newborn **Strategy:** The wording of the question indicates that the correct option is also a true statement of fact. Recall information about gonorrhea and the effects on the neonate to aid in choosing the correct answer. **Reference:** Ladewig, P., London, M., & Davidson, M. (2010). *Contemporary maternal-newborn nursing care* (7th ed.). Upper Saddle River, NJ: Pearson Education, p. 120.

9 **Answer: 4 Rationale:** Rash on the palms of hands and soles of feet as well as chancre sores are associated with syphilis. Crusted ulcers are commonly seen with herpes. A small, soft, papillary swelling is most likely human papilloma virus infection, which can be confirmed by colposcopy and directed biopsy. **Cognitive Level:** Analyzing **Client Need:** Physiological Adaptation **Integrated Process:** Nursing Process: Assessment **Content Area:** Maternal-Newborn **Strategy:** Correlate papilloma in the question with papillary swellings in the correct option to choose correctly. **Reference:** Ladewig, P., London, M., & Davidson, M. (2010). *Contemporary maternal-newborn nursing care* (7th ed.). Upper Saddle River, NJ: Pearson Education, p. 121.

10 **Answer: 3 Rationale:** Early detection and treatment of problems can decrease or eliminate problems for the mother or fetus that may develop or worsen as the pregnancy continues. Concern that a client will not come back is not the reason for performing all tests in one visit. Insurance reimbursement is not the reason for performing all tests in one visit. Referring to the health care provider's level of practice does not address the client's question. **Cognitive Level:** Applying **Client Need:** Health Promotion and Maintenance **Integrated Process:** Communication and Documentation **Content Area:** Maternal-Newborn **Strategy:** The focus of this question is a need for information. The correct answer would be the option that contains a true statement about a point of client education. **Reference:** Ladewig, P., London, M., & Davidson, M. (2010). *Contemporary maternal-newborn nursing care* (7th ed.). Upper Saddle River, NJ: Pearson Education, p. 21.

Posttest

1 **Answer: 2 Rationale:** The red blood cell (RBC) count is a measure of the number of red blood cells per mm^3 of peripheral blood. Within each RBC are molecules of hemoglobin, which are used to carry oxygen. White

blood cells fight infection, so a decreased count could increase the client's risk for infection. Platelets aid in blood clotting so a decreased count could increase the client's risk for bleeding. **Cognitive Level:** Analyzing **Client Need:** Reduction of Risk Potential **Integrated Process:** Nursing Process: Diagnosis **Content Area:** Maternal-Newborn **Strategy:** Correlate oxygen-carrying capacity in the question with red blood cells in the correct option. Eliminate the incorrect options because they are not related to oxygen-carrying capacity. **Reference:** Kee, J. L. (2010). *Laboratory and diagnostic tests with nursing implications* (8th ed.). Upper Saddle River, NJ: Pearson Education, p. 12.

2 **Answer: 4, 5 Rationale:** Toxoplasmosis is caused by a protozoan that is spread by ingestion of contaminated raw meat or poor handwashing after contact with cat litter. It is not spread by sexual contact, body fluids, or droplets. **Cognitive Level:** Analyzing **Client Need:** Safety and Infection Control **Integrated Process:** Nursing Process: Assessment **Content Area:** Maternal-Newborn **Strategy:** Recall that toxoplasmosis is a contact disease with an animal host. Eliminate the incorrect options that do not fit these criteria. **Reference:** Ladewig, P., London, M., & Davidson, M. (2010). *Contemporary maternal-newborn nursing care* (7th ed.). Upper Saddle River, NJ: Pearson Education, p. 365.

3 **Answer: 2 Rationale:** If test results indicate that the mother is Rh negative, she does not have the Rh antigen. If the fetus is Rh positive and fetal blood is mixed into the mother's blood, her immune system will make antibodies against the Rh antigen. This could result in erythroblastosis fetalis. Having the Rh antigen (by being Rh positive) will prevent erythroblastosis from occurring. Blood type (A, B, AB, O) does not determine the occurrence of erythroblastosis fetalis. **Cognitive Level:** Analyzing **Client Need:** Reduction of Risk Potential **Integrated Process:** Nursing Process: Planning **Content Area:** Maternal-Newborn **Strategy:** Recall that erythroblastosis fetalis is related to Rh factor. First, eliminate two options associated with blood group. Next, remember risk is associated with Rh negative status to select the correct answer. **Reference:** Ladewig, P., London, M., & Davidson, M. (2010). *Contemporary maternal-newborn nursing care* (7th ed.). Upper Saddle River, NJ: Pearson Education, p. 306.

4 **Answer: 2 Rationale:** If the nonimmune client contracts rubella, it can cause miscarriage or serious congenital anomalies. The client should not be vaccinated during pregnancy as the fetus can contract rubella from the live-virus vaccine. Immunity can be determined by assessing a rubella titer. Asking the client's mother is a less reliable method than obtaining a rubella titer. **Cognitive Level:** Analyzing **Client Need:** Health Promotion and Maintenance **Integrated Process:** Nursing Process: Planning **Content Area:** Maternal-Newborn **Strategy:** This question provides incomplete data about the client's immunity. The correct answer would be the option that provides for additional assessment and objective data to determine whether or not the client is immune. **Reference:** Ladewig, P., London, M., & Davidson, M. (2010). *Contemporary maternal-newborn nursing care* (7th ed.). Upper Saddle River, NJ: Pearson Education, p. 362.

5 **Answer: 3 Rationale:** The test requires that the client eat a high-carbohydrate diet for three days and then fast for at least eight hours before testing begins. Clients should not consume caffeine as it tends to increase glucose levels. **Cognitive Level:** Analyzing **Client Need:** Reduction of Risk Potential **Integrated Process:** Nursing Process: Evaluation **Content Area:** Maternal-Newborn **Strategy:** The positive wording of the question indicates the correct option is also a true statement. Knowledge of the procedure to follow for having the test done will aid in choosing the correct answer. **Reference:** Ladewig, P., London, M., & Davidson, M. (2010). *Contemporary maternal-newborn nursing care* (7th ed.). Upper Saddle River, NJ: Pearson Education, p. 316.

6 **Answer: 1 Rationale:** Transvaginal ultrasound, used most often in the first trimester, avoids the need to scan through thick abdominal layers of obese clients. Some modest clients are embarrassed by the use of vaginal scanning. Neither abdominal nor vaginal ultrasound has been shown to have harmful effects on the fetus. **Cognitive Level:** Analyzing **Client Need:** Reduction of Risk Potential **Integrated Process:** Nursing Process: Planning **Content Area:** Maternal-Newborn **Strategy:** The critical words in this question are *indication for transvaginal.* Since most pregnancy ultrasounds are done transabdominally, look for an option that makes the abdominal route unlikely. **Reference:** Ladewig, P., London, M., & Davidson, M. (2010). *Contemporary maternal-newborn nursing care* (7th ed.). Upper Saddle River, NJ: Pearson Education, p. 294.

7 **Answer: 4 Rationale:** Scores on the biophysical profile can range from 0 to 10. A score of less than four indicates impending fetal death and a need for immediate delivery. Telling the mother that the test result indicates fetal well-being is false. Rescheduling the mother for a repeat test in a week or the next day delays care and puts both the mother and fetus at risk. **Cognitive Level:** Analyzing **Client Need:** Physiological Adaptation **Integrated Process:** Nursing Process: Implementation **Content Area:** Maternal-Newborn **Strategy:** Recall that a biophysical profile assigns scores on five criteria; the lower the score the greater the risk to the fetus. The correct answer will indicate the greatest fetal risk and need for immediate intervention. **Reference:** Ladewig, P., London, M., & Davidson, M. (2010). *Contemporary maternal-newborn nursing care* (7th ed.). Upper Saddle River, NJ: Pearson Education, p. 299.

8 **Answer: 4 Rationale:** Before 12 weeks, length as measured by crown-rump length is the most accurate measure of gestation age. Biparietal diameter and femur length are

used to monitor fetal growth later in pregnancy. Abdominal circumference can be used to identify some congenital anomalies. **Cognitive Level:** Applying **Client Need:** Health Promotion and Maintenance **Integrated Process:** Nursing Process: Assessment **Content Area:** Maternal-Newborn **Strategy:** The core issue in this question is fetal growth in early pregnancy. Eliminate the incorrect options because they are dependent on more advanced fetal development that occurs later in gestation. **Reference:** Ladewig, P., London, M., & Davidson, M. (2010). *Contemporary maternal-newborn nursing care* (7th ed.). Upper Saddle River, NJ: Pearson Education, p. 295.

9 **Answer: 4 Rationale:** Complications including hemorrhage, damage to the mother's intestines or bladder, infection, and miscarriage can occur but they are very rare. The procedure is not completely safe. Deferring the question to the health care provider does not address the client's concern. Being still does not avoid risks of the procedure and it also places an unnecessary burden on the client. **Cognitive Level:** Applying **Client Need:** Reduction of Risk Potential **Integrated Process:** Nursing Process: Implementation **Content Area:** Maternal-Newborn **Strategy:** Recall the complications of amniocentesis and use the process of elimination to choose the correct answer. **Reference:** Ladewig, P., London, M., & Davidson, M. (2010). *Contemporary maternal-newborn nursing care* (7th ed.). Upper Saddle River, NJ: Pearson Education, p. 302.

10 **Answer: 3 Rationale:** The non-stress test is a measure of fetal well-being. It is not an accurate predictor of ability to withstand labor or of poor outcome. Test results are not related to the woman's stress level. **Cognitive Level:** Applying **Client Need:** Reduction of Risk Potential **Integrated Process:** Teaching and Learning **Content Area:** Maternal-Newborn **Strategy:** The question is worded in a positive manner, indicating the correct option will be a true statement. Recall the uses of the non-stress test to answer this question correctly. **Reference:** Ladewig, P., London, M., & Davidson, M. (2010). *Contemporary maternal-newborn nursing care* (7th ed.). Upper Saddle River, NJ: Pearson Education, p. 298.

References

Corbett, J. (2008). *Laboratory tests and diagnostic procedures with nursing diagnoses* (7th ed.). Upper Saddle River, NJ: Pearson Education.

Davidson, M., London, M. & Ladewig, P. (2012). *Olds' maternal newborn nursing & women's health across the lifespan* (9th ed.). Upper Saddle River, NJ: Pearson Education.

Kee, J. L. (2010). *Laboratory and diagnostic tests with nursing implications* (8th ed.). Upper Saddle River, NJ: Pearson Education.

Ladewig, P., London, M., and Davidson, M. (2009). *Contemporary maternal-newborn nursing care* (7th ed.). Upper Saddle River, NJ: Pearson Education.

Orshan, S. A. (2008). *Maternity, newborn, and women's health nursing: Comprehensive care across the life span.* Philadelphia: Lippincott Williams & Wilkins.

Pagana, K., & Pagana, T. (2009). *Manual of diagnostic and laboratory tests* (4th ed.). St. Louis, MO: Mosby.

Ricci, S. (2009). *Essentials of maternity, newborn, and women's health nursing* (2nd ed.). Philadelphia: Lippincott Williams & Wilkins.

The Universe of Women's Health. Retrieved February 1, 2011, from http://www.obgyn.net/pregnancy-birth/pregnancy-birth.asp?page=/pregnancy-birth/articles/survellance

7 The Complicated Prenatal Experience

Chapter Outline

Nursing Care of the High-Risk Prenatal Client

Pregestational Conditions

Gestational Conditions

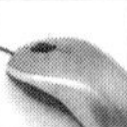

NCLEX-RN® Test Prep

Use the accompanying online resource, NursingReviewsandRationales, to test yourself with hundreds of NCLEX®-style practice questions.

Objectives

- Describe nursing assessments and interventions designed to improve the health of the high-risk prenatal client.
- Describe the effect of preexisting conditions on the health of the pregnant woman and her fetus.
- Delineate nursing responsibilities in the care of the woman with gestational onset complications of pregnancy.

Review at a Glance

abortion spontaneous or induced pregnancy loss before 20 weeks' gestation

abruptio placenta premature separation of normally implanted placenta away from uterine wall

cerclage procedure of looping a suture around cervix to keep it securely closed during pregnancy; used to treat incompetent cervix

chorioamnionitis inflammation and infection in fetal membranes and amniotic fluid

Coombs' test lab test to identify antibodies on RBCs; a direct Coombs' test determines if there are maternal anti-Rh antibodies in fetal cord blood, while an indirect Coombs' identifies anti-Rh antibodies in mother's blood

ectopic pregnancy abnormally placed pregnancy outside uterus

erythroblastosis fetalis destruction of fetal RBCs by maternal anti-Rh antibodies causes production of many immature RBCs (erythroblasts) in fetus

gestational diabetes a disorder of carbohydrate metabolism caused by inability of maternal pancreas to produce additional insulin needed during pregnancy

gestational trophoblastic disease (GTD) rapid reproduction of outermost developing layer of embryo; includes hydatiform mole, invasive mole, and choriocarcinoma

hydrops fetalis generalized fetal edema caused by destruction of fetal RBCs by maternal anti-Rh antibodies

kernicterus yellow staining of basal ganglia and brain from deposit of excessive unbound bilirubin, associated with a poor outcome

macrosomia excessively large body and high birth weight, as in infants of diabetic mothers who experience high glucose levels in utero

placenta previa abnormal implantation of placenta low in uterus near or covering cervical os

PRETEST

1 A client with Class II heart disease is being seen for her first prenatal visit. Which of the following teaching points would the nurse stress for this client? Select all that apply.

1. Avoid all over-the-counter (OTC) medications during pregnancy
2. Regular exercise will help increase cardiac capacity during pregnancy
3. It's important to take prenatal vitamins and iron as prescribed
4. The client's fetus will probably have a similar congenital heart defect
5. Adequate nutrition to prevent anemia and avoid excessive weight gain

2 A client with type 1 diabetes mellitus gives birth. The postpartum nurse monitors the blood glucose level carefully, expecting that the mother's insulin requirements in the first 24 hours after delivery will follow which trend?

1. Drop significantly
2. Gradually return to normal
3. Increase slightly
4. Stay the same as before delivery

3 The nurse is especially interested in the results of which laboratory test that provides the nurse with the best information about ongoing control of type 1 diabetes mellitus in a pregnant adolescent?

1. Fasting blood glucose
2. Glycosylated hemoglobin (HbA1c)
3. Oral glucose tolerance test (OGTT)
4. Post-prandial glucose

4 What would be an appropriate interpretation by the nurse when a substance abusing pregnant woman presents herself for prenatal care?

1. She is ready to stop abusing illegal substances
2. She must be reported to the authorities
3. She recognizes the need for caring interventions
4. She will lack appropriate parenting skills

5 Which nursing action would take priority when caring for a woman with a suspected ectopic pregnancy?

1. Administer oxygen
2. Monitor vital signs
3. Obtain surgical consent
4. Provide emotional support

6 A client is being discharged from the hospital after evacuation of a molar pregnancy. The nurse recognizes that additional discharge teaching is required when the client makes which statement?

1. "I am so sad that I lost this baby."
2. "I may need to have chemotherapy after this."
3. "I will need to see the doctor yearly for follow-up."
4. "I will use contraception for the next year."

7 The charge nurse in the labor and delivery unit has become overwhelmed with admissions and births. For which client can the charge nurse best delegate the needed care to a trusted certified nursing assistant (CNA) who is currently going to school to become a nurse?

1. A client in false labor, who needs teaching about true versus false labor signs
2. A client with preeclampsia who needs evaluation for reflexes and clonus
3. A primigravida in early labor who needs to be helped to the bathroom
4. An obese laboring client who needs to have her fetal monitor adjusted

PRETEST

8 A client with a known placenta previa is admitted at 30 weeks' gestation with painless vaginal bleeding. The nurse weighs the client's peri-pads to monitor blood loss. After noting an increased weight of 50 grams, the nurse would document that this equals approximately _____ mL blood loss.

Fill in your answer below:
_____ mL

9 A client with hyperemesis gravidarum would most likely benefit from nursing care designed to address which nursing diagnosis?

1. Imbalanced Nutrition: More Than Body Requirements related to pregnancy
2. Anxiety related to effects of hyperemesis on fetal well-being
3. Anticipatory Grieving related to inevitable pregnancy loss
4. Ineffective Coping related to unwanted pregnancy

10 The initial laboratory results for a primigravida indicate a hemoglobin of 12 grams/dL, hematocrit of 36%, and a blood group and type of A, Rh-negative. What would be the priority nursing action to promote a healthy pregnancy for this client and her fetus?

1. Plan to determine the blood type of the infant after delivery
2. Encourage the client to eat more dark-green leafy vegetables
3. Provide information on weight gain during pregnancy
4. Suggest an iron supplement in addition to prenatal vitamins

➤ *See pages 150–151 for Answers and Rationales.*

I. NURSING CARE OF THE HIGH-RISK PRENATAL CLIENT

A. Identifying clients at risk

1. Ideally begins even before pregnancy, continues with first prenatal visit, and proceeds through puerperium
2. Risk factors are anything that may be associated with a negative pregnancy outcome including physiological, psychological, sociodemographic, or environmental factors

B. Monitoring of high-risk clients: it is important during pregnancy, labor, and birth, and puerperium to fully assess and monitor closely clients at high risk for complications, so as to improve maternal–fetal outcomes

II. PREGESTATIONAL CONDITIONS

A. Cardiac disease

1. Description and etiology

a. Hemodynamic changes of pregnancy increase workload on heart; cardiac output (CO) increases 30–50% by midpregnancy; a compromised heart with inadequate cardiac capacity and decreased reserves may be unable to adapt to added requirements of pregnancy

b. Treatment options and the likelihood of a positive pregnancy outcome depend on the degree of cardiac compromise as determined by a cardiologist in consultation with the perinatologist; see Table 7-1 for classification of functional capacity for clients with cardiac disease

c. Maternal congenital heart defects that have been effectively treated by modern techniques are being seen more often during pregnancy as this population reaches adulthood; there are decreasing numbers of pregnant women with heart damage from rheumatic fever because of effective treatment of streptococcal infections

Table 7-1 Classification of Functional Capacity for Clients with Cardiac Disease (NYHA, 1994)

Classification	Functional Capacity
I	No limitation on physical activity and no symptoms of cardiac insufficiency (fatigue, palpitations, or dyspnea) with ordinary activity; no anginal pain
II	Slight limitation of physical activity; no symptoms at rest but ordinary activity may cause fatigue, palpitations, dyspnea, or anginal pain
III	Marked limitation of physical activity; no symptoms at rest but less than ordinary activity may cause fatigue, palpitations, dyspnea, or anginal pain
IV	Unable to carry out any physical activity without discomfort; client may experience symptoms even at rest, and they worsen with any activity

! 2. Assessment: most common complication of heart disease during pregnancy is congestive heart failure (CHF)
   a. Edema of varying degree from pedal edema, pitting edema, generalized edema (anasarca), and pulmonary edema
   b. Dyspnea on exertion, increasing fatigue, dyspnea at rest, moist cough, basilar crackles, cyanosis of nail beds, circumoral cyanosis
   c. Tachycardia, irregular pulse, murmurs, chest pain
3. Priority nursing diagnoses: Decreased Cardiac Output; Excess Fluid Volume; Impaired Gas Exchange; Activity Intolerance; Anxiety; Risk for Infection; Deficient Knowledge
4. Implementation and collaborative care
   a. Monitor client and fetal well-being more frequently during pregnancy; changes in maternal vital signs or signs of fetal compromise may indicate inability to handle increasing demands on heart
   b. Coordinate care including both cardiologist and perinatologist, as well as any ancillary departments involved with care such as radiology or rehabilitation
   ! c. Teach adequate nutrition for pregnancy and provide prenatal vitamins and iron to prevent anemia; monitor for signs of infection
   ! d. Instruct client to avoid excessive weight gain or emotional stress, which place added stress on cardiac reserves
   e. Teach client signs of infection to report so treatment may begin early
   f. Diagnostic procedures may include auscultation, electrocardiogram, echocardiogram, and possible cardiac catheterization
   g. Medication therapy in addition to prenatal vitamins and iron may include the following:
      ! 1) Prophylactic antibiotics for any invasive procedures, including dental work, and at time of birth to prevent bacterial endocarditis; penicillin (PCN) is usually prescribed unless client is allergic to it
      2) Cardiac glycosides (digoxin) to increase cardiac contractility and slow heart rate for effective filling
      3) Antidysrhythmia agents for cardiac dysrhythmias
      4) Diuretic such as furosemide (Lasix) to decrease fluid excess; take care to ensure adequate circulating volume to maintain uteroplacental perfusion
      ! 5) Heparin is considered safe for use in pregnancy if an anticoagulant is indicated (Pregnancy Category C); warfarin (Coumadin) is a Pregnancy Category X drug (see Table 7-2 for a listing of drug pregnancy categories)
   h. Teach client to avoid exertion and to plan frequent rest periods to maintain cardiac reserves

Table 7-2 FDA Pregnancy Categories for Prescription Drugs

Category	Risk to the Fetus	Examples of Drugs
A	Controlled studies in women do not demonstrate a risk to fetus in first trimester, and possibility of fetal harm appears remote.	RDA dose of Vitamin C
B	Animal studies have not demonstrated fetal risk but there are no controlled studies in women; animal studies show an adverse effect not confirmed in controlled studies in women in first trimester.	Acetaminophen (Tylenol) Penicillins
C	Animal studies show adverse effects and there are no controlled studies in women; studies in women and animals are not available. Drug should be given only if potential benefit justifies potential risk to fetus.	Zidovudine (Retrovir) Heparin (Liquaemin)
D	Positive evidence of fetal risk in humans but benefits to mother may be acceptable despite risk in certain situations.	Phenobarbitol (Luminal)
X	Risks to fetus clearly outweigh any possible benefit to mother. Drug is contraindicated in women who may become pregnant.	Warfarin (Coumadin) Diethylstilbestrol (DES)

i. Provide adequate pain relief during labor to avoid excessive maternal stress; vaginal delivery is preferred with epidural anesthesia, continuous maternal oxygen administration, and a low-forceps delivery to decrease maternal straining
j. Observe client carefully for complications from hemodynamic changes immediately after delivery as this is known to be a very high-risk time for pregnant cardiac client

5. Evaluation: client experiences a healthy pregnancy, avoids heart failure or cardiac decompensation, and gives birth to a healthy infant

B. Diabetes mellitus (DM)

1. Description
   a. An endocrine disorder with major effects on carbohydrate metabolism; results from insufficient insulin production in beta cells of pancreas or inadequate use of insulin; insulin facilitates movement of glucose from blood into tissue cells for storage or energy use; in a client with type 1 DM, pancreas has all but stopped producing insulin, so client and fetus are at much higher risk than client with gestational diabetes
   b. **Gestational diabetes** mellitus (GMD) results when pancreas is unable to meet increased demands for insulin production during pregnancy
2. Effect of pregnancy on glucose metabolism
   a. During first trimester, insulin needs are low or decreased; although type 1 diabetic clients may experience vast swings in glucose control as compared to their prepregnancy glucose control
   b. Late in first trimester insulin requirements begin to rise as glucose use and glycogen storage by mother and fetus increase
   c. ! Human placental lactogen (hPL) from placenta causes resistance to action of maternal insulin thereby increasing circulating glucose for fetal use and increasing demand on maternal pancreas to produce more insulin
   d. Fetus produces own insulin but obtains glucose from mother across placenta; amount of glucose available in maternal circulation stimulates fetal pancreas to produce insulin
3. Effects of diabetes on pregnancy and fetus relate to degree of control of blood glucose (BG) levels between 70 mg/dL and 110 mg/dL and degree of vascular involvement; complications are more common with type 1 DM and include the following:
   a. Maternal hydraminos (increased volume of amniotic fluid); occurs in 10–20% of type 1 diabetic mothers during pregnancy

   b. Preeclampsia, eclampsia, ketoacidosis, and worsening retinopathy
   c. Dystocia, shoulder dystocia, and stillbirth (usually after 36 weeks)
   d. Neonatal **macrosomia** (large body), hypoglycemia, hyperbilirubinemia, delayed fetal lung maturity resulting in respiratory distress syndrome (RDS), and increased incidence of congenital anomalies including defects of heart or neural tube and sacral agenesis

4. Assessment
   a. Risk factors: family history of diabetes, maternal obesity, previous large-for-gestational age (LGA) infants, previous unexplained stillbirth
   b. Classic symptoms of DM are polyuria, polydipsia, polyphagia
   c. Possibly more frequent urinary tract infections and vaginal candidiasis (yeast) infections caused by altered pH in reproductive tract
   d. Urine testing for glycosuria and ketones as part of routine prenatal care is helpful in assessing glucose control for client with DM and to detect onset of GDM
   e. Diabetes screening should be done around 28 weeks' gestation or earlier if there are risk factors such as history of GDM in previous pregnancies or obesity; client receives a 50-gram oral glucose tolerance test (GTT); if BG is greater than 140 mg/dL at one hour, a three-hour 100-gram oral GTT is performed
   f. Long-term glucose control is estimated with serum glycosylated hemoglobin (HbA_{1c}), which measures percent of hemoglobin with glucose bound to it (glyco-hemoglobin); levels depend on amount of circulating glucose during red blood cell's 120-day lifespan

5. Priority nursing diagnoses: Risk for Imbalanced Nutrition, Maternal and Fetal: More Than Body Requirements; Risk for Injury: Maternal and Fetal; Anxiety; Deficient Knowledge

6. Implementation and collaborative care
   a. Teach client about prescribed ADA diet regulation with no concentrated sweets; dietary regulation usually adequate to control GDM; excessive weight gain should be avoided; caloric needs will increase as pregnancy progresses
   b. Medications: oral hypoglycemic medications such as glyburide (Diabeta) are now used in pregnancy with some clients; insulin (human) more commonly used, must be carefully regulated and adjusted as pregnancy progresses with up to a four-fold dose increase in insulin dose at term
   c. High-risk clients are often hospitalized in order to manage insulin needs, especially in early pregnancy
   d. Instruct client and possibly partner in frequent BG, urine glucose, and ketone testing and keeping a diary of test results and activity levels; also instruct in performing fetal kick counts
   e. Encourage regular nonstrenuous exercise such as walking for control of weight and BG
   f. Monitor fetal well-being: quadruple screen as scheduled, ultrasound for anomalies, amniotic fluid volume, and fetal size; fetal movement counts, weekly non-stress test (NST) from 28 to 32 weeks, possible oxytocin challenge test (OCT), bio-physical profile (BPP), and amniocentesis for lung maturity to assess:
      1) Lecithin/sphingomyelin (L/S) ratio needs to be 1:3 (normal is 1:2)
      2) Phosphatidylglycerol (PG) should be present
   g. Monitor client for development of complications: infection, preeclampsia, and diabetic ketoacidosis
   h. Prepare for possible induction of labor at 38 to 39 weeks with type 1 DM to reduce risk for stillbirth caused by premature placental aging
   i. Prepare for possibility of shoulder dystocia: emergency of second stage of labor, head delivers but fetal shoulders are stuck, risk increased with macrosomia

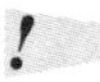

j. Insulin requirements drop dramatically after delivery of placenta and removal of hormonal influences; client may need no insulin or a decreased dose; clients with GDM generally may eat a regular diet

7. Evaluation: HgbA1c levels <7, client maintains BG control during pregnancy and delivers healthy fetus without complications; newborn has normal BG levels

C. Substance abuse

1. Description and etiology
   a. As many as 10% of pregnant women use tobacco, alcohol, or other drugs, often in combination; clients using illegal drugs may delay seeking care for fear of prosecution; all pregnant women should be screened for substance abuse
   b. Substances frequently used in United States are tobacco, alcohol, marijuana, cocaine, crack cocaine, and heroin; methylenedioxymethamphetamine (MDMA or Ecstasy) is most commonly used club drug; effects on pregnancy include spontaneous abortion, intrauterine growth restriction (IUGR), preterm labor, placental abruption, stillbirth, neonatal addiction, and fetal alcohol syndrome (FAS)
2. Assessment
   a. Establish a trusting relationship with client by remaining open, matter-of-fact, and nonjudgmental; women seeking prenatal care (PNC) are interested in improving and safeguarding their health and that of fetus and should be praised for seeking PNC
   b. Encourage client to describe all substances used, amounts, times, and triggers to use, and any previous attempts to discontinue use
   c. Evaluate client's motivation, support systems, and personal strengths that may be elicited to change behaviors
3. Priority nursing diagnoses: Ineffective Health Maintenance; Ineffective Coping; Risk for Impaired Gas Exchange; Risk for Delayed Growth and Development; Deficient Knowledge
4. Implementation and collaborative care
   a. Monitor client for compliance with plan of care and screen for complications: anemia, inadequate nutrition and weight gain, hypertension, preterm labor; random urine toxicology screens may be ordered
   b. Monitor fetal growth and well-being: maternal weight gain, fetal kick counts, fundal height, ultrasound, NST, BPP
   c. Teach client about potential negative effects of substance use on pregnancy and fetus/neonate; teach about need *not* to discontinue methadone during pregnancy and that this can threaten pregnancy
   d. Assist with referrals as indicated: smoking cessation classes, Alcoholics Anonymous, addiction counseling, psychological counseling, and possible hospitalization
   e. Reinforce teaching about nutrition and effects on fetal development; teach danger signs of pregnancy including signs of preterm labor, bleeding or leaking of fluid, and decreased fetal movement
   f. Support client's efforts to change negative behaviors
   g. Client may need to be followed by a perinatologist during pregnancy; an addicted neonate may require intensive care at birth; infants of mothers using methadone or heroin or other opiates will need to be evaluated using a neonatal abstinence scale (NAS) for symptoms of withdrawal and possible treatment with opiates for withdrawal symptoms
   h. Clients with a heroin addiction may be put on methadone rather than the street drug, heroin; however, clients have been known to use both prescribed methadone and street drugs, so toxicology screens may be indicted
   i. Document maternal behaviors and compliance during pregnancy, results of random toxicology screens, and consult with social service; anticipate postpartum issues and possible state intervention evaluating safety of maternal care

Practice to Pass

A client who takes methadone for heroin addiction is in active labor and asking for something for pain. The physician's standing order calls for butorphanol (Stadol), a narcotic agonist–antagonist, to be given IV push. Discuss your concerns about giving this drug to this client.

   j. Maintain strict confidentiality as required by HIPAA and as desired by client, who may not have told partner and/or family about substance abuse
5. Evaluation: client decreases substance abuse during pregnancy and delivers a healthy term neonate; client develops more effective coping mechanisms

D. Human immunodeficiency virus (HIV)/Acquired immunodeficiency syndrome (AIDS)

1. Description and etiology
   a. HIV type 1 (HIV-1) causes condition known as AIDS; HIV is transmitted through contact with infected blood and body secretions, usually during sexual contact or use of contaminated needles; HIV infection progresses to AIDS, characterized by decreased immunity and overwhelming opportunistic infection
   b. Pregnancy does not appear to change course of illness for mother; fetus may contract virus transplacentally or through breast milk, but generally fetal infection is considered to occur during vaginal birth

   c. Current maternal treatment with antiretroviral drugs as described by Centers for Disease Control (CDC), which may include zidovudine (Retrovir) orally during pregnancy and intravenously during labor and delivery, has decreased neonatal transmission to $<7\%$ with vaginal birth and $<1\%$ with cesarean birth
   d. Maternal HIV antibodies cross placenta so all infants of HIV-positive mothers will test positive at birth and until maternal antibodies are depleted at between 15 to 18 months of age

Practice to Pass

When caring for a postpartum HIV positive mother, what precautions would you take? What precautions would you teach the mother to take to protect her newborn?

2. Assessment
   a. Antibodies to HIV are detected with enzyme-linked immunosorbent assay (ELISA) test and results confirmed by Western blot test
   b. All pregnant women should be offered HIV testing because most clients are asymptomatic for an average of 10 years before signs of opportunistic infection occur
3. Priority nursing diagnoses: Risk for Infection: Maternal and fetal; Decisional Conflict; Compromised Family Coping; Anticipatory Grieving; Deficient Knowledge
4. Implementation and collaborative care
   a. Provide emotional support and reproductive counseling to client and family
   b. Evaluate client for other sexually transmitted infections and hepatitis B
   c. Review lab results for signs of anemia, thrombocytopenia, leukopenia, and decreased CD-4 T lymphocytes

   d. Monitor client for signs of opportunistic infection: fever, weight loss, fatigue, candidiasis, cough, skin lesions
   e. Administer prophylactic antiretroviral drugs as ordered during pregnancy and labor and delivery
   f. Monitor fetal growth and well-being

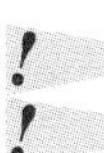

   g. Use standard blood and body fluid precautions with all clients
   h. Protect fetus from maternal secretions
      1) Avoid use of fetal scalp electrode or other invasive devices during labor
      2) Wash infant's eyes and face at birth before administering prophylactic eye drops or ointment; bathe entire newborn as soon as possible after delivery to remove all maternal secretions
      3) Delay any newborn injections or heel-sticks until after bath
      4) Encourage mother to formula-feed newborn to prevent transmission by breast milk
5. Evaluation: client's illness remains stable without opportunistic infection; infant is healthy and tests HIV-negative at 18 months; client and family develop effective coping mechanisms to plan for infant's future

E. Rh sensitization

1. Description and etiology
   a. Rh-negative women who become pregnant with an Rh-positive embryo/fetus (from an Rh-positive father) become sensitized to Rh antigen when there is contact between maternal and fetal blood; other causes of Rh-sensitization might be blood transfusion of Rh-positive blood to an Rh-negative woman, or fetomaternal blood contact during an amniocentesis or other invasive procedure
   b. Sensitized Rh-negative women develop anti-Rh antibodies, which cross placenta in subsequent Rh-positive pregnancies and destroy fetal RBCs
   c. Fetal effects of Rh incompatibility and sensitization are progressively severe
2. Hemolysis of fetal RBCs leads to greatly increased immature RBC production, termed **erythroblastosis fetalis**
3. Continued RBC destruction and anemia results in jaundice and marked fetal edema, known as **hydrops fetalis**, and may lead to fetal congestive heart failure
4. Breakdown of RBCs releases bilirubin, causing jaundice; high levels of circulating bilirubin can cause **kernicterus**, a condition of yellow staining of basal ganglia and brain from bilirubin deposits and may result in permanent neurological damage
5. Assessment
   a. All pregnant women should be tested for blood group, Rh factor, and routine antibody screening; a history of previous miscarriage, blood transfusions, or infants experiencing jaundice should be noted
   b. If client is Rh-negative, father of infant may be tested to determine his Rh status; an Rh-negative father and mother will only produce Rh-negative offspring who will not be affected by Rh-incompatibility
   c. An indirect **Coombs' test** on maternal blood determines whether Rh-negative client has developed antibodies to Rh antigen; serial antibody screening should continue throughout pregnancy to identify increasing antibody production; a direct Coombs' test is done on infant's blood after birth to identify maternal antibodies attached to fetal RBCs
6. Priority nursing diagnoses: Risk for Injury; Deficient Knowledge; Anxiety
7. Implementation and collaborative care
   a. Provide support and education to client and family; client should carry an Rh-negative identification card and recognize that she may need medication RhoGAM with future pregnancies
   b. Unsensitized Rh-negative clients should be given 300 mcg of Rh immune globulin (RhoGAM) IM at 28 weeks, at time of amniocentesis, chorionic villus sampling, abortion, ectopic pregnancy, external fetal version, trauma or possible bleeding internally, and also within 72 hours of delivery if infant has tested to be Rh positive because of risk of maternal exposure to fetal Rh antigen (antibodies in immune globulin bind with any Rh antigens in maternal circulation)
   c. RhoGAM is not given to mothers who are already sensitized and have antibodies (positive indirect Coombs' test)
   d. The Kleihauer-Betke test estimates amount of fetal blood in maternal circulation; is used to determine dose of Rh immune globulin when a larger fetal–maternal bleed is suspected
   e. Evaluate fetus for development of complications using serial ultrasound for amniotic fluid volume, fetal size, enlarged heart, and development of edema
   f. A sinusoidal electronic fetal monitoring pattern indicates severe fetal anemia; biophysical profile (BPP) may be used to identify a compromised fetus
   g. Amniocentesis or percutaneous umbilical cord blood sampling (PUBS) may be used to determine fetal Rh; both procedures carry risk of causing maternal exposure and sensitization, so RhoGAM should be given

h. An early delivery with phototherapy and exchange transfusions may be planned if fetus is developing anemia close to term
i. Intrauterine exchange transfusion may be performed for severely affected fetus until viability is reached

8. Evaluation: Rh-negative client delivers a healthy infant with a negative direct Coombs' test; client receives prophylactic Rh immune globulin to prevent maternal antibody formation that might complicate future pregnancies

III. GESTATIONAL CONDITIONS

A. Hyperemesis gravidarum

1. Description and etiology
   a. Hyperemesis gravidarum, or excessive vomiting during pregnancy, is characterized by extreme nausea and vomiting (N/V) during first half of pregnancy that is associated with dehydration, weight loss, and electrolyte imbalances; emesis is much more severe than common "morning sickness" during early pregnancy and occurs in about 1% of pregnancies
   b. Exact cause of excessive vomiting is not known; hormones including increased levels of hCG are thought to contribute; hyperemesis is rare in developing countries; high levels of hCG, as are found in **gestational trophoblastic disease** (hydatidiform mole, molar pregnancy) and multiple gestation, are associated with severe N/V in pregnancy so therefore may need to be ruled in or out for these clients
   c. Fetus is at risk for abnormal development, IUGR, or death from lack of nutrition, hypoxia, and maternal ketoacidosis
2. Assessment
   a. Intractable vomiting with onset at some time in pregnancy not attributable to other causes
   b. Dehydration with: weight loss of more than 5% of prepregnancy weight, poor skin turgor, dry mucous membranes, possible hypotension, tachycardia, and increased lab values for hematocrit and urine specific gravity
   c. Signs and symptoms of electrolyte or acid–base imbalance (metabolic acidosis): ketosis, confusion, drowsiness, muscle weakness, cramps, clumsiness, tremors, irregular heartbeat, decreased level of consciousness
   d. Signs and symptoms of starvation: weight loss, muscle wasting, ketonuria, jaundice, bleeding gums (vitamin deficiency)
3. Priority nursing diagnoses: Deficient Fluid Volume; Risk for Injury; Imbalanced Nutrition: Less Than Body Requirements; Ineffective Coping
4. Implementation and collaborative care
   a. Client may need hospitalization and IV fluid therapy with glucose, electrolytes, and vitamins to begin treatment and then continue at home once stabilized; nutritional consult is indicated
   b. Monitor daily weight and measure intake and output; assess vital signs as appropriate, hydration, and nutritional status
   c. Administer antiemetics such as phenothiazines or antihistamines as ordered to control N/V
   ! d. Encourage six small feedings a day after acute N/V has passed; clear liquids, such as lemonade and herbal teas, and salty foods are sometimes better tolerated at first
   e. Total parenteral nutrition (TPN) may be required in severe cases when client is unable to tolerate oral feedings
   f. Monitor fetal growth with serial ultrasounds
   g. Counsel client and family that symptoms are not her fault or psychosomatic

! 5. Evaluation: client exhibits signs of adequate hydration: moist mucous membranes, good skin turgor, stable vital signs and intake equal to output; client tolerates adequate nutrition for maternal and fetal requirements and gains appropriate weight during pregnancy

B. ***Ectopic pregnancy***

1. Description and etiology: implantation of a fertilized ovum outside uterus; sites may include ovary or elsewhere in abdominal cavity, but most common site is fallopian tube, which may have been narrowed by scarring or adhesions, ascending infections, pelvic inflammatory disease (PID), use of IUD contraception, or tubal surgery (these are risk factors for tubal damage that may result in an ectopic pregnancy)
2. Assessment
   - **a.** Interview reveals last normal menstrual period (LNMP) consistent with possible pregnancy and possible subjective symptoms of pregnancy such as breast tenderness and nausea
   - ! **b.** Generalized abdominal pain or referred shoulder pain or unilateral lower abdominal pain: may be slowly increasing or sudden and severe with abdominal rigidity and referred right shoulder pain
   - ! **c.** Possible irregular vaginal bleeding or signs of hypovolemic shock if fallopian tube has ruptured; prioritize care accordingly
   - **d.** Laboratory tests: serial quantitative ß-hCG to assess rise of ß-hCG in normally implanted pregnancy
   - **e.** Ultrasound confirms an extrauterine pregnancy
3. Priority nursing diagnoses: Risk for Deficient Fluid Volume; Pain; Fear; Anticipatory Grieving
4. Implementation and collaborative care
   - ! **a.** Monitor blood pressure, pulse, and respirations every 15 minutes, or more frequently if indicated by client condition
   - ! **b.** Start an IV of ordered fluid with at least an 18-gauge needle in case blood products need to be given
   - **c.** Provide oxygen as indicated for shock
   - **d.** Medicate for pain as ordered
   - **e.** Obtain laboratory tests: ß-hCG, CBC, and blood group and type; type and cross-match if hemorrhage is suspected
   - **f.** Prepare client for surgery; if possible, pregnancy will be evacuated and tube preserved for future fertility if desired
   - **g.** Provide routine preoperative care and teaching; offer emotional support to client and family
   - **h.** Provide general postoperative care; facilitate grieving; provide RhoGAM for Rh-negative mothers with an Rh-positive partner; teach client and partner about implications for future pregnancies
5. Evaluation: client experiences evacuation of ectopic pregnancy; vital signs remain stable without signs of hypovolemic shock; fertility is preserved as desired; client and family begin grieving their loss

C. **Gestational trophoblastic disease (GTD)**

1. Description and etiology: abnormal growth of trophoblastic tissue including placenta and chorion
   - **a.** Complete or partial hydatidiform mole or a molar pregnancy is characterized by abnormal development of placenta; chorionic villi grow rapidly into fluid-filled, grapelike clusters; a complete mole develops from an empty ovum that contains no maternal genetic material; a partial mole may have an abnormal embryo that usually spontaneously aborts in first trimester

b. Invasive mole (chorioadenoma destruens) is similar to a complete hydatiform mole but involves uterine myometrium
c. Choriocarcinoma, malignant GTD, is invasive, usually metastatic, and can be fatal; develops following evacuation of a mole in 20% of women

2. Assessment
a. Variable vaginal bleeding usually occurs during first trimester; may be brown, like prune juice, and may contain some grapelike vesicles
b. Unusual uterine growth measured by fundal height; no fetal parts can be palpated and no FHT are heard; "snowstorm" pattern seen on ultrasound
c. Abnormal labs include very high ß-hCG levels and very low MSAFP (maternal serum ß-fetoprotein) levels
d. Complications associated with molar pregnancy include hyperemesis gravidarum (probably associated with high ß-hCG levels), and severe preeclampsia that occurs during first half of pregnancy and is an indication of molar pregnancy; other complications include hyperthyroidism and possible trophoblastic pulmonary embolism

3. Priority nursing diagnoses: Deficient Fluid Volume; Anticipatory Grieving; Fear; Deficient Knowledge

4. Implementation and collaborative care
a. Monitor client for signs of hemorrhage, hypertension, or other complications including disseminated intravascular coagulopathy (DIC)
b. Prepare client and assist with suction uterine evacuation of molar pregnancy; hysterectomy may be chosen for clients who do not want to preserve fertility
c. Provide RhoGAM to appropriate clients (Rh-negative with Rh-positive partners) after procedure
d. Teach client about need for frequent follow-up care during next year to rule out development of cancer (choriocarcinoma)
   1) Frequent ß-hCG levels are done initially with other testing to rule out cancer; reinforce need for diligent follow-up care (one in five women develop cancer)
   2) Client should not become pregnant for one year following a molar pregnancy to allow for assessment via ß-hCG levels; provide contraceptive counseling
e. Provide emotional support for client and family who are grieving loss of pregnancy and living with fear of developing a malignancy

5. Evaluation: molar pregnancy is identified and evacuated; client verbalizes need for follow-up care and uses effective contraception during this period; client remains cancer-free for one year

D. Incompetent cervix

1. Description and etiology
a. Painless cervical effacement and dilatation that is not associated with contractions and usually occurs in second trimester, resulting in spontaneous abortion or very preterm birth
b. Congenital uterine anomalies may be associated with incompetent cervix; other contributing factors may be cervical inflammation or previous cervical trauma

2. Assessment
a. Previous unexplained and asymptomatic second-trimester pregnancy losses may indicate an undiagnosed incompetent cervix
b. Cervical effacement and dilatation without contractions or pain; client may present for care completely dilated with bulging membranes

3. Priority nursing diagnoses: Risk for Injury: Fetal; Anticipatory Grieving; Deficient Knowledge

4. Implementation and collaborative care
   a. Provide emotional support and grief support group referral for client and partner with pregnancy loss from an incompetent cervix
   b. Provide client and partner teaching if client is to be managed on bedrest at home for a cervix just beginning to efface (shorten)
   c. Provide teaching about cervical **cerclage** if this treatment method is chosen; cerclage is a technique of reinforcing closure of cervix with sutures during pregnancy
   d. Monitor client for signs of preterm labor or infection; if labor begins cerclage may be removed to protect cervix from trauma; tocolytics may be administered; antibiotics or anti-inflammatory drugs may be needed; provide appropriate nursing assessments and care related to medication
   e. ! Instruct client and partner to return if contractions begin, as suture will need to be removed before vaginal birth is accomplished
5. Evaluation: client has cervical cerclage placed without complications; pregnancy is continued until fetal viability is reached

Practice to Pass

A client is admitted with the diagnosis of "threatened spontaneous abortion." What would you teach this client about her condition? The client's symptoms continue and she experiences a complete abortion. What communication techniques would be appropriate at this time?

E. Spontaneous *abortion*

1. Description and etiology
   a. An unintended pregnancy loss before 20 weeks' gestation; lay term is *miscarriage*
   b. Abortion is most common cause of bleeding during first trimester and usually results from chromosomal abnormalities in embryo; other causes may be teratogen exposure, inadequate implantation, and maternal endocrine disorders or chronic illness
   c. Late spontaneous abortion may result from incompetent cervix
   d. See Box 7-1 for classification of spontaneous abortion
2. Assessment
   a. Vaginal spotting or bleeding is common; client may pass clots and tissue
   b. Pelvic cramping or dull backache is usually present
   c. Falling hCG levels indicate death of embryo; ultrasound identifies gestational sac and notes whether there is cardiac movement in real time
3. Priority nursing diagnoses: Risk for Deficient Fluid Volume; Anticipatory Grieving; Pain; Deficient Knowledge
4. Implementation and collaborative care
   a. Instruct client who has a threatened abortion and her partner about bedrest at home and when to return if bleeding or cramping worsen
   b. Assess amount of bleeding; instruct client to save all clots and tissue that may be passed for further examination

Box 7-1

Classification of Spontaneous Abortion

Terminology associated with spontaneous abortion helps to classify the clinical condition

- Threatened abortion: Client experiences vaginal bleeding, but cervix remains closed. There may be some mild cramping or backache.
- Inevitable abortion: Client experiences cramping and bleeding. Cervix dilates and membranes may rupture.
- Incomplete abortion: Client experiences bleeding, cramping, and expulsion of part of products of conception. Tissue remains in uterus and cervix is dilated. Hemorrhage is possible.
- Complete abortion: Client experiences bleeding, cramping, and expulsion of all products of conception. Cervix is closed and uterus contracts.
- Missed abortion: Client experiences decreasing signs of pregnancy as fetus has died in utero but has not been expelled. Client may be at risk for DIC if products of conception are not removed.

c. Monitor blood pressure, pulse, and respirations frequently if bleeding is heavy; evaluate client for signs of impending shock
d. Initiate IV therapy with at least an 18-gauge needle as ordered
e. Assist with dilatation and curettage (D&C) as indicated for an incomplete abortion
! f. Provide emotional support, without false hope, to client and family
g. Refer to pregnancy loss or grief support groups
h. Do not underestimate emotional significance of an early pregnancy loss, validate client and partner's emotional responses; tell client and partner that she/they should not feel responsible for this loss; it is extremely unlikely that anything she/they did or did not do caused the loss
i. Give RhoGAM to Rh-negative clients with Rh-positive partners within 72 hours of abortion

5. Evaluation: pregnancy is either maintained or products of conception are expelled without further complication; client and family mourn the loss

F. ***Placenta previa***

1. Description and etiology: placenta is abnormally implanted near to or over internal cervical os; as cervix softens and begins to efface and dilate, placental sinuses are opened causing progressive hemorrhages
a. May be a low implantation near cervix (Figure 7-1a), a partial previa covering part of os (Figure 7-1b), or a complete placenta previa, which covers entire internal cervical os (Figure 7-1c)
b. Incidence of placenta previa is higher with multiple gestation, history of uterine surgery, and multiparity
! c. Delivery of a client with a complete previa is by cesarean section, often with a classical uterine incision to avoid placenta
d. Vaginal birth may be possible with a low-lying placenta if fetal head is down to press against placenta and occlude sinuses

2. Assessment
! a. Episodic painless vaginal bleeding after 20th week of pregnancy without contractions (most frequently first bleeding episode is at about 29 weeks); each successive bleeding episode is often heavier than the last; profuse hemorrhage may occur as cervix dilates under placenta
b. Ultrasound identification of placental location
c. CBC to assess baseline anemia status; blood type, screen, and hold

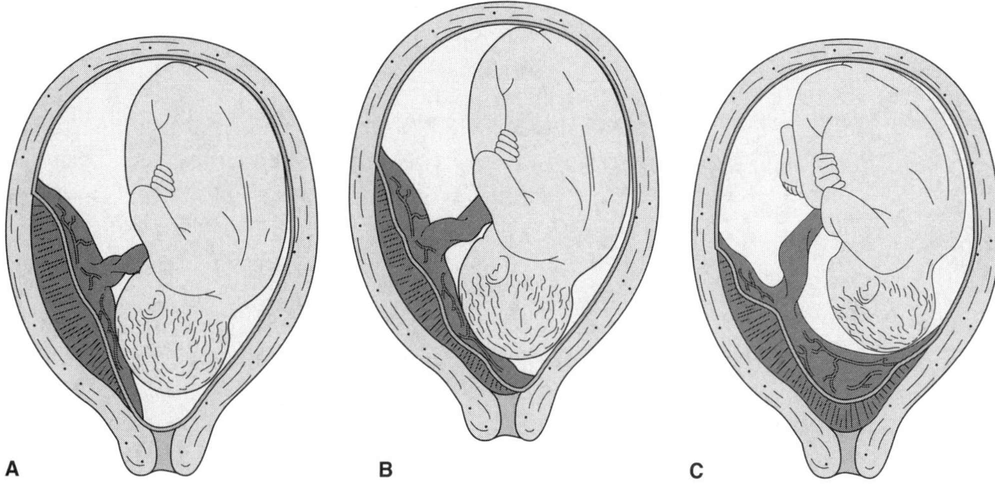

Figure 7-1
Placenta previa. A. Low placental implantation, B. Partial placenta previa, C. Complete placenta previa.

d. Assess fetal maturity and appropriateness of steroid treatment (betamethasone) to assist maturation of lungs before delivery
e. Continuous fetal monitoring assessing for any nonreassuring findings including sinusoidal pattern, late decelerations, or loss of variability

3. Priority nursing diagnoses: Risk for or Actual Deficient Fluid Volume; Risk for Injury: Maternal or Fetal; Fear; Deficient Knowledge
4. Implementation and collaborative care

! a. Never perform a vaginal exam on a pregnant client presenting with painless vaginal bleeding without documented ultrasound localization of placenta, as this may create profuse hemorrhage
b. If ultrasound is not available, pregnancy is near term and profuse bleeding is present, assist with a double setup procedure; physician performs a careful vaginal exam in operating room with equipment and staff ready to perform either a cesarean or a vaginal delivery depending on whether bleeding is caused by placenta previa or is increased bloody show of advanced labor
c. Maintain preterm clients on bedrest with bathroom privileges until fetal maturity is reached or hemorrhage is such that cesarean delivery is imperative; monitor for bedrest-related complications, such as deep vein thrombosis
d. Monitor maternal vital signs to rule out ascending infection or shock
e. Assess blood loss by weighing peripads and bed pads that are bloody; one gram equals one milliliter (1 gram = 1 mL)
f. Monitor serial hemoglobin and hematocrit levels; obtain blood group and type, cross-match as needed
g. Monitor fetal well-being with continuous or intermittent monitoring and other testing as indicated
h. Maintain IV access with at least an 18-gauge needle and provide replacement fluids as ordered
i. Provide emotional support to the client on bedrest; facilitate family visits
j. Promote adequate nutrition with prenatal vitamins and iron as needed to prevent maternal anemia
k. Provide routine pre- and postoperative cesarean teaching and care if indicated; instruct client about location of uterine incision as it relates to future desire for a trial of labor after cesarean (TOLAC)

5. Evaluation: bleeding does not become excessive; client's vital signs remain stable; client delivers a healthy mature newborn

G. Abruptio placenta

1. Description and etiology: premature separation of placenta from uterine wall during pregnancy; quantified in percentages of whole placenta
a. Placenta may separate only at margins, causing vaginal bleeding but perhaps little pain (see Figure 7-2a)
b. A central (concealed) abruption may not result in vaginal bleeding but does cause increasing uterine irritability and tenderness see (Figure 7-2b)
c. A complete (100%) separation from uterine wall results in profuse hemorrhage (Figure 7-2c)
d. Most common identified precipitating factors are maternal hypertension, cocaine abuse, and abdominal trauma
e. A client with an **abruptio placenta** is at increased risk of depleting clotting factors and developing disseminated intravascular coagulopathy (DIC)
2. Assessment

! a. A painful, rigid, boardlike abdomen with vaginal bleeding are classic signs of abruptio placenta; abdomen may increase in size as bleeding continues; ultrasound confirms diagnosis

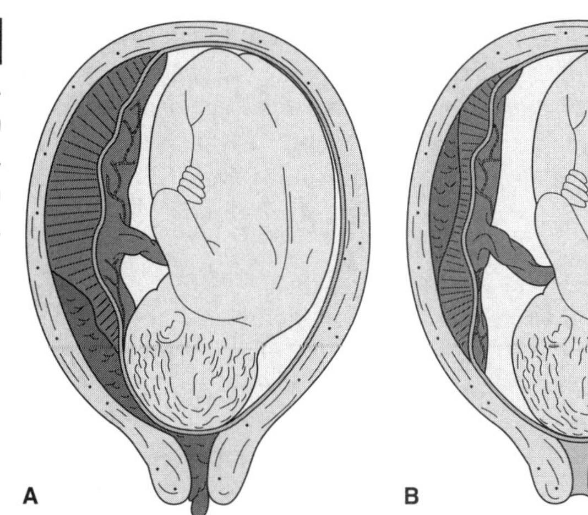

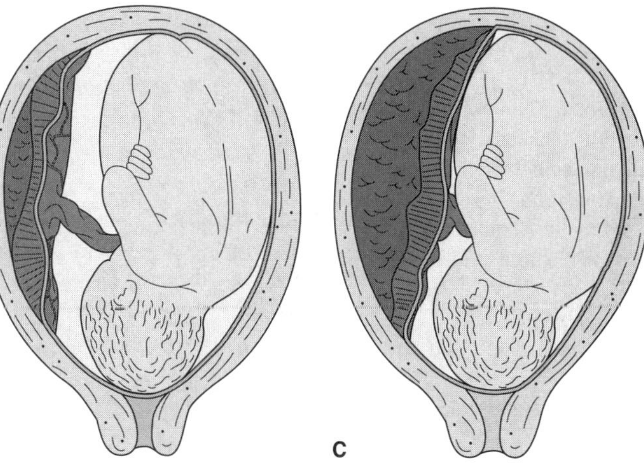

Figure 7-2

Abruptio placenta. A. Marginal abruption with external hemorrhage, B. Central abruption with concealed hemorrhage, C. Complete separation.

   b. A central abruption causes severe pain from bleeding behind placenta and distends uterine muscle with little to no vaginal bleeding; uterus is very irritable and fetus shows consistent late decelerations
   c. Bleeding behind placenta is forced into myometrium and may result in a Couvelaire uterus; uterus becomes bluish-purple, extremely irritable, distended, and rigid; uterus does not contract efficiently after delivery leading to postpartum hemorrhage
   d. Marginal placental abruption may present with more vaginal bleeding but less pain than a concealed abruption
   e. Fetal outcome depends on degree of placental separation and fetal maturity at time of birth
   f. Perform continuous fetal monitoring, assessing for any nonreassuring findings including sinusoidal pattern, late decelerations, or loss of variability
   g. Assess fetal maturity and appropriateness of steroid (betamethasone) treatment to assist maturation of lungs before delivery
3. Priority nursing diagnoses: Deficient Fluid Volume; Risk for Injury: Maternal and fetal; Risk for Impaired Gas Exchange; Deficient Knowledge
4. Implementation and collaborative care

   a. Monitor maternal blood pressure, pulse, and respirations for signs of impending shock
   ! b. Monitor fetus continuously for signs of distress: increased fetal movement, decreased FHR variability, changes in baseline FHR, late decelerations
   c. Assess client for bleeding, uterine activity, and abdominal pain; place on external fetal monitor to evaluate uterine irritability and fetal well-being; palpate uterine tone
   ! d. Measure client's abdominal girth at umbilicus for baseline size and repeat periodically to evaluate occult bleeding
   e. Review lab values to estimate blood loss (hemoglobin and hematocrit) and monitor for potential development of DIC (platelets, fibrinogen, fibrin degradation products, PT, and PTT); review toxicology screen if ordered
   f. Monitor client for signs of developing coagulation defects: unusual bleeding from injection sites, gums, or development of petechiae
   g. Start and maintain IV fluids with at least an 18-gauge needle; monitor intake and output; a Foley catheter may be inserted with expected urine output of 30 mL/hour or greater

Practice to Pass

A client at 37 weeks' gestation has been in an automobile accident. She was wearing her seatbelt and is uninjured but complains of shoulder and abdominal pain. What assessments and interventions would you implement for this client?

h. Provide oxygen as indicated at 8 to 12 L/min via snug face mask
i. Carefully monitor client and fetus if vaginal delivery is attempted; prepare for an emergency cesarean delivery if fetus develops distress
j. Provide ongoing information and emotional support for client and family

5. Evaluation: maternal blood loss is minimized and fetal well-being is maintained; client delivers a healthy infant without further complications

H. Premature rupture of membranes (ROM)

1. Description and etiology
   a. Premature ROM refers to amniotic membrane rupture before labor begins; labor usually begins spontaneously within 24 hours of membrane rupture
   b. Preterm ROM refers to membrane rupture prior to term gestation or before 38 weeks; risk factors include infection, incompetent cervix, and trauma
   c. Prolonged ROM refers to membranes ruptured more than 12 hours before birth; many caregivers will induce labor rather than risk prolonged rupture with possible ascending infection
   d. May or may not be accompanied by preterm labor or incompetent cervix
2. Assessment
   a. Gush of watery, clear, or meconium-stained fluid from vagina with continued leakage

   b. Amniotic fluid turns nitrazine paper blue, indicating an alkaline pH; urine is almost always acidic and does not change the yellow color of nitrazine paper
   c. Amniotic fluid shows characteristic ferning pattern on microscopic examination of a slide with dried fluid on it; urine and vaginal secretions do not display ferning
   d. The unengaged fetus is at risk for a prolapsed cord when the membranes rupture
3. Priority nursing diagnoses: Risk for Infection; Anxiety; Risk for Injury: Maternal or fetal; Deficient Knowledge
4. Implementation and collaborative care
   a. Assess FHR when membranes rupture to rule out prolapsed cord; note time, color, and amount of fluid; obtain a baseline maternal temperature
   b. Evaluate client's temperature every two hours, other vital signs may be routine; assess CBC as ordered to detect elevated WBCs and/or elevated immature WBCs, and/or elevation of erythrocyte sedimentation rate (ESR) as indicators of infection
   c. Avoid vaginal exams to prevent introducing microorganisms that may cause an ascending infection

Practice to Pass

A client reports feeling a sudden wetness as if her water broke. How would you assess the fluid to determine if it is amniotic fluid?

   d. Monitor client for signs of **chorioamnionitis** (inflammation and infection of fetal membranes and amniotic fluid): elevated temperature, abdominal tenderness, increased WBCs, and ESR
   e. Obtain vaginal culture as ordered
   f. Provide client teaching and reassurance that amniotic fluid is continuously produced and that there is no such thing as a "dry birth"
   g. Administer antibiotics and/or analgesics if ordered; some caregivers prefer to wait and treat newborn
   h. Perform fetal monitoring as ordered, assessing for any nonreassuring findings including fetal tachycardia, variable decelerations, late decelerations, loss of variability; also monitor for development of uterine contractions
   i. Assess fetal maturity and appropriateness of steroid (betamethasone) treatment to assist maturation of lungs before delivery
5. Evaluation: client and fetus remain infection-free; umbilical cord does not prolapse; client delivers a healthy infant without complications associated with prematurity

I. Gestational hypertension, preeclampsia, and eclampsia

1. Description and etiology: hypertensive disorders that begin during pregnancy; etiology is unknown, but preeclampsia is associated with vasospasm and reduced renal perfusion; is more common in young primigravidas, women over 35, multiple gestation, DM, and hydatidiform mole; preeclamptic client is at risk for stroke, DIC, renal failure, and hepatic rupture
   - **a.** Gestational hypertension is high blood pressure that occurs during pregnancy and resolves after delivery; it is not associated with proteinuria or edema
   - **b.** Mild preeclampsia is characterized by hypertension of >140/90 after 20 weeks' gestation and proteinuria of 1–2+ (by dipstick)
   - **c.** Sudden onset of severe edema warrants evaluation for preeclampsia or renal disease
   - **d.** Severe preeclampsia is characterized by blood pressure >180/110 on two occasions at least six hours apart while on bedrest and presence of proteinuria of 3–4+ (dipstick)
   - **e.** Eclampsia is term used to describe preeclampsia that has progressed to include maternal tonic-clonic seizures or coma
   - **f.** HELLP syndrome is a subclassification of preeclampsia; tends to occur earlier in gestation and present more severely, name is an acronym for symptoms including Hemolysis, Elevated Liver enzymes, and a Low Platelet count; the client is at risk for hemorrhage, pulmonary edema, and hepatic rupture
2. Assessment: symptoms usually develop during third trimester except in cases of hydatidiform mole; client is at risk for seizures and other complications up to 48 hours after delivery
   - **a.** Mild preeclampsia: hypertension of 140/90 and proteinuria 1+ to 2; weight gain >1.5 kg/month in second trimester or >0.5 kg/week in third trimester may be associated with edema and requires further evaluation
   - **b.** Severe preeclampsia: hypertension >180/110 and proteinuria 3+ or more than 5 grams in a 24-hour urine specimen; sudden large weight gain with facial edema, pitting pretibial edema and possible signs of central nervous system (CNS) irritation
   - **c.** Systemic responses: CNS irritability causes severe or continuous headache, hyperreflexia (greater than +2, baseline, or clonus), or visual disturbance (blurred vision, seeing spots or flashing lights); renal damage is indicated by oliguria (less than 30 mL/hr); portal hypertension may result in epigastric pain and may precede hepatic rupture
   - **d.** Lab values: increased hematocrit (as fluid moves out of intravascular space), serum uric acid, BUN, and liver enzymes (ALT, AST); decreased RBCs and platelets as condition worsens
3. Priority nursing diagnoses: Deficient Fluid Volume; Risk for Injury; Anxiety; Deficient Knowledge
4. Implementation and collaborative care: only cure is delivery; goal of care is to deliver a healthy, viable infant while safeguarding mother's health
   - **a.** Bedrest at home is indicated if preeclampsia is mild; hospitalization if severe until fetus is mature enough to be delivered; bedrest on left side to facilitate uteroplacental perfusion
   - **b.** A quiet, calm environment is maintained to decrease CNS stimulation; siderails should be up and padded for clients with severe preeclampsia who are at risk of progressing to seizures
   - **c.** Assess fetal maturity and appropriateness of steroid (betamethasone) treatment to assist maturation of lungs before delivery
   - **d.** Implement frequent assessments (every 15 minutes to 1–4 hours as indicated by client condition) to include blood pressure, pulse, and respirations, edema, deep

tendon reflexes, and clonus checks; assess client for headache, visual disturbances, and epigastric pain; assessment of fetal heart tracing for signs of fetal compromise and/or signs of labor

e. Foley catheter is inserted to monitor renal function; record strict intake and output; evaluate urine for protein; assess daily weight

f. Monitor fetal well-being by continuous EFM, serial NSTs, BPP, or amniocentesis as indicated

! **g.** Administer magnesium sulfate as ordered for seizure prevention; monitor client for signs of magnesium toxicity

1) Monitor magnesium blood levels: 5 to 8 mg/dL is therapeutic range

2) Decreased urine output (less than 30 mL/hr) can increase risk for toxicity as magnesium sulfate is excreted by kidneys

! **3)** Depressed reflexes and respirations less than 12–14 per minute indicate magnesium toxicity

! **4)** Keep calcium gluconate within reach for emergency administration to counteract magnesium sulfate toxicity

h. Prepare for induction or cesarean birth when fetus is mature or if maternal condition worsens; assess fetal maturity and appropriateness of steroid treatment to assist maturation of lungs before delivery

i. Provide teaching and support to client and family about condition and therapeutic interventions; clients with mild preeclampsia frequently do not feel ill and may have difficulty maintaining bedrest

j. Evaluate newborn for signs of depression related to magnesium sulfate

k. Continue to monitor client for preeclampsia complications for approximately 48 hours after delivery

5. Evaluation: client does not experience eclampsia; client delivers a healthy mature infant without further complications

POSTTEST

Case Study

A 14-year-old primigravida is admitted in early labor with severe preeclampsia at 42 weeks' gestation. The client's blood pressure is 168/102.

1. What other assessment data would you obtain?
2. Describe the complications this client is at risk for.
3. Discuss the medications you expect to administer to this client.
4. What concerns do you have for this fetus? Why?
5. What would you teach this client and her family about her condition?

For suggested responses, see page 304.

POSTTEST

1 A client at 4 weeks' gestation, who has recently emigrated from Japan, comes to the prenatal clinic because she is having some dark brown vaginal spotting and is experiencing severe nausea and vomiting. The nurse interprets that these symptoms are compatible with which condition?

1. Gestational trophoblastic disease
2. Hyperemesis gravidarum
3. Placenta previa
4. Pregnancy-induced psychosis

2 A client who had an incompetent cervix with a previous pregnancy had a Shirodkar cerclage procedure done at 18 weeks in the current pregnancy. The client calls the clinic at 37 weeks' gestation because of irregular contractions occurring every five to seven minutes. Which response by the nurse is most appropriate?

1. "Go to the hospital to have the cerclage removed so your cervix isn't injured and to allow the birth to progress."
2. "Wait and come in when the contractions are closer and harder."
3. "You sound like you are worried about this baby. It must be frightening for you."
4. "You will need to have a cesarean birth with the Shirodkar cerclage in place."

3 A client who had no prenatal care presents to the labor and delivery unit with moderate vaginal bleeding and severe abdominal pain. Fundal height is 34 centimeters. Contractions are every 1.5 minutes, lasting 60 seconds and strong with increasing resting tone. The monitor shows consistent late decelerations. What information obtained from nursing assessment is most consistent with a risk for placental abruption?

1. The client admits to using cocaine a few times weekly
2. The client works part-time in a nearby department store
3. The client is human immunodeficiency virus (HIV)-positive
4. The client is of low income and has a 10th-grade education

4 A client is hospitalized on the antepartum unit with premature rupture of membranes at 37 weeks' gestation. Which routine physician prescription would the nurse question for this client?

1. Bedrest with bathroom privileges
2. Diet as tolerated
3. External fetal monitor prn
4. Vital signs every shift

5 The nurse would question an order for which laboratory test, which is inappropriate to test the current condition of a newborn whose mother who is human immunodeficiency (HIV)-positive?

1. Bilirubin level
2. Blood glucose level
3. ELISA testing
4. Hematocrit

6 A client with heart disease has been prescribed digoxin (Lanoxin) during her pregnancy. The nurse evaluates that client teaching has been effective when the client makes which statement?

1. "I will avoid eating foods high in potassium while taking this medication."
2. "I will check my pulse and not take the medication if it is less than 60."
3. "I will not take antibiotics at the same time as this medication."
4. "I will take this medication with a full glass of water before breakfast."

7 A 34-year-old client comes to the emergency room with cramping and vaginal bleeding. She has missed two menstrual periods. Which statement by the nurse is appropriate when the client is diagnosed with an incomplete abortion? Select all that apply.

1. "I am so sorry. This must be difficult for you."
2. "The doctor will clean out your womb with a D and C."
3. "Did you really want to be pregnant now?"
4. "You'll still be able to have children after this is over."
5. "Would you like to speak with a hospital chaplain or counselor?"

8 A client with preeclampsia is receiving magnesium sulfate and oxytocin (Pitocin) IV to induce labor at 38 weeks. The nurse determines the magnesium sulfate has been effective after noting which effect on the client?

1. Lowered blood pressure
2. Absence of seizures
3. Onset of sedation
4. Stools that are soft

9 The nurse anticipates that which complication of pregnancy would be most consistent with development of a sinusoidal fetal heart rate pattern during labor?

1. Abruptio placenta
2. Chorioamnionitis
3. Preeclampsia
4. Prolapsed cord

10 A client who admits to substance abuse during pregnancy tells the nurse, "I know I am just a really weak person, but I will try to cut down while I'm pregnant." Which response by the nurse would be most therapeutic?

1. "I am concerned about you and your baby. What can I do to help you?"
2. "I don't believe that you are weak at all. You just need to say no to drugs."
3. "I have heard that before. You need to get serious now or your baby will suffer."
4. "That is a very positive plan. Could you tell me more about feeling like a weak person?"

➤ *See pages 152–153 for Answers and Rationales.*

POSTTEST

ANSWERS & RATIONALES

ANSWERS & RATIONALES

Pretest

1 **Answer: 3, 5 Rationale:** Taking prenatal vitamins and iron will help prevent anemia as well as positively affect fetal growth and development. Anemia and excessive weight gain increase the cardiac workload and should be avoided by clients with heart disease. The client should discuss medications with her caregiver, but she may be allowed to take acetaminophen or a few other OTC medications. The client with Class II cardiac disease is slightly compromised with ordinary activity levels and would not tolerate exercise. There is a 2 to 4% chance that the baby will inherit a congenital defect. **Cognitive Level:** Analyzing **Client Need:** Physiological Adaptation **Integrated Process:** Teaching and Learning **Content Area:** Maternal-Newborn **Strategy:** Knowledge of the complications from heart disease during pregnancy will help to answer the question correctly. **Reference:** Ladewig, P., London, M., & Davidson, M. (2010). *Contemporary maternal-newborn nursing care* (7th ed.). Upper Saddle River, NJ: Pearson Education, p. 331.

2 **Answer: 1 Rationale:** The placenta produces human placental lactogen (hPL) and increased amounts of estrogen and progesterone. These hormones interfere with maternal glucose metabolism and require increased insulin production or supplementation. As soon as the placenta is expelled, these hormone levels fall dramatically and the mother may require no insulin at all or a very reduced dose in the first 24 hours. **Cognitive Level:** Applying **Client Need:** Physiological Adaptation **Integrated Process:** Nursing Process: Planning **Content Area:** Maternal-Newborn **Strategy:** This question is time-dependent, as noted by the words *insulin needs within 24 hours of delivery*. Recall that this is the time of rapid and dramatic changes for the woman. Eliminate options that do not meet this criterion. **Reference:** Ladewig, P., London, M., & Davidson, M. (2010). *Contemporary maternal-newborn nursing care* (7th ed.). Upper Saddle River, NJ: Pearson Education, p. 318.

3 **Answer: 2 Rationale:** The glycosylated hemoglobin (HbA1c) test provides an indication of what glucose levels have been over the last four to eight weeks because glucose attaches to the red blood cells (RBC) and remains there for the residual life of the RBC. Increased blood glucose levels will be reflected in an increased percentage of HbA1c. The other tests indicate current blood glucose levels only. **Cognitive Level:** Applying **Client Need:** Reduction of Risk Potential **Integrated Process:** Nursing Process: Assessment **Content Area:** Maternal-Newborn **Strategy:** The critical words in the question are *ongoing control*. This tells you that the correct option identifies a test measurement that does not only reflect current time. Recall laboratory assessment of long-term glucose control to aid in answering the question correctly. **Reference:** Ladewig, P., London, M., & Davidson, M. (2009). *Contemporary maternal-newborn nursing care* (7th ed.). Upper Saddle River, NJ: Pearson Education, p. 318.

4 **Answer: 3 Rationale:** Pregnancy presents an ideal time for nurses to reach out to substance-abusing clients in a caring way since the client herself recognizes that she and her baby will benefit from prenatal care. Believing the client is ready to stop abusing substances is unrealistic. Reporting the client to the authorities is punitive and could prevent the client from seeking care in the future. Assuming the client will lack appropriate parenting skills because of substance abuse is judgmental. It is difficult to predict how the client will respond to pregnancy and motherhood. **Cognitive Level:** Applying **Client Need:** Physiological Adaptation **Integrated Process:** Caring **Content Area:** Maternal-Newborn **Strategy:** Three

options are punitive and should be eliminated. Only one option is a therapeutic response to someone who recognizes the need for prenatal care even though she is abusing drugs. **Reference:** Ladewig, P., London, M., & Davidson, M. (2010). *Contemporary maternal-newborn nursing care* (7th ed.). Upper Saddle River, NJ: Pearson Education, p. 249.

5 **Answer: 2 Rationale:** The client with a suspected ectopic pregnancy may be at risk for the development of hypovolemic shock. Assessment is the first step of the nursing process and airway, breathing, and circulation are the priorities. Administering oxygen and providing emotional support are possible later interventions, and obtaining surgical consent is the surgeon's responsibility. **Cognitive Level:** Analyzing **Client Need:** Physiological Adaptation **Integrated Process:** Nursing Process: Implementation **Content Area:** Maternal-Newborn **Strategy:** The critical word in this question is *suspected*. The correct answer would be the option that provides further assessment of the client's condition. **Reference:** Ladewig, P., London, M., & Davidson, M. (2010). *Contemporary maternal-newborn nursing care* (7th ed.). Upper Saddle River, NJ: Pearson Education, p. 343.

6 **Answer: 3 Rationale:** The client requires frequent monitoring to rule out development of malignancy after experiencing trophoblastic gestational disease. Weekly hCG measurements are done until normal levels are recorded for three weeks. Expressions of sadness are appropriate for any pregnancy loss, even if no fetus developed. Needing chemotherapy is a possibility for this client. The client should use contraception for at least one year during the follow-up care. **Cognitive Level:** Applying **Client Need:** Physiological Adaptation **Integrated Process:** Nursing Process: Evaluation **Content Area:** Maternal-Newborn **Strategy:** The wording of the question reflects a negative stem, and so the correct option will be an option that is false. Knowledge of the complications from hydatiform mole and the required medical regimen will aid in choosing the correct answer. **Reference:** Ladewig, P., London, M., & Davidson, M. (2010). *Contemporary maternal-newborn nursing care* (7th ed.). Upper Saddle River, NJ: Pearson Education, p. 344.

7 **Answer: 3 Rationale:** The registered nurse is responsible for client assessments (such as for preeclampsia and fetal monitoring status) and for client teaching (such as signs of true versus false labor). Helping the client to the bathroom is within the practice abilities of a CNA if the RN has determined that it is safe for this client to get out of bed. **Cognitive Level:** Analyzing **Client Need:** Coordinated Care **Integrated Process:** Nursing Process: Implementation **Content Area:** Maternal-Newborn **Strategy:** Recall that assessment and teaching should not be delegated to unlicensed personnel to eliminate incorrect options. **Reference:** Ladewig, P., London, M., & Davidson, M. (2010). *Contemporary maternal-newborn nursing care* (7th ed.). Upper Saddle River, NJ: Pearson Education, p. 3.

8 **Answer: 50 Rationale:** One mL of blood weighs approximately 1 gram. Thus, 50 mL of blood would weigh approximately 50 grams. **Cognitive Level:** Applying **Client Need:** Physiological Adaptation **Integrated Process:** Nursing Process: Assessment **Content Area:** Maternal-Newborn **Strategy:** The critical information needed to answer the question is that 1 mL is approximately equal to 1 gram. Learn this information now if this question was difficult. **Reference:** Ladewig, P., London, M., & Davidson, M. (2010). *Contemporary maternal-newborn nursing care* (7th ed.). Upper Saddle River, NJ: Pearson Education, p. 890.

9 **Answer: 2 Rationale:** The client with hyperemesis gravidarum is anxious or even fearful about the effects of her condition on the fetus. The etiology of hyperemesis is unknown but the incidence is increased in conditions with increased hCG. The client experiences excessive vomiting and would have the diagnosis of Imbalanced Nutrition: Less Than Body Requirements. With appropriate treatment, the prognosis is favorable for the fetus. There may be an emotional component, but there is no indication that this is an unwanted pregnancy. **Cognitive Level:** Analyzing **Client Need:** Psychosocial Integrity **Integrated Process:** Nursing Process: Diagnosis **Content Area:** Maternal-Newborn **Strategy:** The core focus in this question is the effects of hyperemesis, excessive vomiting, and deficient nutrition. Eliminate one option as it deals with over nutrition. Eliminate two other options for which there are no data to support them. **Reference:** Ladewig, P., London, M., & Davidson, M. (2009). *Contemporary maternal-newborn nursing care* (7th ed.). Upper Saddle River, NJ: Pearson Education, p. 345.

10 **Answer: 1 Rationale:** The Rh-negative client whose infant is Rh-positive would be at risk for Rh-sensitization, which could create risks for future pregnancies. The infant's blood type cannot be obtained until after birth. The client is not anemic based on the hemoglobin and hematocrit values, so encouraging the client to eat more dark-green leafy vegetables and suggesting an iron supplement are incorrect. There is no relationship between the lab values and the client's weight in this scenario. **Cognitive Level:** Analyzing **Client Need:** Physiological Adaptation **Integrated Process:** Nursing Process: Implementation **Content Area:** Maternal-Newborn **Strategy:** Only one option indicates a need that is identified by the scenario. The other answers are incorrect given the normal hemoglobin and hematocrit. In addition, three options are similar (focusing on nutrition) and are therefore, likely to be incorrect. The correct answer is different. **Reference:** Ladewig, P., London, M., & Davidson, M. (2010). *Contemporary maternal-newborn nursing care* (7th ed.). Upper Saddle River, NJ: Pearson Education, p. 360.

Posttest

1 **Answer: 1** **Rationale:** The client has three risk factors of molar pregnancy: Japanese background, brownish "prune juice" vaginal bleeding, and the severe nausea and vomiting at too early a gestational age (associated with excessive hCG found in trophoblastic disease). The client has only one symptom of hyperemesis and this is too early for most women to experience hyperemesis. Placenta previa presents with bright red bleeding usually at a later gestational age. There is no information suggestive of psychosis. **Cognitive Level:** Analyzing **Client Need:** Physiological Adaptation **Integrated Process:** Nursing Process: Assessment **Content Area:** Maternal-Newborn **Strategy:** The core issue of this question is a cluster of symptoms. Eliminate two options because they are characterized by one main symptom. Eliminate another because no psychological symptoms are presented. **Reference:** Ladewig, P., London, M., & Davidson, M. (2010). *Contemporary maternal-newborn nursing care* (7th ed.). Upper Saddle River, NJ: Pearson Education, p. 344.

2 **Answer: 1** **Rationale:** The Shirdkar cerclage is closure of the cervix with suture material to prevent preterm dilatation. When labor ensues, the suture must be cut so the fetus can pass through the birth canal. Waiting for harder contractions will increase the likelihood of cervical damage from the suture. Focusing on possible worries and fear of the client does not address the client's risk, which is the priority. Clients who expect to have several future pregnancies may be delivered by cesarean to avoid repeated cerclage, but there is no necessity to this option. **Cognitive Level:** Applying **Client Need:** Physiological Adaptation **Integrated Process:** Nursing Process: Implementation **Content Area:** Maternal-Newborn **Strategy:** Recall that the placement of a suture in cerclage places a barrier to safe delivery of an infant as the due date approaches. With this in mind, select the option that allows for labor to progress safely, or to begin safely, if the labor is false at this time. **Reference:** Ricci, S. (2008). *Essentials of maternity, newborn, and women's health nursing* (2nd ed.). Philadelphia, PA: Lippincott Williams and Wilkins, p 535.

3 **Answer: 1** **Rationale:** The risk for placental abruption is increased with cocaine abuse. Being HIV-positive and having low income and little education are factors that make the client high risk for complications of pregnancy, but not particularly for abruption. Working part-time does not place the client at any specific risk. **Cognitive Level:** Applying **Client Need:** Physiological Adaptation **Integrated Process:** Nursing Process: Assessment **Content Area:** Maternal-Newborn **Strategy:** Recall the risks of cocaine abuse to aid in answering this question correctly. Eliminate the other answers, which are not factors that increase the risk for placental abruption. **Reference:** Ricci, S. (2008). *Essentials of maternity, newborn, and women's health nursing* (2nd ed.). Philadelphia, PA: Lippincott Williams and Wilkins, p. 601.

4 **Answer: 4** **Rationale:** The client with ruptured membranes prior to the beginning of labor is at increased risk for ascending infection (chorioamnionitis). The client's temperature should be taken every two to four hours to identify early signs of sepsis. Bedrest with bathroom privileges, diet as tolerated, and external fetal monitor prn are routine orders that would be anticipated for the client. **Cognitive Level:** Analyzing **Client Need:** Physiological Adaptation **Integrated Process:** Nursing Process: Implementation **Content Area:** Maternal-Newborn **Strategy:** The core focus of this question is planning care for a client with a complication. The correct answer would be the option that includes additional or more frequent assessment of the client's status. **Reference:** Ricci, S. (2008). *Essentials of maternity, newborn, and women's health nursing* (2nd ed.). Philadelphia, PA: Lippincott Williams and Wilkins, p. 557.

5 **Answer: 3** **Rationale:** The infant of an HIV-positive mother will test positive on an ELISA test for the human immunodeficiency virus because the maternal antibodies cross the placenta during pregnancy. This does not indicate that the newborn has HIV. The diagnosis using the ELISA test for the baby is not made until around 15 months when maternal antibodies are degraded and the infant forms antibodies to HIV if infected. The bilirubin level, blood glucose level, and hematocrit give information about the infant's current condition. **Cognitive Level:** Analyzing **Client Need:** Physiological Adaptation **Integrated Process:** Nursing Process: Planning **Content Area:** Maternal-Newborn **Strategy:** The focus of this question is an immune disorder. The correct answer would be the option that includes a test designed to assess antigen-antibody responses. Knowledge of the care of the newborn exposed to HIV/AIDS and the transmission of maternal antibodies to the newborn will aid in answering correctly. **Reference:** Ricci, S. (2008). *Essentials of maternity, newborn, and women's health nursing* (2nd ed.). Philadelphia, PA: Lippincott Williams and Wilkins, p. 595.

6 **Answer: 2** **Rationale:** Digoxin is a cardiac glycoside that increases cardiac output by increasing the strength of contraction of the myocardium and slowing the heart rate. A pulse rate of less than 60 is a serious adverse effect of the medication and the dose should be held. The client needs adequate potassium for myocardial function. Antibiotics are not contraindicated with digoxin. The drug may be given with or without food. **Cognitive Level:** Analyzing **Client Need:** Pharmacological and Parenteral Therapies **Integrated Process:** Teaching and Learning **Content Area:** Maternal-Newborn **Strategy:** A critical word in the question is *effective*. This indicates the correct option is also a correct statement of fact. Knowledge of the action of digoxin and the side effects will help to choose the correct answer. **Reference:** Ladewig, P.,

London, M., & Davidson, M. (2009). *Contemporary maternal-newborn nursing care* (7th ed.). Upper Saddle River, NJ: Pearson Education, p. 203.

7 **Answer: 1, 5 Rationale:** The nurse should provide emotional support to all clients experiencing perinatal loss. Offering the client an opportunity to talk with another healthcare professional or clergy for additional help is also supportive. Stating the need for a D and C (dilatation and curettage) uses medical jargon that the client may not understand and focuses only on the physiological aspect of the client's care. Questioning whether the client wanted to be pregnant serves no useful purpose and is insensitive to the client's loss. The nurse does not know whether the client will be able to have other children. **Cognitive Level:** Analyzing **Client Need:** Psychosocial Integrity **Integrated Process:** Caring **Content Area:** Maternal-Newborn **Strategy:** Choose options that contain therapeutic communications. Only two options are therapeutic and offer support; the other answers can be eliminated since they are not supportive measures. **Reference:** Ladewig, P., London, M., & Davidson, M. (2009). *Contemporary maternal-newborn nursing care* (7th ed.). Upper Saddle River, NJ: Pearson Education, p. 530.

8 **Answer: 2 Rationale:** Magnesium sulfate is a central nervous system depressant used to prevent seizure activity in the preeclamptic client. Lowered blood pressure, onset of sedation and stools that are soft may occur but are not the intended effect of the drug. **Cognitive Level:** Analyzing **Client Need:** Pharmacological and Parenteral Therapies **Integrated Process:** Nursing Process: Evaluation **Content Area:** Maternal-Newborn **Strategy:** Recall the classification of magnesium sulfate as a CNS depressant, which will help you to recall that it will prevent seizures, the major risk of preeclampsia. The other options are all similar and incorrect, may occur when the drug is used, but are not the primary action of the drug. **Reference:** Ladewig, P., London, M., & Davidson, M. (2009). *Contemporary maternal-newborn nursing care* (7th ed.). Upper Saddle River, NJ: Pearson Education, p. 486.

9 **Answer: 1 Rationale:** A sinusoidal fetal heart rhythm is associated with fetal anemia, which may be associated with an abruption. Chorioamnionitis, preeclampsia and prolapsed cord would result in other signs of fetal distress such as tachycardia, loss of variability, and late decelerations. **Cognitive Level:** Analyzing **Client Need:** Physiological Adaptation **Integrated Process:** Nursing Process: Assessment **Content Area:** Maternal-Newborn **Strategy:** Identify the option that is different from the others. Blood loss from abruptio placenta can cause fetal anemia, which is associated with a sinusoidal fetal heart rhythm. The other options are similar because they can cause fetal distress, but not fetal anemia, and thus, are incorrect. **Reference:** Ladewig, P., London, M., & Davidson, M. (2009). *Contemporary maternal-newborn nursing care* (7th ed.). Upper Saddle River, NJ: Pearson Education, p. 424.

10 **Answer: 4 Rationale:** Indicating the client has a positive plan acknowledges the client's intent to cut down on substance abuse while seeking additional information about the client's self-concept. Stating the nurse is concerned and asking how to help places the emphasis on the nurse instead of the client. Negating the client's belief and stating to just refuse drugs is insensitive and demeaning to the client. Stating the client should get serious is insensitive to the client who has presented for prenatal care, and stating that the fetus may suffer may frighten the client without providing information about actual risks of drug use during pregnancy. **Cognitive Level:** Applying **Client Need:** Psychosocial Integrity **Integrated Process:** Communication and Documentation **Content Area:** Maternal-Newborn **Strategy:** Eliminate two options that are negative and nontherapeutic. Next eliminate the option that does not focus on the client and her needs to explain herself and her feelings. **Reference:** Ladewig,P., London, M., & Davidson, M. (2009). *Contemporary maternal-newborn nursing care* (7th ed.). Upper Saddle River, NJ: Pearson Education, p. 249.

References

Davidson, M., London, M., & Ladewig, P. (2012). *Olds' maternal newborn nursing & women's health across the lifespan* (9th ed.). Upper Saddle River, NJ: Pearson Education.

Ladewig, P., London, M., & Davidson, M. (2009). *Contemporary maternal-newborn nursing care* (7th ed.). Upper Saddle River, NJ: Pearson Education.

Murray, M., & Huelsmann, G. (2009). *Labor and delivery nursing: A guide to evidence-based practice*. New York: Springer Publishing Company.

Orshan, S. A. (2008). *Maternity, newborn, and women's health nursing: Comprehensive care across the life span*. Philadelphia: Lippincott Williams & Wilkins.

Ricci, S. (2009). *Essentials of maternity, newborn, and women's health nursing* (2nd ed.). Philadelphia: Lippincott Williams & Wilkins.

The Universe of Women's Health. Retrieved February 1, 2011, from http://www.obgyn.net/pregnancy-birth/pregnancy-birth.asp?page=/pregnancy-birth/articles/survellance

8 The Normal Labor and Delivery Experience

Chapter Outline

Nursing Care of the Labor and Delivery Client

The Labor Process

The Stages of Labor

Pain Management during Birth

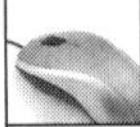

NCLEX-RN® Test Prep

Use the accompanying online resource, NursingReviewsandRationales, to test yourself with hundreds of NCLEX®-style practice questions.

Objectives

- Describe the process of labor in terms of the passenger, passageway, powers, and psyche (also known as the 4 Ps).
- Describe the nursing care needed during each of the four stages of labor.
- Explain the cardinal movements of the fetus during delivery.
- Identify nursing responsibilities during the administration of analgesia and anesthesia for childbirth.

Review at a Glance

accelerations transient increases in fetal heart rate (FHR) accompanying contractions or fetal movement

Apgar score assessment of fetal response to extrauterine life; 0 to 2 points given in each of five areas: color, muscle tone, reflex irritability, respiratory effort, and heart rate

attitude relationship of fetal parts to one another

baseline fetal heart rate average heart rate between contractions; measured in beats per minute (bpm)

cardinal movements individual adaptations that fetus undertakes to maneuver through pelvis during labor and birth

crowning outward bulging and thinning of perineal body and opening of vagina that occurs as fetal head presses downward onto perineum

dilatation opening of cervix from 1 to 10 centimeters

early deceleration gradual deceleration in FHR beginning at onset of a contraction with return to baseline by end of contraction; inversely mirrors contractions; caused by fetal head compression

engagement widest diameter of presenting part has passed through pelvic inlet

effacement thinning and shortening of cervix from 0 to 100%

epidural block very small diameter catheter is inserted into potential space between dural layers of lumbar spine and local anesthetic agent is injected to produce labor analgesia or anesthesia

episiotomy surgical incision into perineum to enlarge vaginal opening

internal fetal scalp electrode fine spiral wire that is attached to epidermis of presenting part to provide a direct ECG of fetal heart rate

intrauterine pressure catheter pressure-sensitive device inserted through cervix and past presenting part into amniotic fluid in uterus to measure intensity of contractions in mm of Hg

late deceleration deceleration of FHR that begins after contraction starts, with nadir occurring after peak of contraction, and returns to baseline after end of contraction; caused by utero-placental insufficiency

lie relationship of longitudinal axis of fetus to longitudinal axis of mother

long-term variability cyclical and rhythmic fluctuations in FHR that occur two to six times per minute

nadir lowest point; can refer to lowest FHR when used to describe FHR decelerations or resting phase of contraction when used in relation to uterine contractions during labor

paracervical block local anesthetic agent injected into lateral aspects of cervix for labor analgesia

position relationship of fetal presenting part to maternal pelvis

presentation fetal part entering pelvis first

pudendal block local anesthetic agent injected near ischial spines and pudendal nerve for delivery anesthesia

short-term variability change in rate between one fetal heart beat and the next

station relationship between widest diameter of presenting part and ischial spines of maternal pelvis

variable deceleration decelerations that occur suddenly, have steep sidewalls, return rapidly to baseline, and are variable in relationship to contractions; caused by compression of umbilical cord

PRETEST

1 The nurse performs a vaginal examination and determines that the fetus is in a sacrum anterior position. The nurse draws which conclusion from this assessment data?

1. The fetal sacrum is toward the maternal symphysis pubis.
2. The fetal sacrum is toward the maternal sacrum.
3. The fetal face is toward the maternal sacrum.
4. The fetal face is toward the maternal symphysis pubis.

2 The client has been having contractions every five minutes for seven hours. Which factor would the nurse use to determine if this is true labor?

1. The cervix is showing a pattern of effacement and dilatation.
2. The client has given birth to three children previously.
3. The contractions increasing in intensity and duration.
4. There was a spontaneous rupture of membranes.

3 Which of the following would be the highest priority of the nurse who is caring for the laboring client?

1. Pain relief measures that are offered are acceptable to the client.
2. Involvement of the client's partner with the labor and delivery.
3. Monitoring of appropriate fluid intake.
4. Assessment of fetal response to the labor.

4 As labor progresses, the nurse expects to assess that a client's contractions are developing which characteristics?

1. More intense, less frequent, and of longer duration
2. More intense, more frequent, and of longer duration
3. Constant in intensity, more frequent, and of shorter duration
4. Constant in intensity and frequency, but of shorter duration

5 The neonate is crying, has a pink body with blue extremities, has flexed arms with clenched fists, heart rate of 154, and gags when the bulb suction is used. The nurse records the Apgar score to be _______. Provide an answer that is a whole number.

Fill in your answer below:

____

6 Which of the following nursing observations would indicate a sign of impending placental separation and expulsion?

1. Steady trickle of blood with an unchanged cord length
2. Lengthening of the cord with associated cord tear
3. Small gush of blood with lengthening of the cord
4. Small gush of blood with an unchanged cord length

7 The nurse determines that a laboring client is exhibiting signs of increased anxiety. The nurse anticipates that this may result in which of the following?

1. A rapid progression of labor
2. Increased pain during the labor process
3. Lack of a support from support person or system
4. The need for an episiotomy

8 Earlier in the day, the baseline fetal heart rate (FHR) on a laboring client's fetus was 140. It is now 170. The nurse considers that which of the following could be an explanation for this change? Select all that apply.

1. Maternal fever
2. Narcotic administration
3. Fetal movement
4. Utero-placental insufficiency
5. Fetal distress

PRETEST

9 The nurse determines teaching has been effective when a laboring client makes which statement?

1. "Effacement is the opening of my cervix."
2. "My cervix will probably efface before it dilates because this is my first pregnancy."
3. "Effacement is measured from 0 to 10 centimeters."
4. "My cervix will efface and dilate at the same time because this is my first pregnancy."

10 The client's vaginal examination reveals: three centimeters dilated, 80% effaced, vertex at zero station. The woman is talkative and appears excited. The nurse determines the client to be in which stage and phase of labor?

1. First stage, latent phase
2. First stage, active phase
3. Second stage, latent phase
4. Third stage, transition phase

➤ *See pages 170–171 for Answers and Rationales.*

I. NURSING CARE OF THE LABOR AND DELIVERY CLIENT

A. **Physiologic safety**: laboring client is actually two clients—mother and newborn; nursing care focuses on physiologic safety of both

B. **Psychological safety**
   1. Nursing care also focuses on mother's psychological safety and includes consideration of fear, comfort, partner involvement, parental attachment to newborn, and past experiences
   2. Primigravida women experience fear of unknown and often have longer labors, while multigravida women can expect a shorter labor with subsequent pregnancies but may have memories of perceived bad experiences from previous births

C. **Maternal history**: assess for abuse, assault, and violence, as these past experiences will often manifest as extreme fear and tension during labor process or vaginal examinations

D. **Cultural background**
   1. Assess and try to understand in order to provide a safe and acceptable birthing environment for childbearing family
   2. Some common nursing actions may be cultural taboos for a particular client and affect parents' view of child throughout life

E. **Preparation for labor by the client and support person(s)**
   1. Can vary from formal prenatal education classes to information passed from generation to generation
   2. Misconceptions about birthing process and expectations of sensations during birth can occur; address them in a nonjudgmental manner that informs and supports birthing family

F. **Electronic fetal monitoring**: provides computer-assisted auditory and visual assessment of fetal heart rate (FHR) and uterine contractions (UC)
   1. FHR monitoring continuously records FHR on upper portion of monitor strip
      a. External monitoring: an ultrasound transducer is placed over fetal back and detects movements of fetal heart; fetal or maternal movement and maternal obesity may interfere with obtaining a continuous reading
      b. Internal monitoring: an **internal fetal scalp electrode** is inserted through cervix (which must be at least 2 cm dilated with ruptured membranes) and attached to epidermis of presenting part providing a direct ECG of fetal heart; unaffected by maternal obesity, maternal or fetal movement; thick fetal hair may prevent adequate insertion on a cephalic presentation

      c. **Baseline fetal heart rate** is average heart rate between contractions; measured in beats per minute (bpm); normal range: 110 to 160, bradycardia: <110, tachycardia: >160
      d. **Short-term variability**: change in rate between one fetal heart beat and the next; creates a jaggedness or zigzag appearance in the baseline FHR; determined by

interplay between the fetal sympathetic and parasympathetic nervous systems; decreased by fetal tachycardia, prematurity, fetal heart and CNS anomalies, and fetal sleep; normal: 2 to 3 bpm; classified as present or absent and can only be evaluated by internal monitoring

!

e. **Long-term variability**: rhythmic fluctuations that occur two to six times per minute; determined by interplay between fetal sympathetic and parasympathetic nervous systems; increased by fetal movement and decreased by fetal sleep or hypoxia and subsequent acidosis; average or moderate: 6 to 25 bpm

f. Periodic changes in FHR are deviations from baseline separate from variability which occur in relationship to or independent of contractions; these may be either accelerations or decelerations

!

g. **Accelerations**: transient increases in FHR
   1) Nonperiodic (spontaneous): symmetric, uniform, not related to contractions; occur in response to fetal movement and indicate fetal well-being
   2) Periodic: occur with contractions and may indicate decreased amniotic fluid or mild umbilical cord compression

!

h. Decelerations are categorized as early, late, or variable
   1) **Early decelerations**: decrease in FHR beginning at onset of a contraction and return to baseline by end of contraction with nadir at its acme (see Figure 8-1)
      a) Uniform shape inversely mirrors contraction

!

      b) Caused by fetal head compression; usually benign
      c) Nursing interventions include performing a vaginal examination to determine if fetus is descending in pelvis, and if fetus is not descending, notify health care provider

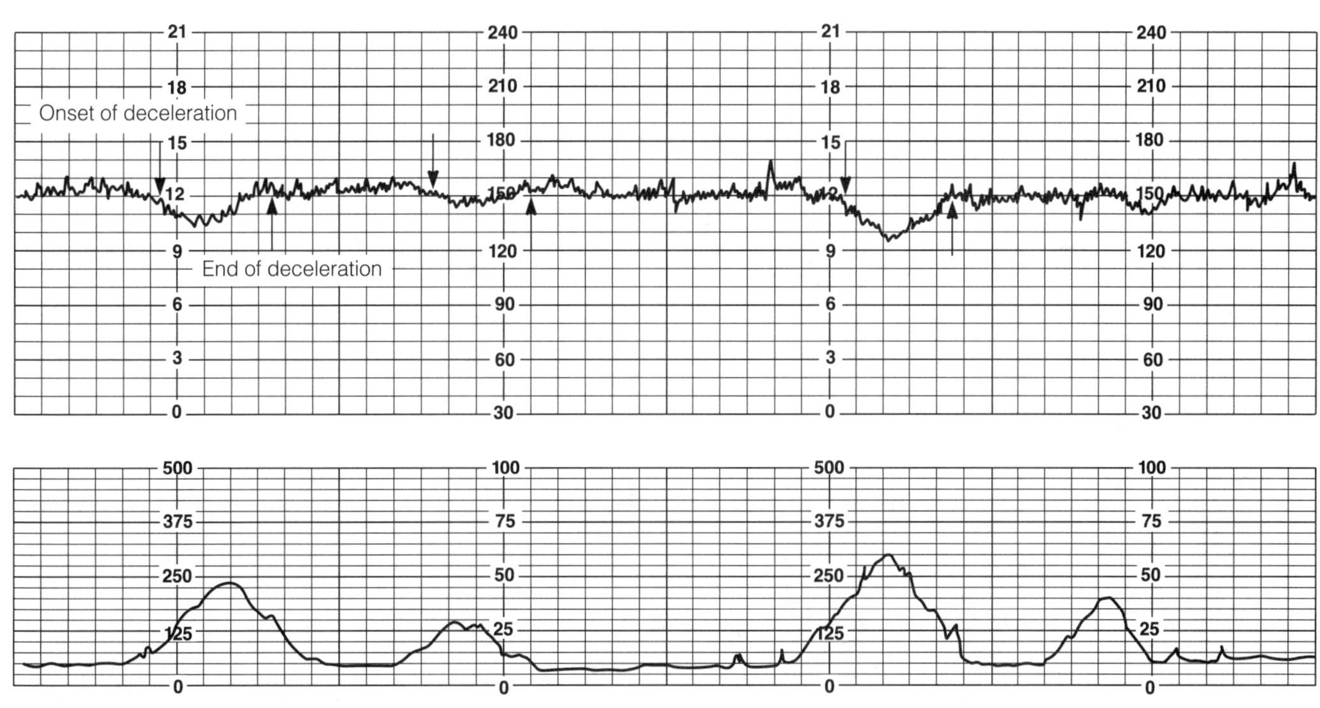

Figure 8-1

Early decelerations. Baseline FHR is 150–155 beats/min. Nadir (lowest point) of decelerations is 130–145 beats/min.

Source: Davidson, M., London, M., & Ladewig, P. (2012). *Olds' maternal newborn nursing & women's health across the lifespan* (9th ed.). Upper Saddle River, NJ: Pearson Education, p. 586.

2) **Late decelerations** begin after contraction starts with nadir occurring after peak of contraction and return to baseline after end of contraction (see Figure 8-2)
   a) Smooth, uniform shape that inversely mirrors contractions but late in onset and recovery
   b) Caused by utero-placental insufficiency; always considered ominous
   c) Nursing interventions focus on maintaining oxygenation by repositioning client to left lateral side, administering oxygen by mask at 7 to 10 L/min, correcting hypotension through increased IV fluid rate or prescribed medications, discontinuing oxytocin if being administered, and reporting to health care provider

Practice to Pass

The FHR baseline was 155 bpm before onset of contraction, decreases to 120 bpm during contraction, and returns to baseline 40 seconds after contraction ends. Describe the nursing interventions the nurse should implement.

3) **Variable decelerations** occur suddenly, vary in duration and intensity, vary in relation to contractions, and resolve abruptly (see Figure 8-3)
   a) Variable shape, usually "U" or "V," with steep sides; may or may not be associated with contractions
   b) Caused by compression of umbilical cord
   c) Categorized as mild, moderate, or severe based on lowest FHR reading and duration of deceleration; repetitive, prolonged, or more severe decelerations with a slow return or overshoot to baseline are ominous and indicate fetal asphyxia
   d) Nursing interventions focus on relieving cord compression through repositioning client until improvement occurs, vaginal examination to detect prolapsed cord, and oxygen if decelerations are severe or uncorrectable
   e) Amnio-infusion (instillation of warmed normal saline through an intrauterine pressure catheter) may be used to recreate cushioning effect on umbilical cord during contractions that is normally provided by amniotic fluid

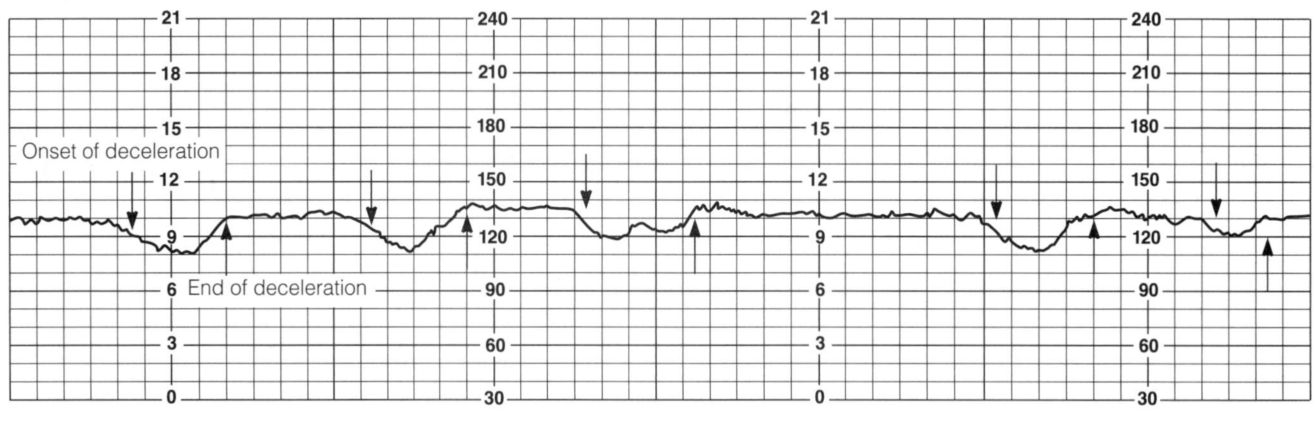

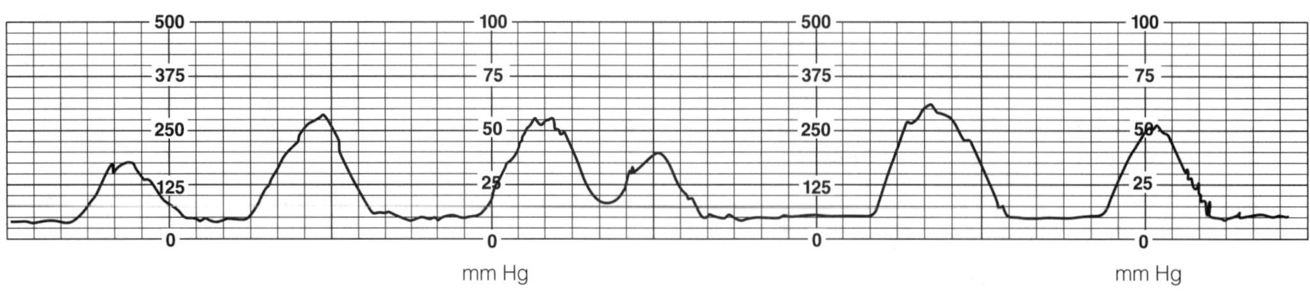

Figure 8-2

Late decelerations. Baseline FHR is 130–148 beats/min. Nadir (lowest point) of decelerations is 110–120 beats/min. Variability is absent.

Source: Davidson, M., London, M., & Ladewig, P. (2012). *Olds' maternal newborn nursing & women's health across the lifespan* (9th ed.). Upper Saddle River, NJ: Pearson Education, p. 587.

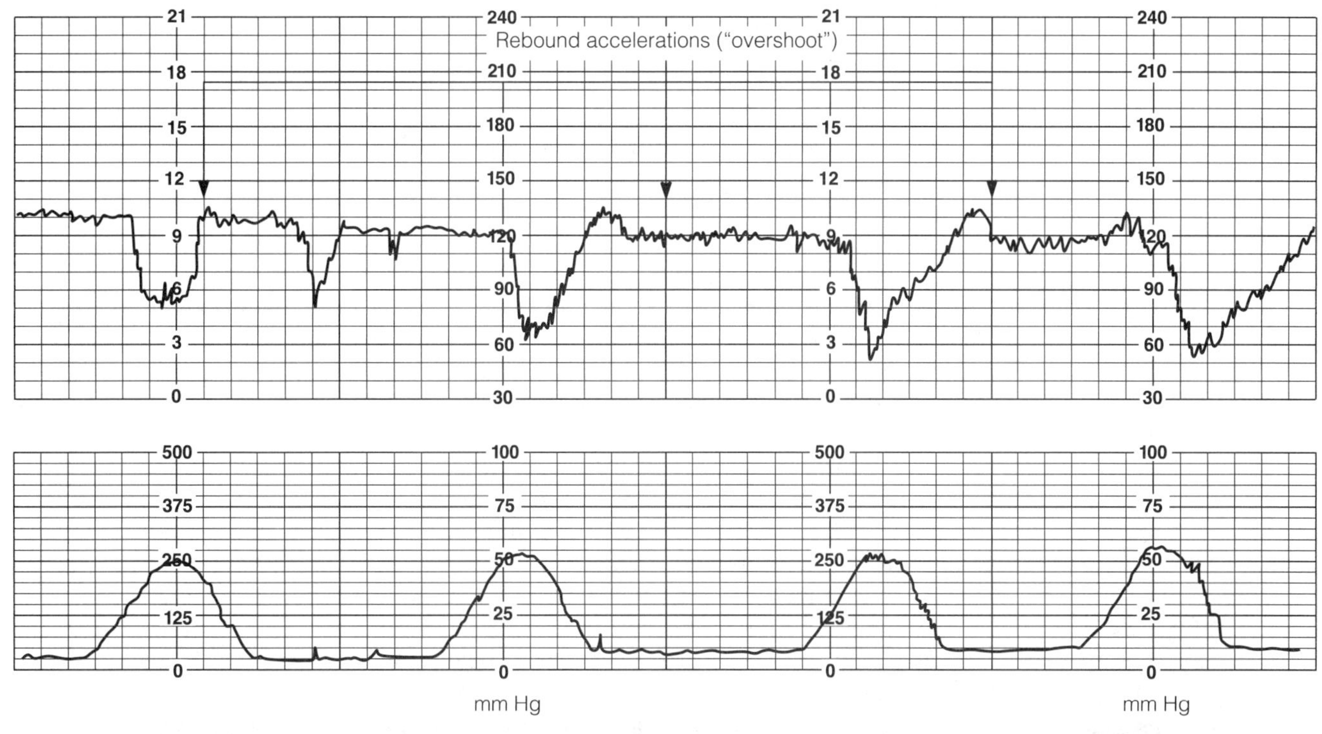

Figure 8-3

Variable decelerations with overshoot. Timing of decelerations is variable, most have sharp declines. A rebound acceleration (overshoot) occurs with most decelerations. Baseline FHR is 115–130 beats/min. Nadir (lowest point) of decelerations is 55–80 beats/min.

Source: Davidson, M., London, M. & Ladewig, P. (2012). *Olds' maternal newborn nursing & women's health across the lifespan* (9th ed.). Upper Saddle River, NJ: Pearson Education, p. 585.

2. Uterine contraction monitoring documents contraction frequency, duration, and intensity; contractions are documented on lower half of monitor strip
   a. External monitoring: pressure-sensitive tocodynamometer is placed on maternal abdomen near fundus; accurate only for documenting contraction frequency and duration; affected by fetal or maternal movement, transverse or oblique lie, and maternal abdominal fat: a thin woman's mild contractions may look strong on monitor strip, while an obese woman's strong contractions may not be detected at all
   b. Internal monitoring is accomplished through an **intrauterine pressure catheter** (IUPC), a wire with pressure gauge on one end or a saline-filled tube, which is inserted through cervix and past presenting part into amniotic fluid in uterus; an increase in intrauterine pressure is detected by IUPC, and measured in mm of Hg; cervix must be at least 2 to 3 cm dilated with ruptured membranes before an IUPC can be inserted

Practice to Pass

The laboring client asks what the intrauterine pressure catheter is for and why it is used. How should the nurse reply?

II. THE LABOR PROCESS

A. **Initiation of labor**: comes about from an interplay of factors including distension of uterus causing irritability and contractility, and hormonal influence of prostaglandins, oxytocin, fetal cortisol, estrogen, and progesterone

! B. **True versus false labor**: differentiated by cervical change: effacement and dilatation

C. **Factors of labor**: the passageway, passenger, powers, and psyche (4 Ps)
   1. Passageway refers to maternal bony pelvis comprised of innominate bones (ilium, ischium, and pubis), sacrum, and coccyx
      a. False pelvis lies above pelvic brim, supports increasing weight of enlarging pregnant uterus and directs presenting part into true pelvis below

b. True pelvis consists of inlet, midpelvis, and outlet, and represents bony limits of birth canal; the adequacy of each part, measured as transverse and anterior–posterior diameters, must be sufficient to allow passage of fetus through passageway
c. Four pelvic types are *gynecoid*, *android*, *anthropoid*, and *platypelloid* (see Table 8-1); type of pelvis and its diameters influence descent of fetus, progression of labor, and type of delivery

2. Passenger refers to fetus
   a. **Attitude** is the relationship of the fetal parts to one another; the normal attitude is flexion of the neck, arms, and legs
   b. **Lie** is the relationship of longitudinal axis of fetus to longitudinal axis of mother; vertex (head first) is most common, but breech (most frequently buttocks first, see presentation that follows), transverse (laterally across uterus), and oblique (diagonally across uterus) lies are possible
   c. **Presentation** refers to fetal part entering pelvis first; most common presentation is cephalic, but frank breech (buttocks), shoulder, footling, and, rarely, full face can also occur
   d. **Position** is relationship of fetal presenting part to maternal pelvis; a three-letter notation is used to describe fetal position
      1) First letter is R for right or L for left, indicating which side of maternal pelvis the presenting part is toward
      2) Second letter indicates landmark of fetal presenting part: O = occiput, M = mentum, S = sacrum, or A = acromion process
      3) Third letter indicates relationship of landmark of presenting part to front, back, or side of pelvis: A = anterior P = posterior, T = transverse; most common positions at delivery are ROA or LOA
   e. **Engagement** occurs when largest diameter of presenting part reaches pelvic inlet and can be detected by vaginal examination
      1) If presenting part is directed toward pelvis but can easily be moved out of inlet, it is floating
      2) When presenting part dips into inlet but can be displaced with upward pressure from examiner's fingers, it is ballotable
      3) If presenting part is fixed in pelvic inlet and cannot be displaced, it is engaged
   f. **Station** is relationship of presenting part to ischial spines of pelvis; measured in centimeters above (–1 to –5 station), at (0 station), or below (+1 to +4 station) the ischial spines (see Figure 8-4)
3. Powers include primary and secondary forces of labor
   a. Primary forces consist of involuntary contractions of uterine muscle fibers, which are stimulated by a pacemaker located in upper uterine segment

Practice to Pass

Describe the attitude, lie, presentation, and position of a fetus listed as frank breech, RSA.

Table 8-1 Pelvic Types

Pelvic Type	Incidence	Inlet	Midpelvis	Outlet	Implications for Birth
Gynecoid	50%	Round, adequate diameters	Round, adequate diameters	Wide transverse and long anterior–posterior diameters	Occiput anterior most common, NSVD favorable
Android	20%	Heart-shaped, angulated	Short anterior–posterior diameter	Short anterior–posterior diameter	Slow descent, arrest of labor, operative birth more common
Anthropoid	25%	Ovoid, long anterior–posterior diameter	Rounded, adequate diameters	Narrow transverse	Occiput anterior or posterior, NSVD favorable
Platypelloid	5%	Ovoid, wide transverse diameter	Rounded, wide transverse diameter	Wide transverse, short anterior–posterior diameter	Occiput posterior more common, NSVD not favorable

Note: NSVD = Normal sterile vaginal delivery

Figure 8-4

Stations of fetal descent in labor

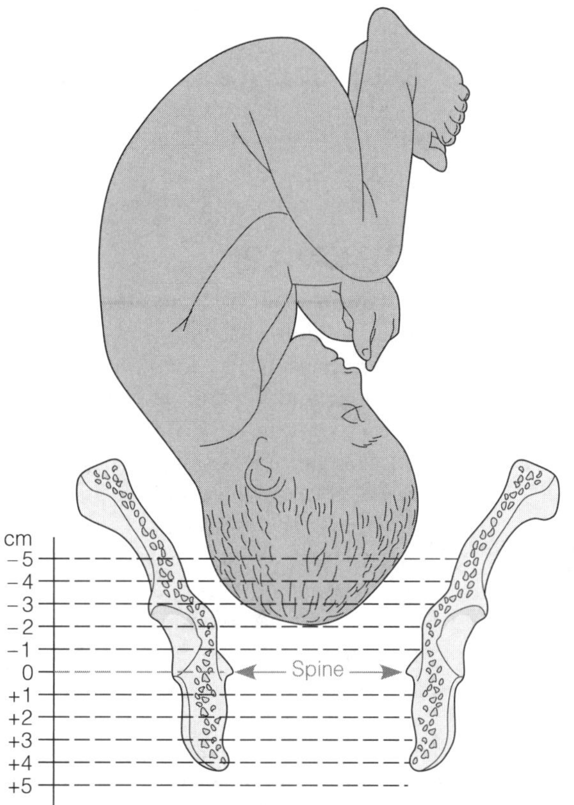

1) Contractions consist of increment (building-up phase), acme (peak), and decrement (letting-up phase) and are followed by a resting phase (**nadir**) to facilitate utero-placental–fetal reoxygenation
2) Frequency of contractions is time in seconds or minutes from onset of one contraction to onset of next contraction
3) Intensity is strength of contraction at the acme (peak), which can be palpated as mild, moderate, or strong, or detected with a fetal monitor externally or measured internally in mm Hg
4) Duration is length of contraction measured in seconds from beginning of increment to end of decrement
5) With each contraction, muscles of upper uterine segment shorten and exert longitudinal traction on cervix causing **effacement**, a thinning and drawing up of internal os and cervical canal into uterine side walls; measured from 0 to 100%; in primigravidas effacement usually precedes dilatation; in multigravidas effacement and dilatation normally occur simultaneously
6) As uterus elongates with contractions, fetal body straightens and exerts pressure against lower uterine segment and cervix; **dilatation** (opening of cervix) results and is measured from 0 to 10 cm; this allows for birth of fetus

b. Secondary powers consist of voluntary use of abdominal muscles during second stage of labor to facilitate fetal descent and delivery

4. Psyche represents psychological component of childbearing; excitement, fear, perceived loss of control, and anxiety are common emotions during labor and birth process

a. Extreme emotions such as fear result in muscular tension, which can create more pain from friction between working uterus and tense abdominal muscles, or impede fetal descent when pelvic and perineal muscles are tense rather than relaxed when pushing

b. Psyche can also be manifested physiologically; increased blood pressure, pulse, and respiratory rates occur with fear, excitement, and anxiety
c. Lack of knowledge and preparation for childbirth can negatively affect psyche
d. Women with altered thought processes, inability to understand the spoken language, or who have lower IQs can be negatively affected by labor/birth process

III. THE STAGES OF LABOR

A. **First stage**: extends from onset of true labor to complete dilatation of cervix (0 to 10 cm) and is divided into three phases

1. Latent phase: 0 to 3 centimeters dilated, little descent occurs; contractions usually begin irregularly and become more regular, with frequency becoming closer, duration increasing, and intensity increasing from mild to moderate; woman is usually relieved labor has started, may be anxious, happy, excited, or talkative, and may change position without reminder; average length is 8.6 hours for nullipara and 5.3 hours for multiparas
2. Active phase: 4 to 7 centimeters dilated, progressive effacement and descent, contractions usually every 2 to 3 minutes, 60 seconds in duration, and moderate to strong intensity; woman is usually serious, intense, has a need for increased concentration, and answers questions in short phrases only between contractions; fatigue increases and woman becomes more dependent; pain increases, relaxation becomes more difficult, and she may need reminders to change positions; average length is 4.6 hours for nulliparas and 2.4 hours for multiparas
3. Transition phase: 8 to 10 centimeters dilated, effacement is completed, and descent increases; contractions every 1½ to 2 minutes, lasting 60 to 90 seconds, strong intensity; woman is working hard with intense concentration and gives one-word answers to questions only between contractions; anxiety increases, fears loss of control and abandonment, senses helplessness and may state, "I can't do this anymore"; relaxation is difficult as contraction time exceeds resting phase between contractions; may experience intense low abdominal, pelvic, and rectal discomfort from descent of fetus; nausea and vomiting are common; may need reminders to empty bladder and change position; average length is 3.6 hours for nulliparas and 30 minutes for multiparas
4. Assessment
   a. Upon admission: review medical, obstetric and prenatal history; labor status (contractions, vaginal examination if indicated), fetal status (heart rate, variability, periodic changes), status of membranes (intact or if ruptured, length of time and amount, color, odor), maternal vital signs, laboratory testing if ordered (Hgb and UA), desired birth plan including cultural considerations, preparation for childbirth, level of comfort and coping, and support system
   b. First stage of labor
      1) Latent phase: blood pressure, pulse, respirations every hour if normal; temperature q4h if normal or membranes intact, if abnormal or membranes ruptured q2h; contractions q30 min; FHR every hour for low-risk women or q30min if high-risk or nonreassuring pattern
      2) Active phase: blood pressure, pulse, respirations, temperature, contractions same as latent phase; FHR q30min for low-risk women or q15min for high-risk women or nonreassuring pattern
      3) Transition phase: blood pressure, pulse, respirations q30min; temperature same as latent phase; contractions q15min, FHR q15min
5. Priority nursing diagnoses: Anxiety; Fear; Deficient Knowledge; Pain; Compromised Family Coping

6. Implementation and collaborative care
   a. Orient to environment, expected assessments, and procedures
   b. Encourage ambulation (if presenting part is engaged) unless contraindicated
   c. ! Provide comfort through frequent position change, effleurage, focal point, hydrotherapy, caregiver presence, therapeutic touch, sacral pressure, back rub, or administration of analgesia as requested by client and ordered by health care provider
   d. Encourage voiding q2h
   e. Monitor labor progress and fetal well-being
   f. Provide ice chips and clear liquids to prevent dehydration
   g. Teach, reinforce, or support use of relaxation, visualization, or breathing patterns
   h. Encourage rest between contractions
   i. Document in client record and provide continuing status reports to health care provider
7. Evaluation: client states she is able to cope with contractions; maternal and fetal well-being is maintained throughout labor

! B. **Second stage**: extends from complete cervical dilatation to delivery of fetus; accompanied by involuntary efforts to expel fetus characterized by low-pitched, guttural, grunting sounds; many women initially feel renewed energy because they can voluntarily work with contractions to push out fetus; over time can be exhausting work; normal length for nulliparas is up to 3 hours and up to 30 minutes for multiparas

1. ! **Cardinal movements**: adaptations that fetus undertakes to maneuver through pelvis during labor and birth; a mnemonic phrase to assist in remembering these movements is created by using first letter (shown in boldface type) of each cardinal movement to begin a word (shown in italics), these words are used to create a phrase: ***E**very **d**arn **f**ool **i**n **R**otterdam **e**ats **r**otten **e**gg **r**olls **e**veryday*; in occipital (most common) presentation, movements occur in this order:
   a. *Engagement* of presenting part occurs
   b. *Descent* of fetus into pelvis
   c. *Flexion* of fetal head; (descent and flexion often occur simultaneously)
   d. *Internal rotation* of fetal head must take place to accommodate maternal pelvis and occurs so that anterior–posterior diameter of fetal head, largest diameter of fetus, aligns with anterior–posterior dimension of maternal pelvis
   e. *Extension* of fetal head occurs as it comes under maternal symphysis pubis and emerges from vagina
   f. ***R**estitution* occurs as fetal head turns 45° to untwist neck after head has delivered
   g. *External **r**otation* is viewed as head turns an additional 45° as second-largest fetal diameter (lateral diameter of fetal shoulders) rotates into alignment with anterior–posterior dimension of maternal pelvis
   h. *Expulsion* occurs as anterior shoulder slips beneath symphysis pubis to facilitate delivery of body
2. ! **Crowning**: outward bulging and thinning of perineum and opening of vagina as fetal presenting part presses downward onto perineum and becomes visible prior to delivery; this process is slower in nulliparous client than multiparous client
3. Assessment
   a. Blood pressure, pulse, and respirations every 5 to 15 minutes
   b. Contractions palpated continuously
   c. Fetal heart rate q15min if low risk, q5min if high risk, and if nonreassuring pattern, monitor continuously
   d. Monitor fetal descent, cardinal fetal movements and crowning
4. Priority nursing diagnoses: Pain; Fear; Deficient Knowledge; Ineffective Coping
5. Implementation and collaborative care

a. Position comfortably for pushing and birth; encourage rest and relaxation between contractions
b. Comfort measures: cool cloth to forehead, support legs while pushing, provide encouragement to push
c. Ice chips and clear fluids to prevent dehydration
d. Empty bladder, straight catheter if bladder distended or unable to void
e. Local infiltration of anesthetic agent for birth by health care provider

!

f. **Episiotomy**: a surgical incision into perineum to enlarge vaginal opening (see Figure 8-5); usually done during or just prior to crowning; medically indicated in presence of fetal distress, but often performed to prevent tearing of perineal tissues because lacerations have irregular edges and are more difficult to repair

1) Midline episiotomy: 1- to 3-centimeter incision is made straight back from vagina toward rectum; advantage: muscle fibers are split lengthwise allowing faster and less painful healing; disadvantage: 30% will extend into 3rd- or 4th-degree lacerations
2) Mediolateral episiotomy: 4- to 5-centimeter incision is made from vagina obliquely toward one buttock; advantage: larger episiotomy possible and rectal structures avoided; disadvantage: muscle fibers are cut across causing more pain during healing

Practice to Pass

The laboring client asks the nurse if she will need an episiotomy or have a laceration. How should the nurse respond?

g. Lacerations to perineum or surrounding tissues may occur during childbirth; 3rd- and 4th-degree lacerations most commonly occur after midline episiotomy is performed
1) 1st degree: involves only epidermal layers, if no bleeding may not need repair
2) 2nd degree: epidermal and muscle/fascia involvement that requires suturing
3) 3rd degree: extends into rectal sphincter
4) 4th degree: extends through rectal wall (mucosa)
h. Document in client record: time of birth, gender, position, nuchal cord (umbilical cord around the neonate's neck), if present, and medications administered

6. Evaluation: client states is able to cope with contractions and pushing; maternal and fetal well-being is maintained through delivery

C. Third stage: extends from birth of the newborn to delivery of placenta; average length is 30 minutes for nulliparas and multiparas

1. Maternal assessment
a. Blood pressure, pulse, and respirations q5min

Figure 8-5
Locations for episiotomy

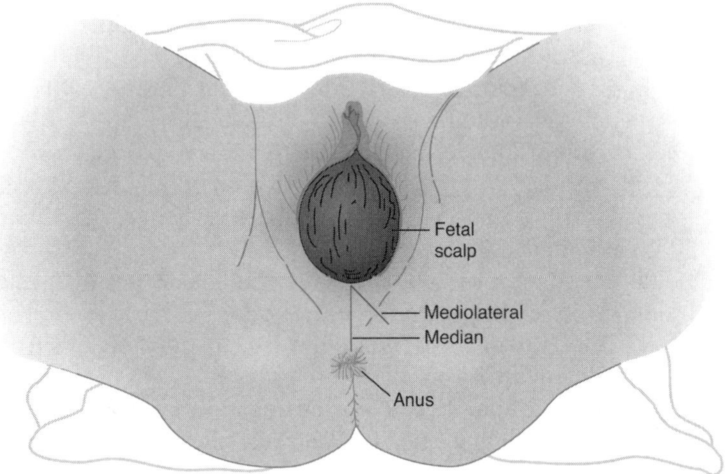

b. Uterine fundus maintains tone and contraction pattern to deliver placenta by decreasing surface volume of uterus and shearing placenta from uterine wall
c. Monitor for signs of placental separation: uterus rises up in abdomen, uterine volume shrinks from contractions, creating a gush of blood vaginally as uterine contents are expelled; as placenta is separating and beginning to be expelled, umbilical cord protrudes further from vagina and appears to lengthen

2. Fetal assessment
   a. **Apgar score**: a quick method to assess fetal adaptation to extrauterine life (see Table 8-2); five criteria are scored at 1 and 5 minutes after birth with 0, 1, or 2 points given for each criteria; five criteria include color, heart rate, reflex irritability, muscle tone, and respiratory effort; Apgar scores of 8 or greater indicate newborn needs minimal intervention (nasopharyngeal suction and oxygen near face); scores of 4 to 7 indicate a need for intervention through oropharyngeal suctioning, tactile stimulation, and oxygen administration; and scores of 3 or less indicate a need for resuscitation
   b. Respirations: normally 30 to 60, may be irregular
   c. Apical pulse: 110 to 160, may be irregular and may increase to 180 transiently while crying
   d. Temperature: skin temperature above 97.8°F (36.5°C)
   e. Umbilical cord: normally two arteries and one vein (note that one artery with one vein can occur)
   f. Gestational age assessment: consistent with expected date of delivery
   g. Physical assessment: abbreviated examination is conducted to detect presence of visible congenital anomalies
3. Priority nursing diagnoses: Pain; Fear; Deficient Knowledge; Ineffective Coping
4. Implementation and collaborative care
   a. Encourage mother to rest and relax while awaiting delivery of placenta

   b. Immediate care of newborn includes placing in a modified Trendelenburg position, suctioning nose and oropharynx (bulb syringe or DeLee mucus trap), providing and maintaining warmth (dry immediately with warm blankets, skin-to-skin contact with mother covered with warm blankets, radiant heat source, cap)

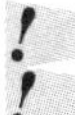

   c. Assist parents to see and hold newborn to begin attachment
   d. Document time of placental delivery, appearance and intactness of placenta, mechanism of placental expulsion and estimated delivery blood loss (averages 250 to 500 mL)
      1) If placenta separates from edge progressing toward center and rough maternal side of placenta is visible, it is called a dirty Duncan mechanism of delivery
      2) If placenta separates from center progressing outward and membrane-covered fetal side of placenta is visible, it is called a shiny Schultze mechanism of delivery
   e. Administer oxytocic agent as ordered
   f. Consider cultural practices in disposal of placenta
5. Evaluation: mother and newborn experience a safe labor and birth

Table 8-2 Apgar Scoring

	Color (Appearance)	Heart Rate (Pulse)	Reflex Irritability (Grimace)	Muscle Tone (Activity)	Respiratory Effort (Respirations)
0 Points	Blue, pale	Absent	Absent	Absent	Absent
1 Point	Blue extremities, pink body	<100	Grimace	Some flexion of extremities	Slow, irregular
2 Points	Completely pink	≥100	Vigorous cry	Active motion	Good cry

D. Fourth stage (immediate recovery phase): includes first one to four hours after delivery; the term is misleading because labor and birth are completed with delivery of placenta; this stage is actually part of postpartal period but client usually remains in birthing suite for nursing care if not already in an LDRP (labor, delivery, recovery, postpartum) room

1. Assessment: blood pressure, pulse, respirations, fundus, lochia and perineum *per agency protocol*; usually q15min for 1 hour; q30min for 2 hours; q60min for 1 hour
2. Priority nursing diagnoses: Pain; Deficient Knowledge; Interrupted Family Processes
3. Implementation and collaborative care
   a. Episiotomy or lacerations are repaired
   b. Provide comfort: clean gown, warm blanket, position of comfort, ice to perineum if sutures or edema are present, analgesia as requested and ordered
   c. Assist parents to explore their newborn and initiate breastfeeding, if desired and mother and baby are stable
   d. Provide fluids and regular diet as tolerated; consider cultural preferences
4. Evaluation: maternal and newborn well-being are maintained; family unit is supported and participates in birth process as desired

IV. PAIN MANAGEMENT DURING BIRTH

A. Analgesia and anesthesia: can be given to decrease or eliminate pain during birthing process when nonpharmacologic methods of pain relief are ineffective

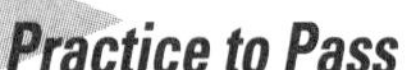

Practice to Pass

The nulliparous client is experiencing a normal progression of labor. She is currently 4 cm dilated, 100% effaced, vertex, at a 0 station, with contractions of moderate intensity every 4 minutes lasting 60 seconds. She asks what she can do for pain relief. How should the nurse respond?

B. Type of analgesia or anesthesia: determined by client's obstetric history, stage and phase of labor, rate of progression in labor, and preferences of client and health care provider; regional differences in use of particular methods or medications exist

C. Nonpharmacologic methods of pain relief

1. Position changes to decrease weight of fetus from area of most intense pain
2. Hydrotherapy by standing or sitting in a warm shower or reclining in a tub
3. Breathing techniques to prevent breath holding and to facilitate oxygen and carbon dioxide exchange; use of a focal point for concentration
4. Relaxation through verbal instruction, massage, soft music, or therapeutic touch

D. Pharmacological methods of pain relief

1. Analgesics decrease amount of pain perceived; goal is maximum pain relief with minimal risk to woman and fetus; must consider effect on woman, fetus and contractions
2. All systemic drugs cross placental barrier in varying amounts; analgesia given too early may prolong labor and depress fetus; analgesia given too late may cause neonatal respiratory depression with no benefit to woman

3. Intravenous opioids: nalbuphine hydrochloride (Nubain) and butorphanol tartrate (Stadol) most commonly used in active phase of first stage of labor
   a. Advantages: RN administration, rapid onset of pain relief, ease of administration, relatively short duration
   b. Disadvantages: may decrease contraction frequency and intensity, crosses placenta resulting in neonatal respiratory depression, and short duration may not give adequate pain control during nulliparous or prolonged labor

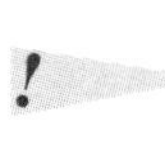

   c. Nursing implications: nalbuphine is a narcotic agonist–antagonist and should never be given to a client with narcotic dependency or abuse as immediate withdrawal will occur that can stimulate seizures

4. Regional analgesia and anesthesia provide temporary and reversible loss of sensation by injecting an agent into an area with direct contact to nervous tissue (see Table 8-3 for summary of types of methods)

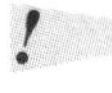

   a. Lumbar **epidural block**: a needle is placed into epidural space at L4–L5 or L5–S1 level, a very small diameter catheter is threaded into space, and local anesthetic agents such as bupivacaine hydrochloride (Marcaine) or lidocaine hydrochloride (Xylocaine) are injected; depending on dose injected, can provide either analgesia or anesthesia

Table 8-3 Summary of Common Regional Blocks Used During Labor

Type of Block	Areas Affected	Use During Labor and Birth	Nursing Actions
Lumbar epidural	Uterus, cervix, vagina, and perineum	Given in first stage and second stage of labor	Assess woman's knowledge regarding the block. Act as advocate to help her obtain further information if needed. Monitor maternal blood pressure to detect the major side effect, which is hypotension. Provide support and comfort.
Combined spinal-epidural	Uterus, cervix, vagina, and perineum	Spinal analgesia may be given in latent phase for pain relief. Epidural is given when active labor begins.	Assess woman's knowledge regarding the block. Monitor maternal vital signs and fetal heart rate (FHR) status. Provide comfort measures.
Pudendal	Perineum and lower vagina	Given in the second stage just before birth to provide anesthesia for episiotomy or for low forceps birth.	Assess woman's knowledge regarding the block. Act as advocate to help her obtain further information if needed.
Local infiltration	Perineum	Administered just before birth to provide anesthesia for episiotomy or after birth for repair of a laceration.	Assess woman's knowledge regarding the block. Provide information as needed. Provide comfort and support. Observe perineum for bruising or other discoloration in the recovery period.
Spinal	Uterus, cervix, vagina, and perineum	Given during first stage for pain relief. Provides immediate onset of anesthesia.	Assess woman's knowledge regarding the block. Monitor maternal vital signs and FHR status.

Source: Davidson, Michele; London, Marcia L.; Ladewig, Patricia W., *Olds' maternal-newborn nursing & women's health across the lifespan*, 9th Ed., ©2012. Reprinted and Electronically reproduced by permission of Pearson Education, Inc., Upper Saddle River, New Jersey.

1) Advantages: excellent pain relief, redosing of medication into epidural catheter is possible, no neonatal respiratory depression results, may provide a few hours of postpartum pain relief as well as during labor and delivery
2) Disadvantage: time involved with set-up and administration make it undesirable for rapidly progressing labors or in transition phase, must be inserted by anesthesia personnel, usually causes numbness of lower extremities limiting mobility, decreases contraction frequency and intensity thus requiring pharmacologic augmentation, contraction intensity difficult to detect and may require use of IUPC, little or no urge to push is felt, relaxation of musculature below injection site often results in failure of fetus to accomplish internal rotation necessitating an operative birth
3) ! Nursing implications: monitor urinary output as retention requiring indwelling urinary catheter may result; monitor blood pressure as maternal hypotension commonly results from vasodilation; avoid supine position

b. Intrathecal opioids (not commonly used): preservative-free morphine sulfate (morphine) or fentanyl citrate (fentanyl) injected into L4–L5 or L5–S1 subarachnoid space

1) Advantages: excellent pain control within several minutes that lasts several hours; rarely results in neonatal respiratory depression; easier and faster injection method than epidural
2) Disadvantages: set-up and administration time prevent use in rapidly progressing labors or transition phase; may eliminate urge to push; spinal headache may occur from leakage of CSF through dura at injection site; may lead to maternal urinary retention and with morphine, possibly delayed respiratory depression
3) ! Nursing implications: monitor for common side effects including nausea, pruritus, urinary retention, muscle spasms at injection site

c. **Paracervical block**: local anesthetic agent is injected into lateral aspects of cervix during active or transition phases
   1) Advantages: rapid onset of pain relief, no neonatal respiratory depression, can be administered during transition, relative ease of administration
   2) Disadvantages: systemic drug absorption can occur through vascular cervix, excessive bleeding from cervix may result, or woman may experience a decreased or absent urge to push
   3) ! Nursing implications: monitor FHR as bradycardia can result from systemic absorption
d. **Pudendal block**: local anesthetic agent is injected into lateral vaginal walls near ischial spines to anesthetize pudendal nerve; administered during second stage in preparation for cutting and repairing an episiotomy
   1) Advantages: excellent anesthesia of the perineum, rarely need readminstration, provides a few hours of postpartum pain relief
   2) Disadvantages: must inject along presenting part creating increased vaginal pressure and discomfort for client; eliminates urge to push
   3) ! Nursing implications: monitor client safety as decreased sensation in lower extremities affects mobility
e. Local infiltration: local anesthetic agents are injected into perineal tissues to provide anesthesia for episiotomy incision or repair and suturing of lacerations
   1) Advantage: ease of administration, provides a few hours of postpartum pain relief
   2) Disadvantages: reinjection may be needed to obtain complete anesthesia with extensive lacerations or large episiotomies
   3) ! Nursing implications: loss of sensation may decrease urge or ability to urinate

Case Study

The client is a nullipara at 5 centimeters dilation, 100% effacement, 0 station, vertex presentation, LOP position, with intact membranes. Contractions are occurring every 3 minutes lasting 60 seconds with strong intensity. The health care provider orders continuous external electronic fetal monitoring.

1. How often should the nurse assess maternal vital signs and fetal well-being?
2. Where might the client be feeling discomfort and why?
3. What interventions should the nurse use to promote the client's comfort at this stage and phase of labor?
4. When the client asks what to expect as labor progresses, how should the nurse respond?
5. The client states she has experienced a healthy pregnancy and asks why continuous fetal monitoring is necessary. How should the nurse respond?

For suggested responses, see page 304.

POSTTEST

1 The nurse is planning to teach a class of expectant parents about the cardinal movements, or changes in position, that occur as the fetus passes through the birth canal. The nurse plans to teach the positional changes in the sequence in which they occur when the fetus is in a cephalic presentation. Place the cardinal movements in the correct sequence.

1. Expulsion
2. External rotation
3. Flexion
4. Internal rotation
5. Restitution

2 Which statement would indicate that the laboring client needs further education?

1. "Because this is my first labor, I will need an epidural."
2. "Labor can be long and difficult sometimes."
3. "I should keep taking at least ice chips throughout labor."
4. "My partner can help me stay relaxed and focused."

3 The nurse anticipates that assessment of a normal episiotomy immediately post-delivery is most likely to reveal which of the following?

1. Gaping between the sutures
2. Slight yellow brown bruising
3. Purulent drainage from the suture line
4. Edema at the episiotomy site making the tissue appear shiny

4 Fourth-stage nursing care for a client with an episiotomy includes which of the following? Select all that apply.

1. Application of ice beginning four hours after delivery
2. Ice pack to the perineum for up to 60 minutes (min) per application
3. Inspection every 15 min during the first hour after birth
4. Instructions to avoid intercourse for at least 12 weeks
5. Ice packs to be applied for 20–30 min and removed for at least 20 min

5 The nurse would formulate what general goal when developing childbirth education classes for pregnant women in the community?

1. Provide education for all pregnant clients.
2. Ensure a normal spontaneous vaginal delivery.
3. Assist clients to know what to expect during labor.
4. Prepare the couple for any possible complications.

6 After performing a vaginal exam the nurse discussed the results with the client and her partner. The nurse later concludes that client teaching was effective when the partner shouts, "She must be crowning; this means it will be soon," after viewing which of the following?

1. A little of the baby's head is pushing through the cervical opening.
2. The baby's head recedes upward between pushing contractions.
3. The perineum is thin and stretching around the occiput.
4. The mouth and nose are being suctioned.

7 The nurse notes on the antepartal history that the pregnant client has an android pelvis. The nurse concludes that this client is at an increased risk for which of the following?

1. A prolonged labor
2. Occiput posterior position
3. Precipitous delivery
4. Postpartum hemorrhage

8 The maternal newborn nurse would use which description of the fetal position when explaining to the mother the occurrence of a frank breech position?

1. "Both the hips and the knees are flexed."
2. "The hips are extended and the knees are flexed."
3. "The hips are flexed and the knees are extended."
4. "Both the hips and the knees are extended."

9 The fetal head is determined to be presenting in a position of complete extension. The maternal newborn nurse should anticipate which type of labor and delivery?

1. Precipitous labor and delivery
2. Prolonged labor and possible cesarean delivery
3. Normal labor and spontaneous vaginal delivery
4. Forceps-assisted vaginal delivery

10 The pregnant client is seven cm dilated, 100% effaced, and at a +1 station. The fetus is in a face presentation. The nurse concludes that client teaching has been effective when the client's husband makes which statement?

1. "Our baby will come out face first."
2. "Our baby will come out facing one hip."
3. "Our baby will come out buttocks first."
4. "Our baby will come out with the back of the head first."

➤ *See pages 171–173 for Answers and Rationales.*

ANSWERS & RATIONALES

Pretest

1 **Answer: 1** **Rationale:** The presenting part is given first when describing fetal position. The second half of the fetal position description refers to the maternal pelvis. In this client, it is the sacrum presenting, and the fetal sacrum is toward the maternal anterior pelvis. The fetal sacrum is not a standard reference point. In this question, the sacrum (not the face) is being described. The maternal sacrum is also the posterior part of the maternal pelvis. The fetal sacrum (not the fetal face) is being described in this question. **Cognitive Level:** Analyzing **Client Need:** Health Promotion and Maintenance **Integrated Process:** Nursing Process: Assessment **Content Area:** Maternal-Newborn **Strategy:** The critical words in this question are *sacrum anterior*. Eliminate two options that do not refer to the sacrum. Recall that the first locator, sacrum, refers to the fetus and the second locator, anterior, refers to the mother. The correct answer would be the option that refers to the fetal sacrum closest to the anterior maternal reference point, the symphysis. **Reference:** Ladewig, P. A., London, M. L., & Davidson, M. R. (2010). *Contemporary maternal-newborn nursing care* (7th ed.). Upper Saddle River, NJ: Pearson Education, pp. 379–381.

2 **Answer: 1** **Rationale:** Changes in the cervix, showing a pattern of continuous dilatation and effacement, is the only indicator of true labor. Being a multipara, increased intensity and duration of contractions, and spontaneous rupture of membranes do not correlate as closely as the cervical changes. **Cognitive Level:** Applying **Client Need:** Health Promotion and Maintenance **Integrated Process:** Nursing Process: Assessment **Content Area:** Maternal-Newborn **Strategy:** The critical words in this question are *true labor*. Recalling that true labor is only defined by cervical change, eliminate options that do not include change in the cervix. **Reference:** Ladewig, P. A., London, M. L., & Davidson, M. R. (2010). *Contemporary maternal-newborn nursing care* (7th ed.). Upper Saddle River, NJ: Pearson Education, p. 387.

3 **Answer: 4** **Rationale:** The fetal heart rate response to contractions is a physiologic assessment that indicates the presence or absence of fetal well-being. Providing pain relief measures, assessing partner involvement, and monitoring fluid intake are appropriate for the laboring client, but safety of the fetus and the mother are the highest priorities. **Cognitive Level:** Analyzing **Client Need:** Management of Care **Integrated Process:** Nursing Process: Planning **Content Area:** Maternal-Newborn **Strategy:** Recall that the goal for every birth is a safe outcome for mother and baby. The correct answer will be the option that includes a true statement about maintaining safe passage. Remember that there are two clients in the question: the fetus and the mother, so the correct answer will refer to one or both. **Reference:** Ladewig, P. A., London, M. L., & Davidson, M. R. (2010). *Contemporary maternal-newborn nursing care* (7th ed.). Upper Saddle River, NJ: Pearson Education, pp. 387–393.

4 **Answer: 2** **Rationale:** As labor progresses, contractions will become more intense, occur more frequently (shorter resting phase between contractions), and have an increasing duration. Less frequent or shorter duration contractions can impede labor progress. **Cognitive Level:** Applying **Client Need:** Health Promotion and Maintenance **Integrated Process:** Nursing Process: Assessment **Content Area:** Maternal-Newborn **Strategy:** The focus of this question is the relationship of contractions to birth. Recall that contractions are the powers to facilitate birth; the work gets harder over time. The correct answer would be the option that makes a true statement about increasing intensity, frequency, and duration of contractions. **Reference:** Ladewig, P. A., London, M. L., & Davidson, M. R. (2010). *Contemporary maternal-newborn nursing care* (7th ed.). Upper Saddle River, NJ: Pearson Education, pp. 387–389.

5 **Answer: 9** **Rationale:** Apgar scores are based on 0, 1, or 2 points in each of the five categories: respiratory effort, color, muscle tone, heart rate, and reflexes. This neonate would score 2 points in each category except color, where the presence of acrocyanosis would warrant a score of 1 point. **Cognitive Level:** Applying **Client Need:** Health Promotion and Maintenance **Integrated Process:** Nursing Process: Assessment **Content Area:** Maternal-Newborn **Strategy:** Recall that the Apgar score includes 0–2 points on five criteria. The data given in the question includes one exception statement, making a perfect score of 10 unlikely and leading you to subtract one point. **Reference:** Ladewig, P. A., London, M. L., & Davidson, M. R.

(2010). *Contemporary maternal-newborn nursing care* (7th ed.). Upper Saddle River, NJ: Pearson Education, pp. 453–454.

6 **Answer: 3 Rationale:** As the uterus contracts and the placenta begins to shear off the uterine wall for expulsion, there is a small gush of blood resulting from the uterine contractions emptying the uterus. In addition, the cord will lengthen as the placenta is released from the uterine wall and moves toward the cervix prior to expulsion. There should not be an associated cord tear. **Cognitive Level:** Analyzing **Client Need:** Health Promotion and Maintenance **Integrated Process:** Nursing Process: Assessment **Content Area:** Maternal-Newborn **Strategy:** The critical words in this question are *separation* and *expulsion*. As the placenta and cord are expelled, more of the umbilical cord becomes visible. Eliminate two options because they do not include a true statement about cord change. Recall that the umbilical cord should not tear to eliminate that option. **Reference:** Ladewig, P. A., London, M. L., & Davidson, M. R. (2010). *Contemporary maternal-newborn nursing care* (7th ed.). Upper Saddle River, NJ: Pearson Education, pp. 456–457.

7 **Answer: 2 Rationale:** Anxiety commonly increases the perception of pain, and childbearing is no exception to this. Decreasing anxiety through education and support will facilitate the birthing process. Anxiety will not hasten the labor process. The client's anxiety level is not expected to reduce or eliminate the support from a support person or system. The need for an episiotomy would be determined by the status of the perineum, not the client's anxiety. **Cognitive Level:** Applying **Client Need:** Psychosocial Integrity **Integrated Process:** Nursing Process: Diagnosis **Content Area:** Maternal-Newborn **Strategy:** Recall the four P's of labor; the psyche influences the experience and progress of birth. Recall the fear-tension-pain cycle; anxiety and pain are directly related. This should help to eliminate incorrect options and select the correct answer. **Reference:** Ladewig, P. A., London, M. L., & Davidson, M. R. (2010). *Contemporary maternal-newborn nursing care* (7th ed.). Upper Saddle River, NJ: Pearson Education, pp. 443–444.

8 **Answer: 1, 5 Rationale:** An increase in FHR baseline can be an indication of fetal distress and can also occur with maternal fever. Narcotics may decrease the short-term variability but do not affect the baseline. Fetal movement will create an acceleration of the fetal heart rate. Utero-placental insufficiency causes late decelerations. **Cognitive Level:** Analyzing **Client Need:** Physiological Adaptation **Integrated Process:** Nursing Process: Diagnosis **Content Area:** Maternal-Newborn **Strategy:** Eliminate options that are obviously incorrect. Recall that narcotics are CNS depressants, movement temporarily increases heart rate, and utero-placental insufficiency causes periodic late decelerations. **Reference:** Ladewig, P. A., London, M. L., & Davidson, M. R. (2010). *Contemporary maternal-newborn nursing care* (7th ed.). Upper Saddle River, NJ: Pearson Education, pp. 426–427.

9 **Answer: 2 Rationale:** Effacement is the thinning of the cervix from 0 to 100%. The opening of the cervix from 0 to 10 centimeters is called dilatation. In primigravidas effacement usually precedes dilatation while in multigravidas these processes usually occur concurrently. **Cognitive Level:** Analyzing **Client Need:** Health Promotion and Maintenance **Integrated Process:** Teaching and Learning **Content Area:** Maternal-Newborn **Strategy:** The positive wording of the question indicates that the correct option is also a true statement of fact. Recall definitions of effacement, dilatation, and when they occur for the primipara and multipara to aid in answering the question correctly. **Reference:** Ladewig, P. A., London, M. L., & Davidson, M. R. (2010). *Contemporary maternal-newborn nursing care* (7th ed.). Upper Saddle River, NJ: Pearson Education, pp. 387–391.

10 **Answer: 1 Rationale:** The first stage of labor is from the onset of labor to complete dilatation, and is divided into latent (0 to 3 centimeters), active (4 to 7 centimeters), and transition (8 to 10 centimeters) phases. The second stage of labor has no phases and extends from complete dilatation until delivery of the newborn. The third stage has no phases and extends from delivery of the newborn to delivery of the placenta. **Cognitive Level:** Applying **Client Need:** Health Promotion and Maintenance **Integrated Process:** Nursing Process: Assessment **Content Area:** Maternal-Newborn **Strategy:** Recall that the first stage of labor is from 0 to 10 cm dilatation and is divided into phases. **Reference:** Ladewig, P. A., London, M. L., & Davidson, M. R. (2010). *Contemporary maternal-newborn nursing care* (7th ed.). Upper Saddle River, NJ: Pearson Education, pp. 387–392.

Posttest

1 **Answer: 3, 4, 5, 2, 1 Rationale:** The cardinal movements (position changes) of the fetus occur in the order of engagement, descent, flexion, internal rotation, extension, restitution, external rotation, and expulsion. These movements represent the normal adaptation of the fetus in a cephalic presentation to the maternal pelvis and facilitate vaginal birth. **Cognitive Level:** Analyzing **Client Need:** Health Promotion and Maintenance **Integrated Process:** Nursing Process: Planning **Content Area:** Maternal-Newborn **Strategy:** Recall the memory aid "Every darn fool in Rotterdam eats rotten egg rolls everyday." The first letter of each word in the memory aid represents the first letter of the cardinal movements of the fetus in a cephalic position. **Reference:** Ladewig, P. A., London, M. L., & Davidson, M. R. (2010). *Contemporary maternal-newborn nursing care* (7th ed.). Upper Saddle River, NJ: Pearson Education, pp. 390–391.

2 **Answer: 1 Rationale:** Analgesia and anesthesia methods are used for pain relief during labor as indicated by the client's response to pain, what phase and stage of labor the woman is in, how fast labor is progressing, and the fetal response to contractions. Parity alone does not

determine what analgesia or anesthesia is indicated. The other responses are all accurate. **Cognitive Level:** Applying **Client Need:** Health Promotion and Maintenance **Integrated Process:** Nursing Process: Evaluation **Content Area:** Maternal-Newborn **Strategy:** Recall the labor process and its effect on the client to choose correctly. Eliminate options that are correct responses and choose the response that indicates the need for further teaching. **Reference:** Ladewig, P. A., London, M. L., & Davidson, M. R. (2010). *Contemporary maternal-newborn nursing care* (7th ed.). Upper Saddle River, NJ: Pearson Education, pp. 471–472.

3 **Answer: 2** **Rationale:** Moderate ecchymosis and edema are a normal response to the trauma of childbirth, as well as to the presence of sutures. As this heals, the bruising takes on a slight yellow brown appearance. Sutures should be closely aligned without gaps. There should be no purulent-like drainage, which would indicate infection. Edema severe enough to cause the tissue to look shiny or taut is abnormal. **Cognitive Level:** Applying **Client Need:** Physiological Adaptation **Integrated Process:** Nursing Process: Assessment **Content Area:** Maternal-Newborn **Strategy:** Critical words are *normal* and *immediately post-delivery*. Knowledge of episiotomy management and care will help to answer the question correctly. **Reference:** Ladewig, P. A., London, M. L., & Davidson, M. R. (2010). *Contemporary maternal-newborn nursing care* (7th ed.). Upper Saddle River, NJ: Pearson Education, pp. 547–548.

4 **Answer: 3, 5** **Rationale:** Frequent inspection for redness, swelling, tenderness, and hematoma is essential to fourth-stage nursing care. Pain relief begins with immediate application of ice. Ice packs should be applied for 20 to 30 minutes and removed for at least 20 minutes. If ice is applied for more than 30 minutes, vasodilation and edema may occur. Clients are usually advised to wait until bleeding stops and stitches heal (about three weeks) before resuming sexual activity, but this teaching would be part of the client's discharge instructions, and is not appropriate during the fourth stage of labor. **Cognitive Level:** Applying **Client Need:** Health Promotion and Maintenance **Integrated Process:** Nursing Process: Implementation **Content Area:** Maternal-Newborn **Strategy:** The critical issue in this question is time related. The fourth stage of labor is a time of critical physiologic adaptation and requires frequent assessment. The correct answer is the option that includes a true statement about nursing action at this time. **Reference:** Ladewig, P. A., London, M. L., & Davidson, M. R. (2010). *Contemporary maternal-newborn nursing care* (7th ed.). Upper Saddle River, NJ: Pearson Education, pp. 547–548.

5 **Answer: 3** **Rationale:** The goal of childbirth education classes is to teach pregnant women and their support person(s) the birth process, strategies to cope with the pain of labor and to facilitate an easier labor, what to expect during childbirth, an understanding of operative delivery (use of forceps, vacuum extraction, and cesarean birth), and common procedures that may be performed throughout the birthing process. Many pregnant families get the information they need about the childbearing process by reading or from friends and extended family members. Childbirth preparation cannot prevent complications and thus cannot ensure vaginal deliveries for all clients. **Cognitive Level:** Applying **Client Need:** Health Promotion and Maintenance **Integrated Process:** Nursing Process: Planning **Content Area:** Maternal-Newborn **Strategy:** Knowledge of the goals of childbirth education will help to choose the correct answer. Eliminate the three options that are unrealistic and unattainable. **Reference:** Ladewig, P. A., London, M. L., & Davidson, M. R. (2010). *Contemporary maternal-newborn nursing care* (7th ed.). Upper Saddle River, NJ: Pearson Education, pp. 175–177.

6 **Answer: 3** **Rationale:** Crowning is the point in time when the perineum is thin and stretching around the fetal head both between and during contractions. Delivery is imminent when crowning occurs. **Cognitive Level:** Applying **Client Need:** Health Promotion and Maintenance **Integrated Process:** Nursing Process: Evaluation **Content Area:** Maternal-Newborn **Strategy:** The question is worded in a positive way. The correct answer will be the option that is a true statement about a point of client education. **Reference:** Ladewig, P. A., London, M. L., & Davidson, M. R. (2010). *Contemporary maternal-newborn nursing care* (7th ed.). Upper Saddle River, NJ: Pearson Education, p. 389.

7 **Answer: 1** **Rationale:** An android pelvic structure is narrow in both the anterior-posterior diameter and the lateral diameter, and can cause prolonged labor if there is a large fetus or a malpositioned fetus. An android pelvic structure does not increase the likelihood of occiput posterior position, precipitous delivery, or postpartum hemorrhage. **Cognitive Level:** Analyzing **Client Need:** Physiological Adaptation **Integrated Process:** Nursing Process: Assessment **Content Area:** Maternal-Newborn **Strategy:** Recall the four P's of labor; pelvic size and shape influence labor outcome. The correct answer is the option that delays or slows the birth process. **Reference:** Ladewig, P. A., London, M. L., & Davidson, M. R. (2010). *Contemporary maternal-newborn nursing care* (7th ed.). Upper Saddle River, NJ: Pearson Education, p. 377.

8 **Answer: 3** **Rationale:** Frank breech position is when the sacrum of the baby is presenting, the hips are flexed, and the feet are extended upward toward the fetal head. Both hip and knee flexion occurs with a complete breech. Hip extension with knee flexion is characteristic of a kneeling breech. And both hip and knee extension occur with a double footling breech. **Cognitive Level:** Applying **Client Need:** Physiological Adaptation **Integrated Process:** Teaching and Learning **Content Area:** Maternal-Newborn **Strategy:** The correct answer is the option that contains a true statement. Knowledge of the types of breech presentations is necessary to choose the correct answer. **Reference:** Ladewig, P. A., London, M. L., & Davidson, M. R. (2010). *Contemporary maternal-newborn nursing care* (7th ed.). Upper Saddle River, NJ: Pearson Education, p. 382.

9 **Answer: 2** **Rationale:** The normal attitude of the fetal head is one of moderate flexion. Changes in fetal attitude, particularly the position of the head, present larger diameters to the maternal pelvis, which contributes to a prolonged and difficult labor and increases the likelihood of cesarean delivery. **Cognitive Level:** Analyzing **Client Need:** Physiological Adaptation **Integrated Process:** Nursing Process: Planning **Content Area:** Maternal-Newborn **Strategy:** The critical words in this question are *complete extension*. Recall that flexion is the preferred fetal attitude for birth. The correct answer would be the option that contains a statement about a delayed or impossible vaginal birth. **Reference:** Ladewig, P. A., London, M. L., & Davidson, M. R. (2010). *Contemporary maternal-newborn nursing care* (7th ed.). Upper Saddle River, NJ: Pearson Education, pp. 378–379.

10 **Answer: 1** **Rationale:** Presentation refers to the part of the fetus that is coming through the cervix and birth canal first. Thus, a face presentation occurs when the face is coming through first. This is considered a position of caution as the face is a large part of the head. It must be dealt with cautiously. **Cognitive Level:** Applying **Client Need:** Physiological Adaptation **Integrated Process:** Teaching and Learning **Content Area:** Maternal-Newborn **Strategy:** The wording of the question indicates the correct option is a true statement that matches the information in the stem of the question. Use knowledge of the fetal presentation and presenting part to make a selection. **Reference:** Ladewig, P. A., London, M. L., & Davidson, M. R. (2010). *Contemporary maternal-newborn nursing care* (7th ed.). Upper Saddle River, NJ: Pearson Education, pp. 378–379.

References

Davidson, M., London, M., & Ladewig, P. (2012). *Olds' maternal newborn nursing & women's health across the lifespan* (9th ed.). Upper Saddle River, NJ: Pearson Education.

Ladewig, P., London, M., & Davidson, M. (2009). *Contemporary maternal-newborn nursing care* (7th ed.). Upper Saddle River, NJ: Pearson Education.

Murray, M., & Huelsmann, G. (2009). *Labor and delivery nursing: A guide to evidence-based practice.* New York: Springer Publishing Company.

Perry, S. E., Hockenberry, M. J., Lowdermilk, D. L., & Wilson, D. (2010). *Maternal child nursing care* (4th ed.). St. Louis, MO: Mosby.

Ricci, S. (2009). *Essentials of maternity, newborn, and women's health nursing* (2nd ed.). Philadelphia: Lippincott Williams & Wilkins.

9 The Complicated Labor and Delivery Experience

Chapter Outline

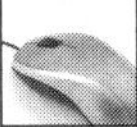

NCLEX-RN® Test Prep

Use the accompanying online resource, NursingReviewsandRationales, to test yourself with hundreds of NCLEX®-style practice questions.

Objectives

- Discuss nursing assessments that lead to early recognition of complications during labor and delivery.
- Describe nursing interventions to promote maternal and fetal well-being during a complicated labor and delivery.
- Summarize nursing care needed by the client experiencing a cesarean delivery.

Review at a Glance

amnioinfusion (AI) infusion of warmed, sterile saline or Ringer's Lactate solution into uterine cavity to replace amniotic fluid and prevent fetal distress

amniotomy artificial breaking of amniotic sac to hasten labor

augmentation of labor stimulating uterine contractions by pharmacologic means to hasten labor and delivery

Bishop score a means of measuring readiness of cervix for induction of labor

cephalopelvic disproportion (CPD) pelvic size is too small to allow descent and passage of fetal head

cesarean section delivery of fetus through an abdominal incision

dystocia difficult labor caused by factors of pelvis, fetus, or abnormal or uncoordinated uterine contractions

external cephalic version external manipulation of fetus from a breech to a vertex presentation

hypertonic uterine dysfunction frequent, painful uterine contractions that are uncoordinated and do not efface or dilate cervix; often occurs in latent phase of labor

hypotonic uterine dysfunction weak, ineffective uterine contractions; often occurs in active phase of labor and is associated with cephalopelvic disproportion (CPD)

induction of labor process of causing onset of labor through administration of pharmacologic agents or amniotomy

intrauterine resuscitation an emergency procedure instituted during labor to treat fetal distress by stopping uterine contractions with a tocolytic agent and allowing restoration of maternal–fetal circulation so that fetus can recover from distress

malpresentation abnormal presentation occurring when any other fetal part besides flexed head enters pelvis

malposition abnormal position of presenting part of fetus in relation to maternal pelvis occurring when any other position besides flexed fetal head in an occiput anterior position presents

precipitate labor and birth rapid labor and delivery of less than three hours from beginning of dilatation to birth of infant; often results in unattended or nurse attended delivery

premature labor onset of regular contractions between 20 to 37 weeks' gestation with or without cervical change

tocolytic agents pharmacologic agents that suppress or stop uterine contractions

trial of labor (TOL) observation period to determine if a laboring woman with a borderline or small pelvis can progress to a vaginal birth

uterine inversion prolapse of uterine fundus through cervix and vagina during or following third stage of labor; associated with massive bleeding and shock and requires emergency intervention

uterine rupture tearing open or separation of uterine wall; associated with severe hemorrhage and shock necessitating hysterectomy

PRETEST

1 Following amniotomy, the nurse would carry out which interventions as important nursing actions? Select all that apply.

1. Assist the mother into a lithotomy position for delivery.
2. Place clean bedding/underpads on the bed.
3. Assess and document fetal heart tones.
4. Observe and document the color and consistency of the amniotic fluid.
5. Take vital signs every four hours to monitor for infection.

2 The nurse concludes that a fetus in which of the following positions has a right occiput anterior (ROA) position?

1. 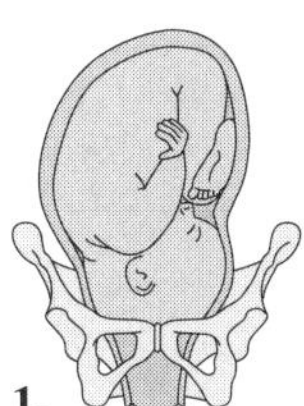
2. 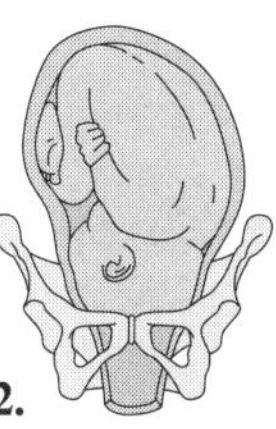
3. 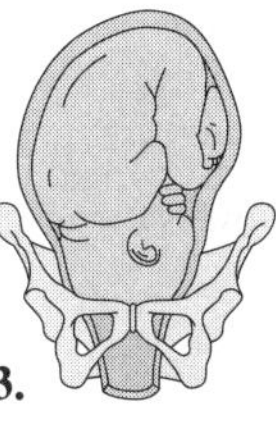
4. 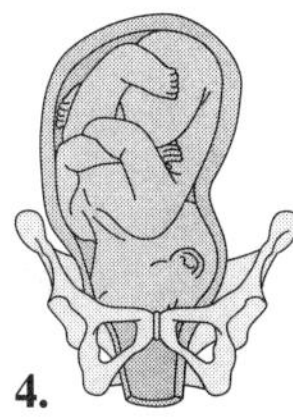

3 A nulliparous client has not made any progress in cervical dilatation or station since she was 7 cm and 0 station over two hours ago. The nurse interprets that this client is most likely experiencing which of the following?

1. Prolonged deceleration phase
2. Protracted active phase
3. Arrest of descent
4. Secondary arrest of dilatation

4 A client's amniotic fluid is greenish-tinged. The fetal presentation is vertex. Fetal heart rate (FHR) and uterine activity have remained within normal limits. At the time of delivery, the nurse should anticipate the need for which equipment?

1. An infant laryngoscope and suction catheters
2. Forceps
3. A transport isolette
4. Emergency cesarean setup

5 A client who is 34 weeks' gestation has been having contractions every 10 minutes regularly. In addition to instructing her to lie down and rest while continuing to time contractions, the nurse should also tell her to do which of the following?

1. Refrain from eating or drinking anything.
2. Take slow, deep breaths with each contraction.
3. Go to the hospital if contractions continue for more than one hour.
4. Drink three to four cups of water.

6 The client who has had a previous cesarean birth asks about trial of labor after cesarean (TOLAC). Which of the following factors from her history is a contraindication for TOLAC?

1. Previous cesarean was for breech presentation.
2. Client had a classic uterine incision.
3. The abdominal incision was vertical rather than transverse.
4. An induction of labor is planned for this delivery.

7 Which statement by the nurse is most therapeutic in talking with a client and her family following emergency cesarean birth?

1. "I'm sorry that you couldn't have a normal delivery."
2. "Your baby was really in danger. I think he is doing better now."
3. "You did so well throughout the delivery. I'm sorry I didn't have more time to explain things."
4. "I know you never expected this to happen. Maybe things will work out better next time."

PRETEST

8 The pregnant client is receiving oxytocin (Pitocin) to induce labor. The nurse should monitor the client for which adverse maternal effects? Select all that apply.

1. Bradycardia
2. Decreased urine output
3. Dehydration
4. Jaundice
5. Uterine hyperstimulation

9 A pregnant client is receiving a tocolytic drug to stop contractions and prevent premature labor. What assessments for side/adverse drug effects should the nurse monitor for in this client? Select all that apply.

1. Lung sounds
2. Flushing and headache
3. Eye movements
4. Excessive energy and euphoria
5. Deep tendon reflexes

10 The nurse is monitoring a client during a vaginal delivery of a breech infant. Which of the following would the nurse consider to be the greatest risk during delivery?

1. Umbilical cord prolapse
2. Intracranial hemorrhage
3. Meconium aspiration
4. Fracture of the clavicle

➤ *See pages 194–196 for Answers and Rationales.*

I. NURSING CARE OF THE HIGH-RISK LABOR AND DELIVERY CLIENT AND FAMILY

A. **High-risk factors**: may develop at any time during labor in a client who has been otherwise healthy throughout pregnancy and may be related to the 4 Ps
   1. The *passenger* or fetus
   2. The *passageway* or pelvic bones and other pelvic structures
   3. The *powers* or uterine contractions
   4. The client's *psyche* or psychological state

B. **Client response to onset of high-risk factors in labor**
   1. Stress, fear, and anxiety brought about by unexpected complications during labor may have profound effects on maternal and fetal outcome
   2. Maternal anxiety can increase tension, produce higher pain perception, and may make labor contractions less effective
   3. Catecholamines released during stress produce vasoconstriction that may negatively affect uterine blood flow

C. **Family members**: may be overwhelmed with concern and less capable of providing needed emotional support for client

D. **Nursing care**: in addition to basic intrapartal care, nursing care during complicated labor requires special knowledge and skill in assessing and caring for mother and fetus

II. PROBLEMS WITH THE PASSENGER

A. **Fetal *malposition***: ideal fetal position is flexed with occiput in right or left anterior quadrant of maternal pelvis
   1. Types of malpositions
      a. Occiput posterior (OP) position
         1) Right or left OP position occurs in about 25% of all term pregnancies but usually rotates to occiput anterior (OA) as labor progresses
         2) Failure to rotate is termed persistent occiput posterior; may be related to small maternal pelvis, poor contractions, inadequate pushing (such as with epidural anesthesia), abnormal flexion of head, or large fetus
         3) Maternal risks include prolonged labor, potential for operative delivery, extension of episiotomy, or 3rd- or 4th-degree laceration of perineum

!
4) Maternal symptoms include intense back pain in labor, dysfunctional labor pattern, prolonged active phase, secondary arrest of dilatation, and/or arrest of descent

b. Occiput transverse (OT) position
1) Incomplete rotation of OP position to OA results in fetal head being in a horizontal or transverse position (OT)
2) Persistent occiput transverse position occurs as a result of ineffective contractions or a flattened bony pelvis
3) If pelvic structure is adequate, vaginal delivery can be accomplished by stimulating contractions with oxytocin (Pitocin) and application of forceps for delivery

2. Nursing care
a. Nursing diagnoses: Pain; Ineffective Coping
b. Planning and implementation

!
1) Encourage mother to lie on her side opposite from fetal back, which may help with rotation
2) Knee–chest position may facilitate rotation (provides downward slant to vaginal canal)
3) Pelvic rocking may help with rotation

!
4) Apply sacral counterpressure with heel of hand to reduce back pain
5) Continue support and encouragement
a) Keep client and family informed of progress
b) Encourage relaxation with contractions
c) Praise client's efforts to maintain control
6) Anticipate forceps rotation and forceps-assisted birth

c. Evaluation: client's discomfort is decreased and coping abilities are strengthened

3. Medical management
a. Forceps: metal instruments applied to fetal head to facilitate delivery
1) Provides traction or a means of rotating fetal head
2) Risks are fetal ecchymosis or facial edema, transient facial paralysis, maternal lacerations, or episiotomy extensions

b. Vacuum extraction: a suction cup applied to fetal head to facilitate delivery
1) Provides traction to shorten second stage of labor
2) Risks are newborn cephalohematoma, retinal hemorrhage, and intracranial hemorrhage

Practice to Pass

A client asks you if forceps will leave a mark on her baby's head or face. How will you answer this question?

B. Fetal *malpresentation*

1. Cephalic (vertex) malpresentations result from failure of fetus to assume a flexed attitude; normal presentation is occipital; cephalic malpresentations include brow, face, and sinciputal (military)

a. Brow presentation
1) Fetal forehead is presenting part; 50% convert to vertex or face presentation
2) Maternal risks include longer labor and possible cesarean birth; neonatal risks include facial edema, bruising, exaggerated molding of head, increased risk of cerebral and neck compression, and damage to trachea and larynx

b. Face presentation
1) Fetal head is hyperextended more than in brow presentation; there is increased risk for prolonged labor
2) Anticipate vaginal delivery if pelvis is adequate and chin (mentum) is in anterior position

!
3) Anticipate cesarean delivery if mentum is posterior or signs of fetal distress occur

!
4) Fetal monitor electrode should not be placed on presenting part (infant's face); requires external fetal heart rate (FHR) monitoring

!
5) Edema and bruising of face, eyes, and lips are common occurrences; prepare client for this possibility before seeing infant for first time

c. Sinciputal presentation (military attitude)
   1) Larger diameter of fetal head is presented
   2) Labor progress is slowed with slower descent of fetal head
2. Breech presentations
   a. Three types (see Figure 9-1)
      1) Complete breech: sacrum is the presenting part, knees flexed
      2) Frank breech: sacrum is the presenting part, legs are extended
      3) Incomplete (footling) breech: one or both feet are presenting, increasing the risk of umbilical cord prolapse
   b. Maternal risks
      1) Prolonged labor due to decreased pressure exerted by breech on cervix
      2) Premature rupture of membranes may expose client to infection
      3) Cesarean or forceps delivery
      4) Trauma to birth canal during delivery from manipulation and forceps to free fetal head
      5) Intrapartum or postpartum hemorrhage
   c. Fetal risks
      1) ! Compression or prolapse of umbilical cord
      2) ! Entrapment of fetal head in incompletely dilated cervix
      3) Aspiration and asphyxia at birth
      4) Birth trauma from manipulation and forceps to free fetal head
   d. Vaginal delivery of breech
      1) ! Fetal body may pass through an incompletely dilated cervix entrapping larger fetal head that follows
      2) ! Delivery of fetal head must be done quickly to avoid hypoxia
      3) Piper (long handle) forceps may be applied to the after-coming fetal head
   e. **Cesarean section**: increased fetal morbidity and mortality has convinced most physicians not to attempt vaginal delivery; most breech presentations are delivered by planned cesarean section, or abdominal delivery

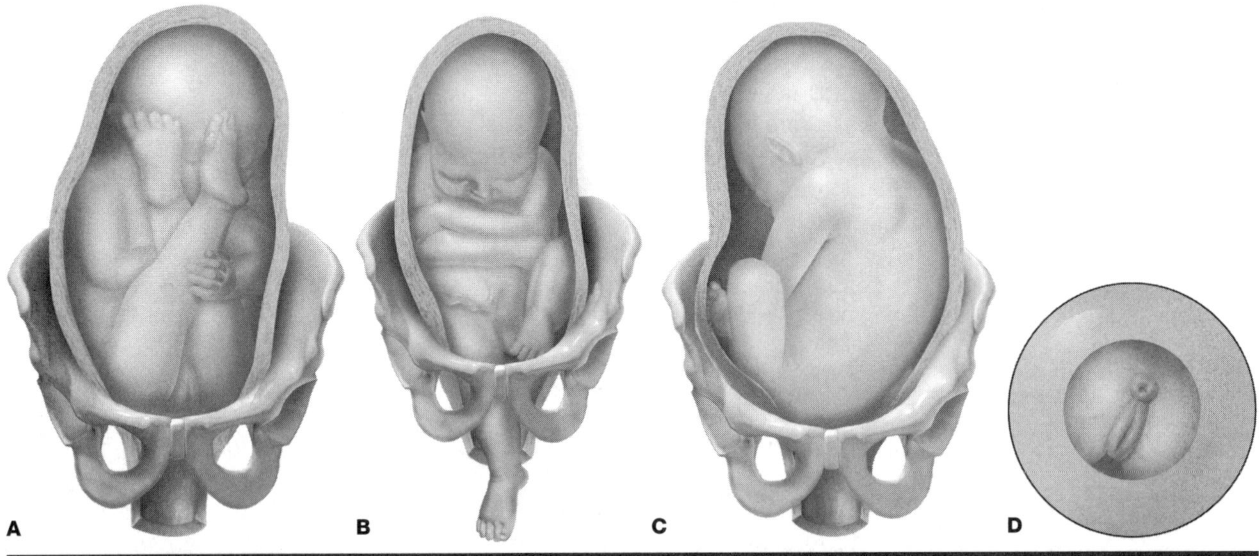

Figure 9-1

Breech presentation. A. Frank breech, B. Incomplete footling breech, C. Complete breech in left sacral anterior (LSA) position, D. On vaginal examination, the nurse may feel the anal sphincter. The tissue of the fetal buttocks feels soft.

Source: Davidson, M., London, M., & Ladewig, P. (2012). *Olds' maternal newborn nursing & women's health across the lifespan* (9th ed.). Upper Saddle River, NJ: Pearson Education, p. 709.

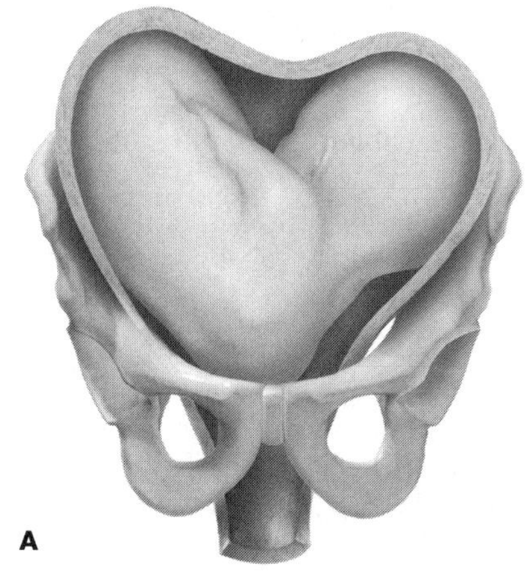

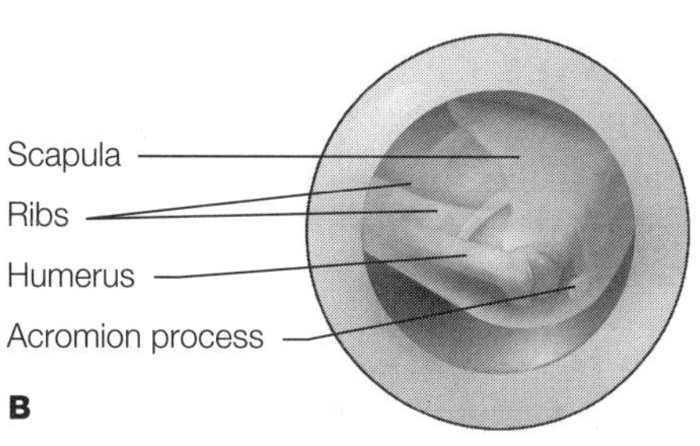

Figure 9-2

Transverse lie. A. Shoulder presentation; frontal view, B. Vaginal view.

Source: Davidson, M., London, M., & Ladewig, P. (2012). *Olds' maternal newborn nursing & women's health across the lifespan* (9th ed.). Upper Saddle River, NJ: Pearson Education, p. 710.

f. **External cephalic version**: manipulation of fetus through abdominal wall from a breech or shoulder to a vertex presentation prior to onset of labor; is usually attempted at about 36 weeks or shortly thereafter
   1) Client is placed on external fetal monitor
   2) IV fluids are started
   3) Terbutaline (Brethine) is administered via a piggybacked IV line to relax uterine muscle
   4) FHR is closely monitored during version attempt
   5) Version is discontinued if undue maternal or fetal distress is noted

3. Shoulder presentation (transverse lie): acromion process is presenting part (see Figure 9-2)
   a. External cephalic version is attempted at 36–37 weeks, because of risk of prolapsed umbilical cord; is followed by labor induction if successful
   b. Vaginal delivery is not considered possible in term infant; cesarean birth is preferred method of delivery
4. Compound presentations: more than one part of fetus presents
   a. Most common type is a hand or arm prolapsing beside head
   b. Risk of cord compression and prolapse is increased
   c. Vaginal versus cesarean delivery depends on size of fetus, presence of fetal distress, and progress in labor
5. Nursing care of clients with malpresentations
   a. Assessment and nursing diagnoses
      1) Leopold's maneuvers may help detect abnormal presentation; accomplished by examiner placing both hands on uterus and moving hands down maternal abdomen tracing fetal outline; helps to estimate fetal weight as well as position in utero
      2) Priority nursing diagnoses: Risk for Injury; Anxiety; Fear; Deficient Knowledge; Ineffective Coping; Ineffective Family Coping
   b. Planning and implementation
      1) Observe closely for abnormal labor patterns
      2) Monitor fetal heart rate (FHR) and contractions continuously
      3) Provide client and family teaching
      4) Provide client support and encouragement
      5) Anticipate forceps-assisted birth
      6) Anticipate cesarean birth for incomplete breech or shoulder presentation
      7) Be prepared for childbirth emergencies such as cesarean section, forceps-assisted delivery, and neonatal resuscitation
   c. Evaluation
      1) Client and fetus have a safe labor and delivery
      2) Client verbalizes understanding of implications of malpresentation

Practice to Pass

In doing Leopold's maneuvers, what findings would make you suspect that the fetus is in a breech presentation?

C. Fetal distress: insufficient oxygen supply to meet demands of fetus

1. Causes
   a. Umbilical cord compression
   b. Uteroplacental insufficiency caused by placental abnormalities or maternal condition
2. Signs and symptoms
   a. Meconium-stained amniotic fluid (excluding breech presentation)
   b. Changes in FHR baseline
      1) Tachycardia (above 160): early sign of distress
      2) Bradycardia (below 110): late sign of distress
   c. Decreased or absence of variability of heart rate
      1) Heart rate varies less than two to five beats per minute causing a flattened appearance to heart rate
      2) Indicates depression of autonomic nervous system that controls heart rate
      3) Fetal sleep, sedation, and hypoxia may affect variability
   d. Late deceleration pattern (see also Chapter 8)
      1) FHR slows following peak of a contraction and slowly returns to baseline rate during resting phase
      2) Indicates fetal response to hypoxia from uteroplacental insufficiency
      3) Considered an ominous pattern regardless of depth of FHR deceleration and requires immediate intervention
   e. Severe variable deceleration pattern
      1) Fetal heart rate repeatedly decelerates below 90 beats per minute for over 60 seconds before returning to baseline
      2) Indicates interference of fetal blood flow from cord compression
      3) Leads to fetal hypoxia and low APGAR scores unless corrective steps are taken
3. Nursing care
   a. Assessment and nursing diagnoses
      1) Assess FHR baseline, variability, and pattern of periodic changes
      2) Assess contraction pattern and maternal response to labor
      3) Priority nursing diagnoses: Decreased Cardiac Output (fetal), Impaired Gas Exchange (fetal), Anxiety (maternal)
   b. Planning and implementation
      1) Institute emergency measures to correct fetal hypoxia based on FHR pattern (see Box 9-1); for late deceleration, take steps to improve uteroplacental blood flow and for severe variable deceleration, initiate actions to relieve cord compression
      2) Provide appropriate information and emotional support to the client and family
      3) Maintain continuous monitoring of FHR, uterine activity, and labor progress

Box 9-1

Nursing Management of Fetal Distress

Late decelerations (uteroplacental insufficiency)
The goal is to improve maternal blood flow to the placenta

- Reposition the mother on her left side
- Administer O_2 by face-mask at 8–10 L/min
- Increase IV fluids
- Discontinue oxytocin infusion, if labor is being induced
- Notify the health care provider immediately

Severe variable decelerations or prolonged bradycardia (cord compression)
The goal is to relieve pressure on the umbilical cord

- Reposition the mother on either side
- If not corrected, reposition to opposite side
- Administer O_2 by face mask at 8–10 L/min
- Trendelenburg or knee–chest position, if not corrected
- Perform vaginal examination and apply upward digital pressure on the presenting part to relieve pressure on the umbilical cord

c. Evaluation
   1) FHR remains in normal range with adequate variability and absence of ominous periodic changes
   2) Client verbalizes that anxiety is decreased
   3) Family coping strategies are strengthened

4. Medical management
   a. **Amnioinfusion (AI)**: amniotic fluid may be replaced with warmed sterile saline or Ringer's lactate solution through an intrauterine catheter when signs of cord compression are present during labor
      1) FHR monitoring is continued
      2) Intrauterine catheter is inserted
      3) Warmed sterile saline or Ringer's lactate is delivered via catheter using an infusion pump
      4) Infusion is continued until signs of cord compression disappear
   b. **Intrauterine resuscitation**: administration of terbutaline (Brethine), a tocolytic agent, to stop uterine contractions and provide an opportunity for uteroplacental circulation to improve when fetal distress is present during first stage of labor; is suggested for short term use because it can cause tachycardia, palpitations, and other side effects (see Table 9-2 later in chapter)
   c. Prevention of meconium aspiration
      1) If meconium is present during labor (green-tinged amniotic fluid), amnioinfusion may be used to dilute large amounts of meconium, and steps to prevent aspiration at time of delivery should be taken
      2) Nasopharynx of the infant may be suctioned prior to delivery of chest and abdomen, but this practice is currently under study
      3) Visualization of larynx and vocal cords with deep suction is performed immediately after delivery and before first breath is taken

D. Prolapsed umbilical cord

1. Cause: fetus is not firmly engaged, allowing room for cord to move beyond (prolapse) or alongside presenting part (occult prolapse)

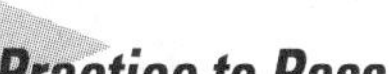

Practice to Pass

Following several late decelerations, a client asks you why she needs to lie on her left side. How will you answer her?

2. Contributing factors
   a. Rupture of membranes before engagement of presenting part
   b. Small fetus
   c. Breech presentation
   d. Multifetal pregnancy
   e. Transverse lie (shoulder presentation)
3. Assessment and nursing diagnoses
   a. Identify client at risk for prolapsed umbilical cord; keep woman with ruptured membranes in a horizontal position
   b. Priority nursing diagnoses: Risk for Impaired Gas Exchange; Risk for Injury; Fear
4. Planning and implementation: actions to relieve pressure on cord and restore fetal oxygenation
   a. Place mother's hips higher than her head
      1) Knee–chest position
      2) Trendelenburg position
   b. Perform sterile vaginal exam pushing fetal presenting part upward with fingers to relieve pressure on cord
   c. If cord protrudes through vagina, determine that pulsation is present and apply sterile saline soaked dressing to prevent drying
   d. Administer O_2 by face mask at 8 to 10 L/min
   e. Maintain continuous electronic fetal monitoring
   f. Prepare for rapid delivery vaginally or by cesarean section

5. Evaluation
    a. FHR remains within normal range and without ominous signs
    b. Fetus is safely delivered
    c. Client and family verbalize understanding of implications of prolapsed umbilical cord and need for emergency management

III. PROBLEMS WITH THE PASSAGEWAY

A. Abnormal pelvic size or shape

1. Contracted pelvic inlet: anterior–posterior diameter less than 10 centimeters; transverse diameter less than 12 centimeters
    a. Makes engagement difficult
    b. Influences fetal position and presentation
2. Contracted mid-pelvic plane: interspinous diameter less than 9.5 centimeters
    a. Hampers internal rotation of fetal head
    b. Secondary arrest of dilatation or arrest of descent of fetal head occurs
3. Contracted pelvic outlet: interischial tuberous diameter less than 8 centimeters
4. **Trial of labor (TOL)**: physician may allow labor to continue or even stimulate labor with oxytocin when pelvic measurements are borderline to see if fetal head will descend making vaginal delivery possible; if progressive changes in dilatation and station do not occur, a cesarean delivery is performed

B. *Cephalopelvic disproportion (CPD)*

1. Fetal head is too large to pass through bony pelvis
2. ! Signs and symptoms: fetal head does not descend even though there are strong contractions
3. Maternal risks include prolonged labor, exhaustion, hemorrhage, and infection
4. Fetal risks include hypoxia and birth trauma
5. Cesarean birth is necessary

! **C. Shoulder dystocia**: an obstetric emergency resulting from difficulty or inability to deliver shoulders

1. Fetal macrosomia increases risk of shoulder dystocia
2. Inability to deliver shoulders leads to fetal hypoxia and death
3. Maternal risks
    a. Lacerations and tears of birth canal
    b. Postpartum hemorrhage
4. Neonatal risks
    a. Hypoxia
    b. Fractures of clavicle
    c. Injury to neck and head
    d. Brachial plexus palsy

D. Nursing care

1. Assessment and identification of client at risk for shoulder dystocia
    a. Obesity
    b. Increased fundal height
    c. History of macrosomia
    d. Maternal diabetes or gestational diabetes
    e. Prolonged second-stage labor
2. Priority nursing diagnoses: Risk for Injury; Fear; Deficient Knowledge
3. Planning and implementation
    a. ! Assist with positioning during delivery: McRoberts maneuver (see Figure 9-3)
        1) Woman flexes thighs on her abdomen
        2) Position changes angle of pelvis, increases pelvic diameters, and facilitates delivery of shoulders
    b. Assess for maternal and newborn injury following delivery

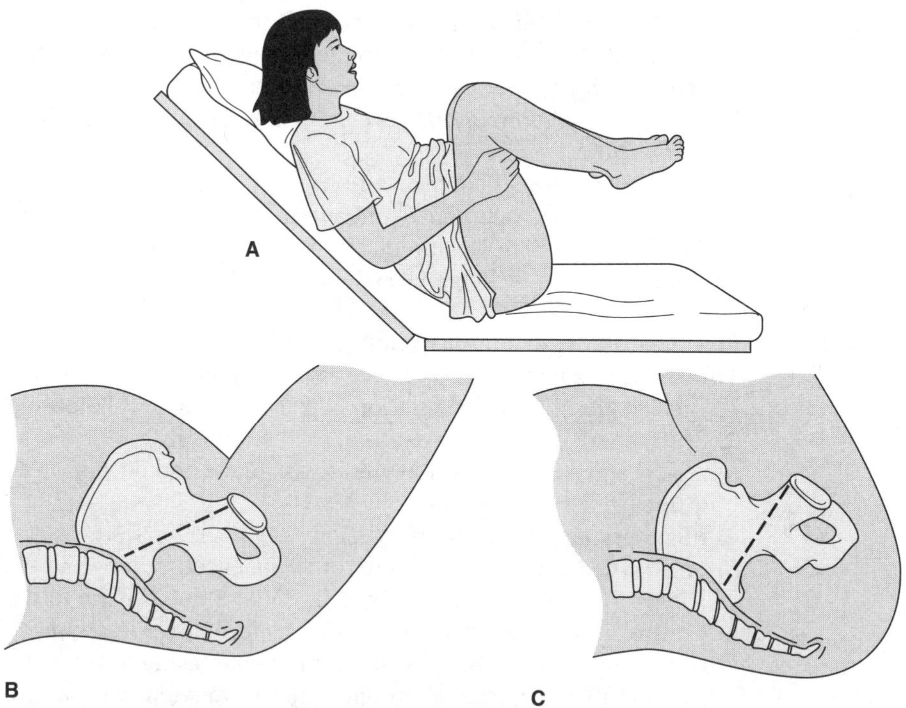

Figure 9-3

McRoberts maneuver. A. Thighs flexed onto abdomen, B. Angle of maternal pelvis prior to maneuver, C. Angle of pelvis with maneuver.

Source: Davidson, M., London, M., & Ladewig, P. (2012). *Olds' maternal newborn nursing & women's health across the lifespan* (9th ed.). Upper Saddle River, NJ: Pearson Education, p. 712.

4. Evaluation
   a. Client and fetus experience a safe delivery without injury
   b. Client indicates that fear is diminished
   c. Client is able to verbalize increased understanding of pelvic disproportion and dystocia, its causes, and implications for delivery

IV. PROBLEMS WITH THE POWERS

A. ***Induction of labor***: pharmacological (see Table 9-1) and nonpharmacological measures to initiate contractions and cervical change
   1. Methods of induction
      a. Cervical ripening
         1) Prostaglandins (PGE_2) gel (Cervidil), dinoprostone (Prepidil)
         2) Laminaria (hydrophilic agent): when inserted into cervix, it absorbs water from cervical mucus, expands, and dilates cervix

Table 9-1 Drugs Used for Induction of Labor

Drug	Route/Action	Side Effects and Potential Complications
Prostaglandin gel (Cervidil), dinoprostone (Prepidil)	Intravaginally close to cervix Causes softening and effacement or cervical ripening	Abdominal cramping, nausea, vomiting, diarrhea
Misoprostol (Cytotec)	Synthetic prostaglandin administered orally or intravaginally to produce contractions	Sudden onset of hypertonic contractions and elevated resting tone of the uterus which may lead to fetal distress
Oxytocin (Pitocin)	Synthetic oxytocin administered IV in small amounts and titrated to produce contractions that mimic normal labor	Uterine tetany and fetal distress are major concerns; can lead to water intoxication, hyponatremia, and hypochloremia

b. **Amniotomy** or artificial rupture of membranes (AROM)
   1) Auscultate FHR prior to and immediately after AROM to detect prolapse of umbilical cord or fetal distress
   2) Take maternal temperature every 1 to 2 hours following AROM to detect signs of infection
c. Misoprostol (Cytotec) administration
   1) A synthetic prostaglandin agent administered intravaginally and/or orally at doses of 25 to 50 mg to stimulate onset of contractions
   2) Continuous monitoring of FHR, uterine activity, and maternal vital signs is essential
d. Oxytocin (Pitocin) administration (see Box 9-2)
   1) **Bishop score** may be used to assess maternal readiness for induction by determining dilatation, effacement, station, cervical consistency, and position of cervix
   2) Prior to induction, begin external fetal monitoring
   3) Assess and record maternal vital signs, intake and output, and contraction frequency and intensity
   4) Begin primary intravenous infusion
   5) Mix oxytocin in 500 to 1000 mL of IV balanced-saline fluid such as lactated Ringer's and piggyback into primary IV at a site as close to client as possible
   6) Control and titrate oxytocin solution using an infusion pump
   7) Begin at 0.5 to 2 milliunits per minute, increasing at increments of 1 to 2 milliunits every 15 to 60 minutes up to a maximum of 40 milliunits according to hospital protocol and until contractions occur regularly
   8) Continue to monitor contractions and FHR closely and stop infusion immediately if contractions are closer than 2 minutes, last longer than 90 seconds, or if there is any indication of fetal distress

2. Absolute contraindications to induction of labor
   a. Complete placenta previa, vasa previa, or abruptio placenta
   b. Acute fetal distress or bradycardia
   c. Prior classic uterine incision, transfundal uterine surgery, or myomectomy
   d. Pelvic structure abnormality
   e. Prolapsed umbilical cord

Box 9-2

Oxytocin (Pitocin) Administration

Hospital protocols for mixing Pitocin with IV fluids vary. Therefore, the nurse should be familiar with the institution's policies and procedures regarding induction of labor. Pitocin is administered IV beginning with 0.5 to 2 milliunits/min and is increased by 1 to 2 milliunits every 15 to 60 min to a maximum of 32 to 40 milliunits/min (per protocol) or until contractions are regular and effective.

Pitocin 10 units in 1000 mL = Pitocin 10,000 milliunits in 1000 mL or 10 milliunits in 1 mL

Set infusion pump to deliver the following:

3 mL/hour = 0.5 milliunits/min
6 mL/hour = 1.0 milliunits/min
12 mL/hour = 2.0 milliunits/min

Increase in increments of 3 to 6 mL to a maximum of 32 to 40 milliunits/min

- Pitocin infusion is stopped and the physician notified if:
  - Contractions are closer than 2 min or last longer than 90 sec
  - There are signs of fetal distress (late decelerations, severe variable decelerations, or bradycardia)
- Pitocin given in an electrolyte-free solution or at a rate exceeding 20 milliunits/min increases the risk of water intoxication
  Signs include: nausea, vomiting, hypotension, tachycardia, and cardiac arrhythmia

f. Active genital herpes infection
g. Invasive cervical cancer

B. ***Dystocia* or difficult labor**

1. **Hypertonic uterine dysfunction**: frequent contractions with decreased intensity and increased uterine tone
   a. Maternal risks are prolonged or nonprogressive labor, pain, and fatigue
   b. Fetal risks include hypoxia caused by decreased uteroplacental blood flow
   c. Medical treatment includes sedation aimed at stopping contractions, promoting rest, and allowing a normal labor pattern to develop
   d. Hydration, monitoring intake and output, and promoting relaxation are important nursing interventions
2. **Hypotonic uterine dysfunction**: infrequent contractions with decreased intensity
   a. Maternal and fetal risks are related to nonprogressive labor, which is often associated with prolonged rupture of membranes, and frequent vaginal examinations leading to infection
   b. More commonly occurs in active phase of labor
   c. Medical treatment includes ruling out CPD and **augmentation of labor**, or stimulation of contractions, with oxytocin
3. **Abnormal progress in labor**: a labor graph may be used to identify deviations from normal progress in labor by plotting cervical dilatation and descent of fetal head over time; progress is plotted and compared to expected pattern called Friedman's curve
   a. Prolonged latent phase: >20 hours in a nulliparous client or >14 hours in a multiparous client
      1) May indicate CPD
      2) May be caused by false labor
      3) Medical treatment is sedation and rest
   b. Protracted active phase: dilatation <1.2 centimeters in a nulliparous client or <1.5 centimeters in a multiparous client
      1) May be caused by malposition
      2) CPD and fetal presentation and position is assessed
   c. Protracted descent: <1 centimeter per hour change in station in a nulliparous client or <2 centimeters per hour in a multiparous client
      1) CPD is ruled out
      2) Contraction intensity and duration are assessed
      3) Labor may be augmented with oxytocin
   d. Secondary arrest of dilatation: cessation of dilatation for >2 hours in a nulliparous client or >1 hour in a multiparous client
      1) CPD is ruled out
      2) If no CPD, labor is augmented with oxytocin
   e. Arrest of descent: no progress in fetal station for >1 hour
      1) CPD is assessed
      2) Labor is augmented, if no CPD
4. Retraction rings
   a. Physiologic retraction ring: boundary between upper uterine segment and lower uterine segment that normally forms during labor
      1) Upper segment contracts and becomes thicker as muscle fibers shorten
      2) Lower segment distends and becomes thinner
   b. Bandl's ring: a pathological retraction ring that forms when labor is obstructed caused by CPD or other complications
      1) Upper segment continues to thicken
      2) Lower segment continues to distend

3) Risk of uterine rupture increases if contractions continue
4) Cesarean delivery is indicated

c. Constriction ring
1) Retraction ring forms and impedes fetal descent
2) Relaxation of constriction ring with analgesics, anesthetics, or both allows vaginal delivery

C. ***Premature labor***: contractions occurring between 20 to 37 weeks' gestation

1. Client teaching for every woman about signs and symptoms of premature labor
   a. Contractions occurring every 10 minutes or less with or without pain
   b. Low abdominal cramping with or without diarrhea
   c. Intermittent sensation of pelvic pressure, urinary frequency
   d. Low backache (constant or intermittent)
   e. Increased vaginal discharge, may be pink-tinged
   f. Leaking amniotic fluid

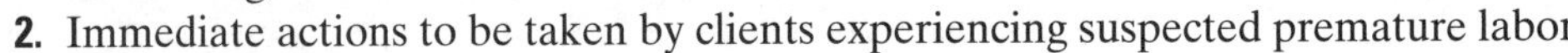

2. Immediate actions to be taken by clients experiencing suspected premature labor
   a. Empty bladder
   b. Assume a side-lying position, left preferred
   c. Drink three to four cups of water
   d. Palpate abdomen for uterine contractions; if 10 minutes apart or closer, contact health care provider
   e. Rest for 30 minutes and slowly resume activity, if symptoms disappear
   f. If symptoms do not subside within one hour, contact health care provider
3. Medical management
   a. Bedrest
   b. Continued monitoring of uterine activity and FHR
   c. Administration of **tocolytic agents**, drugs to stop contractions, if labor continues (see Table 9-2)
      1) Ritodrine (Yutopar)
      2) Terbutaline (Brethine)

Table 9-2 Drugs Used in Premature Labor

Drug	Type/Purpose	Major Side Effects	Nursing Concerns
Ritodrine (Yutopar)	Beta adrenergic/ tocolysis	Maternal or fetal tachycardia, shortness of breath, pulmonary edema, nervousness, tremors, nausea and vomiting, hyperglycemia, hypokalemia	Assess vital signs, breath sounds, fetal heart rate, contractions, and maternal response (not widely used because of cardiac effects)
Terbutaline (Brethine)	Beta adrenergic/ tocolysis	Nervousness, palpitations, maternal or fetal tachycardia, nausea and vomiting, pulmonary edema	Assess vital signs, breath sounds, fetal heart rate, contractions, and maternal response
Magnesium Sulfate	CNS depressant/ tocolysis	Lethargy, heat sensation, respiratory depression, depressed reflexes and cardiac arrest, if high serum level (>10 to 12 mg/dL)	Assess respiratory rate, deep tendon reflexes, and hourly urinary output; monitor serum magnesium levels
Nifedipine (Adalat, Procardia)	Calcium channel blocker/ tocolysis	Headache, dysrhythmias, congestive heart failure, peripheral edema, flushing, hypotension	Monitor pulse and blood pressure, breath sounds, intake and output
Betamethasone (Celestone) or Dexamethasone	Corticosteroid/ stimulates fetal lung maturation by stimulating surfactant production	Increased risk of infection and poor wound healing, produces hypoglycemia, increased risk of pulmonary edema when given with a beta adrenergic agent	Must be given 24 to 48 hours before delivery to be effective; commonly used between 24 to 34 weeks' gestation unless fetal lung maturity can be documented

3) Magnesium sulfate
4) Nifedipine (Adalat), a calcium channel blocker

d. Administration of betamethasone (Celestone) or dexamethasone to stimulate fetal lung maturity

4. Nursing assessment and diagnoses
   a. Identify clients at risk for premature labor
   b. Priority nursing diagnoses: Deficient Knowledge; Fear; Ineffective Coping
5. Planning and implementation
   a. Provide client and family teaching regarding signs and management of premature labor
   b. Promote bedrest encouraging left lateral position
   c. Monitor uterine activity and FHR
   d. Administer tocolytics and monitor for adverse reactions
   e. Provide emotional support encouraging client and family to express feelings and concerns
6. Evaluation
   a. Client can identify signs and symptoms of premature labor to report to health care provider
   b. Client can identify self-care measures to initiate, if premature labor is suspected
   c. Client's coping strategies are strengthened
   d. Client and fetus are delivered safely

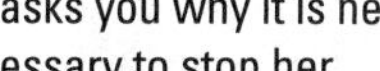

Practice to Pass

A client who is at 34 weeks' gestation asks you why it is necessary to stop her labor instead of just letting the baby be born. What explanation would you give her?

D. ***Precipitate labor and birth***: rapid labor (<3 hours) resulting in precipitous (unattended or nurse attended) birth; some precipitous births can be sudden and overwhelming to mother

1. Maternal risks
   a. Cervical, vaginal, or rectal lacerations
   b. Hemorrhage
2. Fetal risks
   a. Hypoxia caused by decreased perfusion to intervillous spaces
   b. Intracranial hemorrhage due to rapid passage through birth canal
   c. Injury at birth
   d. Pneumothorax because of rapid descent
3. Nursing assessment and diagnoses
   a. Identify client at risk for precipitous labor and birth, who is often a client with a history of precipitous labor (less than three hours)
   b. Priority nursing diagnoses: Risk for Injury; Anxiety; Fear
4. Planning and implementation
   a. Do not leave client; send someone or call for help
   b. Don sterile gloves, if time allows
   c. Instruct client to pant or blow to decrease urge to push
   d. Support perineum with a sterile towel as crowning occurs
   e. Apply gentle pressure on fetal head to prevent rapid delivery
      1) Lacerations of perineum can occur
      2) Subdural or dural tears may occur with sudden expulsion of infant's head
   f. After delivery of head, suctioning of infant's mouth then nose with bulb syringe may be performed; this practice is under study
   g. Check around infant's neck for a possible tight umbilical cord; if present, cord must be clamped and cut before delivery
   h. Place hands on each side of infant's head and instruct client to push
   i. Gentle downward pressure facilitates birth of anterior shoulder
   j. Gentle upward traction facilitates birth of posterior shoulder
   k. Support infant's body with a towel as it is expelled from birth canal
   l. Suction and dry infant thoroughly

Practice to Pass

A client is about to deliver a breech infant. As the nurse in attendance, what steps should you take, how would these differ from a vertex presentation, and what are your major concerns?

m. Place infant on mother's abdomen as soon as stable
n. Clamp and cut umbilical cord
o. Observe for signs of placental separation
   1) Gush of bright blood
   2) Lengthening of cord
p. *Very* gently pull on cord while massaging fundus to deliver placenta
q. Continue to massage fundus to prevent hemorrhage or put infant to breast
r. Inspect perineum for lacerations or tears

5. Evaluation
   a. Client's fear and anxiety are reduced
   b. Client and fetus are safely delivered

E. Uterine prolapse

1. Vigorous massage of fundus and pulling on umbilical cord to speed placental separation may cause prolapse of cervix and lower uterine segment through introitus
2. **Uterine inversion**: turning inside out of uterus
   a. Complete inversion
      1) Inverted uterus is visible outside introitus
      2) Life threatening because of severe hemorrhage and shock
      3) Uterus must be immediately replaced manually to stop blood loss
   b. Partial inversion
      1) Is not visible but can be palpated
      2) Uterine fundus is partially inverted, hampering contraction and control of hemorrhage
      3) Corrected by health care provider using a bimanual technique

F. *Uterine rupture*: tearing open or separation of uterine wall

1. Rare but serious complication, occurring in 1 in 1500 to 2000 births
2. Most common causes
   ! a. Separation of scar from previous classical cesarean incision
   b. Uterine trauma
   c. Intense uterine contractions
   d. Overstimulation of labor with oxytocin
   e. Difficult forceps-assisted birth
   f. External cephalic or internal version
3. Risk factors for uterine rupture
   a. Multiparity
   b. Overdistension of uterus (multifetal pregnancy)
   c. Malpresentation
   d. Previous uterine surgery
4. Types
   a. Complete: extends through uterine wall into peritoneal cavity
   b. Incomplete: extends into peritoneum but not into peritoneal cavity
      1) Partial separation of cesarean scar
      2) May go unnoticed until repeat cesarean is performed
5. Medical management depends on type of rupture
   a. Complete rupture requires management of shock, replacement of blood, and hysterectomy
   b. Incomplete rupture may require laparotomy, repair, and blood transfusion
6. ! Nursing assessment: signs and symptoms may be silent or dramatic
   a. Sudden, sharp, lower abdominal pain
   b. Tearing sensation
   c. Signs of shock

d. Cessation of contractions
e. FHR ceases
f. Blood loss is often concealed
g. Fetal parts may be easily palpated through abdominal wall

7. Priority nursing diagnoses: Risk for Injury; Impaired Gas Exchange; Deficient Fluid Volume
8. Planning and implementation
   a. Prevention is best
      1) Identify clients at risk
      2) Avoid hyperstimulation of uterus during induction
9. Evaluation
   a. Client and infant are delivered without injury
   b. Client's fluid volume is restored to normal

V. PROBLEMS WITH THE PSYCHE

A. Factors influencing psyche of client in labor

1. Fear and anxiety
2. Perception of problem
3. Self-image
4. Preparation for childbirth
5. Support systems
6. Coping ability
7. Lack of understanding of spoken language
8. Intelligence (lowered IQ)
9. Altered mental state (alcohol or drug intoxication)

B. Effect of fear and anxiety on labor progress

1. Epinephrine secretion in response to stress
2. Vascular changes divert blood from uterus to skeletal muscles
3. Decrease in oxygen and glucose supply with accumulation of lactic acid in uterine muscle
4. Higher perception of pain
5. Decrease in available energy supply to support effective contractions
6. Labor progress is slowed

C. Nursing assessment

1. Determine client's past experiences with, preparation for, and expectations of labor and birth
2. Determine client's current coping behaviors and their effectiveness with current situation

D. Priority nursing diagnoses: Ineffective Coping; Fear; Anxiety; Deficient Knowledge

E. Planning and implementation

1. Establish a trusting relationship with client and family
2. Remain at bedside with client and family during labor
3. Encourage relaxation
4. Keep client and family informed about progress and procedures
5. Encourage positive coping behaviors and discourage negative behaviors
6. Promote self-image by praising efforts

F. Evaluation

1. Client coping strategies are strengthened
2. Client's fear and anxiety are reduced
3. Client verbalizes increased understanding of labor and birth process

VI. CESAREAN DELIVERY

A. Delivery of infant by an abdominal incision: purpose is to facilitate delivery to preserve health of mother and fetus
1. Number of cesarean births continues to increase partially because of increase in number of labor inductions and women being able to choose to have a primary elective cesarean delivery
2. 2008 cesarean delivery rate as reported by National Center for Health Statistics has risen to 32.3%

B. Major indications for cesarean delivery
1. Dystocia or CPD
2. Fetal distress
3. Breech presentation
4. Previous cesarean birth
5. Fetal abnormalities may increase rate of cesarean delivery

C. Maternal risks
1. Aspiration
2. Hemorrhage
3. Infections
4. Injury to bowel or bladder
5. Thrombophlebitis
6. Pulmonary embolism

D. Fetal/neonatal risks
1. Prematurity
2. Injury at birth
3. Respiratory problems related to delayed absorption of fetal lung fluid

E. Surgical techniques
1. Skin incisions
   a. Vertical
   b. Pfannenstiel's (transverse lower abdominal incision)
2. Uterine incisions
   a. Classical: through upper uterine segment
   b. Low cervical transverse: lower uterine segment
   c. Lower uterine segment vertical

F. Nursing assessment
1. Determine reason for cesarean delivery
2. Determine client's understanding of indication, procedure, and implications for recovery from abdominal delivery

G. Priority nursing diagnoses: Deficient Knowledge; Fear; Anxiety; Disturbed Self-Esteem, Disturbed Body Image

H. Planning and implementation
1. Discuss cesarean birth in childbirth preparation classes
   a. Clients and families cope better if they have time to learn about cesarean birth
   b. Emergency cesarean birth increases anxiety and alters couple's expectations about childbirth

! 2. Preoperative care
   a. Assess NPO status (mother should have had nothing by mouth, if possible, to prevent aspiration)
   b. Explain procedure so that client and family will know what to expect
   c. Obtain client signature on consent form
   d. Perform abdominal prep
   e. Insert indwelling urinary catheter to prevent bladder trauma during surgery

f. Start IV fluids using a large-bore catheter
g. Administer an antacid either IV or PO to decrease risk of lung damage from aspirating acidic gastric contents during surgery
h. Administer antibiotics, as ordered
i. Assist with positioning and administration of regional anesthesia, if used

3. Intraoperative care
   a. Provide heated crib and supplies to receive newborn
   b. Provide immediate care to newborn or assist nursery personnel as needed
   c. Provide assistance to surgical team and immediate care for mother
4. Postoperative care

   a. Begin post-anesthesia (recovery room) monitoring of vital signs, pulse oximetry, and cardiac monitoring; monitor vital signs every 15 minutes for first hour and until stable

   b. Assess fundus for firmness and location (if boggy, massage until firm)
   c. Assess vaginal bleeding
   d. Assess abdominal dressing
   e. Assess catheter and urine output
   f. Apply and maintain sequential compression devices (SCDs) to legs to prevent deep vein thrombosis
   g. Administer medications for pain, as needed
   h. Turn, cough, and deep breathe hourly
   i. Promote maternal–infant contact and bonding

Practice to Pass

As the childbirth education instructor, you are discussing emergency cesarean delivery. A client asks what she can do to avoid having an emergency cesarean section. How will you answer her?

I. Evaluation

1. Client experiences a safe and satisfying delivery of a healthy infant
2. Client's fear and anxiety are decreased
3. Client's coping strategies are strengthened
4. Client is able to express feelings regarding delivery
5. Client verbalizes understanding of indication for and plan of care following cesarean delivery

VII. TRIAL OF LABOR AFTER CESAREAN (TOLAC)

A. Labor and vaginal birth after a previous cesarean is considered a safe option, if indication for cesarean delivery is not likely to be repeated

B. Contraindications

1. Previous classical incision into uterus
2. Large infant (>4000 grams)
3. Malpresentation
4. Inadequate pelvic measurements
5. Any fetal or placental problem that may require cesarean section
6. Delivery in an alternative birth setting: unless there is access to a facility where emergency cesarean may be performed

C. Assessment of risks versus benefits

1. Risks
   a. Possible uterine rupture and hemorrhage: less likely to occur if previous uterine incision was in lower uterine segment; risk of rupture is approximately 1%
   b. Failure of trial of labor requiring a repeat cesarean delivery
2. Benefits
   a. Ability to experience labor and vaginal delivery, which is desired by some clients; success rates are approximately 70%
   b. Vaginal delivery is less costly than cesarean delivery with faster, easier recovery period and less risk of complications
   c. TOLAC does not preclude induction or augmentation of labor

D. **Priority nursing diagnoses**: Risk for Injury; Anxiety; Fear; Deficient Knowledge

E. **Planning and implementation**

1. Monitor uterine activity and progress in labor; identify deviations from normal progress in labor and report to health care provider as essential care
2. Monitor FHR and response to contractions; identify and report indications of fetal distress quickly
3. Provide teaching before onset of labor that early period of labor carries greatest risk of uterine rupture for TOLAC clients
4. Observe for indications of uterine rupture
   a. Signs of shock or hemorrhage
   b. Report of "ripping or tearing" sensation or sharp uterine pain
   c. Abrupt cessation of contractions
   d. Abrupt onset of fetal distress
   e. Fetus may be palpated more easily than before, because lying outside uterus
5. Be alert and prepared for possible emergency cesarean delivery
6. Provide support and encouragement for client attempting TOLAC

F. **Evaluation**

1. Client and fetus are delivered safely
2. Client's anxiety and fear are decreased
3. Client is able to verbalize risks and benefits of TOLAC and signs and symptoms to be reported immediately to nurse or health care provider

POSTTEST

Case Study

A nulliparous client was admitted to the birthing unit nine hours ago. She progressed from 3 centimeters and 0 station to 6 centimeters and +1 station, but has not made any additional progress for almost two hours. FHR is in the normal baseline range with moderate variability. There are no decelerations. Contractions are presently q3 minutes, 40 seconds duration, and of strong intensity.

1. Following the vaginal examination, what other assessments will you make at this time?
2. During the vaginal examination, you determine that the small triangular fontanel is toward the mother's back on the right side. What is the fetal position?
3. The client's husband asks you why labor has not progressed very much. How will you answer him?
4. What nursing interventions will be most helpful to this client at this time?
5. Should you notify her physician at this time? If so, what information will you give and what medical interventions do you anticipate?

For suggested responses, see pages 304–305.

POSTTEST

1 A multiparous client who has been in labor for almost three hours suddenly announces that the baby is coming. The nurse sees the infant crowning. What is the initial nursing action?

1. Ask the woman to pant while preparing to place gentle counterpressure on the infant's head as it is delivered.
2. Quickly obtain sterile gloves and a towel and drape the perineum.
3. Retrieve the precipitous delivery tray from the nursing station.
4. Telephone the physician using the bedside phone.

2 The nurse determines that a client has an understanding of the planned cesarean delivery when the client makes which statement? Select all that apply.

1. "An indwelling urinary catheter will be inserted before surgery."
2. "My husband can be present during birth."
3. "I may be given an antacid before surgery."
4. "I will receive a blood transfusion during surgery."
5. "I will not need an IV since I will have an epidural anesthesia."

3 The nurse notes a deceleration of the fetal heart rate from 130 to 70 beats per minute with contractions followed by a rapid return to a normal baseline rate. The nurse concludes that this is most likely a client's response to which of the following?

1. Umbilical cord compression
2. Fetal head compression
3. Severe fetal hypoxia
4. Utero-placental insufficiency

4 The nurse determines that fetal distress is occurring after noting which of the following signs?

1. Moderate amount of bloody show
2. Pink-tinged amniotic fluid
3. Meconium-stained amniotic fluid
4. Acceleration of fetal heart rate with each contraction

5 On performing Leopold's maneuvers on a multiparous client in early labor, the nurse finds no fetal parts in the fundus or above the symphysis. The fetal head is palpated in the right mid quadrant. The nurse notifies the admitting physician and anticipates which event?

1. An external version
2. An internal version
3. A cesarean delivery
4. Prolonged labor

6 The nurse discovers a loop of umbilical cord protruding through the vagina when performing a vaginal examination on a client in labor. What is the priority nursing intervention at this time?

1. Call the physician immediately.
2. Place a moist, clean towel over the cord to prevent drying.
3. Immediately turn the client on her side and listen to the fetal heart rate.
4. Continue with the vaginal examination and apply upward digital pressure to the presenting part while having the mother assume a knee-chest position.

7 The client has refused sedation ordered by the physician for hypertonic contractions and prolonged latent-phase labor for fear that her labor will stop. The nurse may help by providing which explanation to the client?

1. Sedation helps to provide needed rest and allows time for the uterine contractions to become coordinated so that labor is progressive.
2. If the woman is experiencing true labor, contractions will not stop even with sedation.
3. If contractions continue without cervical effacement and dilatation, the fetus is at risk for hypoxia.
4. Sedation will stop contractions that are uncoordinated and provide more time to determine if a cesarean delivery is needed.

8 The client is receiving intravenous magnesium sulfate at two grams/hr to stop premature labor. The nurse determines that the most important nursing assessments of this client to determine toxicity include which of the following?

1. Intake and output, level of consciousness, and blood pressure
2. Blood pressure, pulse, and uterine activity
3. Deep tendon reflexes, hourly urine output, and respiratory rate
4. Intake and output, blood pressure, and reflexes

9 During augmentation of labor with intravenous oxytocin (Pitocin), a multiparous client becomes pale and diaphoretic and reports severe lower abdominal pain with a tearing sensation. Fetal distress is noted on the monitor. What complication should the nurse should suspect?

1. Precipitate labor
2. Amniotic fluid embolus
3. Rupture of the uterus
4. Uterine prolapse

10 During a vaginal examination on a pregnant client, the nurse palpates the fetal head and a large diamond-shaped fontanelle. The nurse documents which of the following as the fetal presentation?

1. Breech
2. Shoulder
3. Vertex
4. Brow

➤ *See pages 196–197 for Answers and Rationales.*

ANSWERS & RATIONALES

Pretest

1 **Answer: 2, 3, 4** **Rationale:** Placing a clean underpad on the bed and repositioning the mother is important in providing comfort and can be done after assuring fetal status and documentation. The risk of umbilical cord compression or prolapse increases when amniotic fluid is released. Listening to fetal heart tones after amniotomy will quickly detect the presence of cord compression. Observing and documenting color and consistency of the fluid should be done after fetal assessment is completed. It is unnecessary to position the mother for delivery at this time. Temperature should be monitored every one to two hours for signs of infection. **Cognitive Level:** Analyzing **Client Need:** Reduction of Risk Potential **Integrated Process:** Nursing Process: Implementation **Content Area:** Maternal-Newborn **Strategy:** Recall care of the client undergoing amniotomy and the resulting complications such as umbilical cord compression and infection. The correct answers will be options that best promote the safety of mother and fetus. Eliminate options that could pose a risk to safety. **Reference:** Ladewig, P. A., London, M. L., & Davidson, M. R. (2010). *Contemporary maternal-newborn nursing care* (7th ed.). Upper Saddle River, NJ: Pearson Education, pp. 507–536.

2 **Answer: 3** **Rationale:** In a right occiput anterior (ROA) position, the right side of the occiput (back of the head) is facing front (anterior). In a right occiput transverse (ROT) position, the right side of the occiput is sideways when viewed from the anterior. In a left occiput anterior (LOA) position, the left side of the occiput is facing front (anterior). In a right mentum anterior (RMA) position, the right side of the face is anterior. **Cognitive Level:** Applying **Client Need:** Physiological Adaptation **Integrated Process:** Nursing Process: Assessment **Content Area:** Maternal-Newborn **Strategy:** Recall the various positions at delivery and recall the meanings of the terms occiput and mentum to aid in making the correct selection. **Reference:** Ladewig, P. A., London, M. L., & Davidson, M. R. (2010). *Contemporary maternal-newborn nursing care* (7th ed.). Upper Saddle River, NJ: Pearson Education, pp. 381–382.

3 **Answer: 4** **Rationale:** Dilatation has stopped (arrested) after considerable progress. Causes may be hypotonic uterine contractions, malposition, or cephalopelvic disproportion. Prolonged means that progress occurs at a very slow rate, while this client has stopped progressing. Protracted means that progress occurs at a very slow rate, while this client has stopped progressing. Arrest of descent occurs when the station rather than cervical dilatation does not change. **Cognitive Level:** Analyzing **Client Need:** Physiological Adaptation **Integrated Process:** Nursing Process: Assessment **Content Area:** Maternal-Newborn **Strategy:** The core focus in this question is progress to 7 cm dilatation followed by no change in two hours. Eliminate two options because prolonged and protracted mean that progress occurs at a very slow rate. Eliminate option the third that focuses on the station rather than cervical dilatation. **Reference:** Ladewig, P. A., London, M. L., & Davidson, M. R. (2010). *Contemporary maternal-newborn nursing care* (7th ed.). Upper Saddle River, NJ: Pearson Education, p. 512.

4 **Answer: 1** **Rationale:** Meconium from the fetus causes amniotic fluid to be greenish-tinged. Although there is no evidence of fetal distress at this point in labor, the infant is at risk for aspirating meconium at the time of delivery. Steps to prevent aspiration include visualization of the vocal cords with a laryngoscope and thorough suctioning of the nasopharynx to remove

meconium particles before the first breath. The presence of meconium does not require the assistance of forceps for delivery. A transport isolette would be needed if the neonate had distress at the time of birth and required transportation to an intensive care setting. Meconium in the amniotic fluid does not prevent a vaginal delivery. **Cognitive Level:** Analyzing **Client Need:** Physiological Adaptation **Integrated Process:** Nursing Process: Planning **Content Area:** Maternal-Newborn **Strategy:** Recall the ABC's; meconium in the amniotic fluid can interfere with a clear airway and effective breathing. The correct answer will include an action to clear the airway prior to the newborn's first breath. **Reference:** Ladewig, P. A., London, M. L., & Davidson, M. R. (2010). *Contemporary maternal-newborn nursing care* (7th ed.). Upper Saddle River, NJ: Pearson Education, pp. 763–764.

5 **Answer: 4 Rationale:** Hydration has been shown to decrease premature labor contractions. Therefore, drinking water or other non-caffeinated beverages is recommended. It is unnecessary for the client to stop eating and hydration may help to decrease the contractions. Taking slow deep breaths may comfort the client but will not reduce or stop the contractions. If contractions continue at 10 minutes apart or less for an hour with rest, the client should call her healthcare provider. **Cognitive Level:** Applying **Client Need:** Physiological Adaptation **Integrated Process:** Nursing Process: Implementation **Content Area:** Maternal-Newborn **Strategy:** Knowledge of the nursing care of the premature labor client will help to answer the question correctly. The wording of the question is positive, indicating that the correct option is a true statement of fact. **Reference:** Ladewig, P. A., London, M. L., & Davidson, M. R. (2010). *Contemporary maternal-newborn nursing care* (7th ed.). Upper Saddle River, NJ: Pearson Education, pp. 488–489.

6 **Answer: 2 Rationale:** A classical incision involves the upper uterine segment and is more likely to separate or rupture with subsequent uterine contractions. The reason for the previous cesarean delivery is not of concern, although the current presentation is of interest. The type of abdominal incision is not a concern, since it is not affected by uterine contractions. Induction is not a contraindication if managed judiciously. **Cognitive Level:** Analyzing **Client Need:** Physiological Adaptation **Integrated Process:** Nursing Process: Assessment **Content Area:** Maternal-Newborn **Strategy:** Focus on safety of the mother and infant with this question. The greatest risk during a TOLAC is uterine rupture; potential for rupture is influenced by location of the previous uterine scar. Eliminate three incorrect options because they do not address the prior uterine incision. **Reference:** Ladewig, P. A., London, M. L., & Davidson, M. R. (2010). *Contemporary maternal-newborn nursing care* (7th ed.). Upper Saddle River, NJ: Pearson Education, p. 554.

7 **Answer: 3 Rationale:** Promoting a positive feeling about how well she was able to cope with an emergency cesarean delivery will influence the client's self-image and feelings about her ability to handle future pregnancies and births. In addition, providing an opportunity for the client and her family to ask questions and to express feelings helps in dealing with any disappointment, anger, or guilt they may feel. Statements in the other options indicate that the birth was not normal and can promote negative feelings about the infant or the experience. **Cognitive Level:** Applying **Client Need:** Psychosocial Integrity **Integrated Process:** Communication and Documentation **Content Area:** Maternal-Newborn **Strategy:** This question focuses on therapeutic communication. The correct answer would be the option that best supports the client's feelings and behaviors. Eliminate nontherapeutic responses as incorrect. Only one option is therapeutic and promotes a positive feeling about client's coping through the delivery. **Reference:** Ladewig, P. A., London, M. L., & Davidson, M. R. (2010). *Contemporary maternal-newborn nursing care* (7th ed.). Upper Saddle River, NJ: Pearson Education, p. 554.

8 **Answer: 2, 5 Rationale:** The antidiuretic effect of oxytocin decreases water exchange in the kidney and reduces urinary output. Oxytocin (Pitocin) stimulates uterine contractility; exceeding maximum doses or increasing doses too rapidly can result in uterine hyperstimulation. Blood pressure, not pulse, may initially decrease but after prolonged drug administration, blood pressure may increase 30% above baseline. The antidiuretic effect of oxytocin leads to fluid overload rather than dehydration. Jaundice is not an adverse maternal effect of oxytocin. **Cognitive Level:** Applying **Client Need:** Pharmacological and Parenteral Therapies **Integrated Process:** Nursing Process: Assessment **Content Area:** Maternal-Newborn **Strategy:** The focus of this question is adverse maternal effects of oxytocin (Pitocin). Recall that the drug stimulates uterine smooth muscle of the uterus and blood vessels and has an antidiuretic effect. **Reference:** Ladewig, P. A., London, M. L., & Davidson, M. R. (2010). *Contemporary maternal-newborn nursing care* (7th ed.). Upper Saddle River, NJ: Pearson Education, pp. 542–543.

9 **Answer: 1, 2 Rationale:** Lung sounds should be assessed as pulmonary edema is an adverse effect of tocolytics, leading to lung crackles. Flushing and headache are side effects of tocolytics. Nystagmus (oscillation of the eyes) is an adverse effect of tocolytics. Excessive energy and euphoria are not side effects of tocolytics. Monitoring of deep tendon reflexes would be needed if the client is receiving magnesium sulfate. **Cognitive Level:** Applying **Client Need:** Pharmacological and Parenteral Therapies **Integrated Process:** Nursing Process: Assessment **Content Area:** Maternal-Newborn **Strategy:** The focus of the question is the action of tocolytics. Specific information is needed to answer the question. Note that the style of the question indicates that more than one option is correct. **Reference:** Ladewig, P. A., London, M. L., & Davidson, M. R. (2010). *Contemporary maternal-newborn*

nursing care (7th ed.). Upper Saddle River, NJ: Pearson Education, p. 485.

10 **Answer: 1** **Rationale:** With breech presentation, fetal parts do not completely fill the lower uterine segment, allowing more opportunity for the umbilical cord to proceed through the cervix or become compressed by the fetus, especially following rupture of membranes. The incidence of intracranial hemorrhage, meconium aspiration, or fractured clavicle is no higher in breech than it is with vertex presentation. **Cognitive Level:** Analyzing **Client Need:** Physiological Adaptation **Integrated Process:** Nursing Process: Assessment **Content Area:** Maternal-Newborn **Strategy:** Remember ABC's related to safety of the infant at birth. The correct option would include jeopardizing the safety of the infant by interfering with normal oxygenation and circulation through the umbilical cord. **Reference:** Ladewig, P. A., London, M. L., & Davidson, M. R. (2010). *Contemporary maternal-newborn nursing care* (7th ed.). Upper Saddle River, NJ: Pearson Education, pp. 516–517.

Posttest

1 **Answer: 1** **Rationale:** Nursing action should be directed toward preventing a rapid and uncontrolled delivery of the infant's head. Directing the client to pant prevents pushing. If time allows, the nurse may don gloves or obtain a towel or blanket to support the fetal head. Delivery is imminent, so there may not be time to obtain sterile gloves or contact the physician. The client should not be left alone, so going to the nursing station to get the precipitous delivery tray is not an option. Delivery is imminent, so there may not be time to contact the physician. **Cognitive Level:** Applying **Client Need:** Physiological Adaptation **Integrated Process:** Nursing Process: Implementation **Content Area:** Maternal-Newborn **Strategy:** This question focuses on the imminent delivery of the infant in a safe manner. Eliminate two options because they decrease safety by leaving the client's bedside. Eliminate another because the action is desirable but not required in an emergency. **Reference:** Ladewig, P. A., London, M. L., & Davidson, M. R. (2010). *Contemporary maternal-newborn nursing care* (7th ed.). Upper Saddle River, NJ: Pearson Education, p. 390.

2 **Answer: 1, 2, 3** **Rationale:** An indwelling urinary catheter is inserted to prevent bladder damage during surgery. The client's husband or primary support person is usually present at the birth except in extreme emergencies. An antacid is administered to prevent aspiration of acidic gastric contents, thus reducing the risk of lung damage. Blood transfusions are not routinely given during cesarean sections. Although blood typing and screening is often ordered prior to surgery, it is seldom necessary for a client to receive a blood transfusion. IV lines are necessary for instillation of fluid, medications, and potential blood products during surgery. **Cognitive Level:** Analyzing **Client Need:** Reduction of Risk Potential **Integrated Process:** Nursing Process: Evaluation **Content Area:** Maternal-Newborn **Strategy:** The wording of the question indicates that correct options are true statements. Use knowledge of the care of the client undergoing a cesarean section to aid in determining the appropriate options. **Reference:** Ladewig, P. A., London, M. L., & Davidson, M. R. (2010). *Contemporary maternal-newborn nursing care* (7th ed.). Upper Saddle River, NJ: Pearson Education, pp. 550–556.

3 **Answer: 1** **Rationale:** The pattern described is a variable deceleration, which is associated with umbilical cord compression. During variable decelerations, the FHR drops below 90 beats a minute very quickly as fetal blood flow through the umbilical cord is interrupted. FHR returns rapidly to baseline as soon as the cord compression is relieved. FHR patterns associated with fetal head compression (early deceleration) and uteroplacental insufficiency (late deceleration) have a shallower appearance since they do not drop as precipitously. Variable deceleration, unless severe (lasting longer than 60 seconds), does not indicate severe hypoxia. **Cognitive Level:** Analyzing **Client Need:** Physiological Adaptation **Integrated Process:** Nursing Process: Diagnosis **Content Area:** Maternal-Newborn **Strategy:** The key words in this question are *deceleration with rapid return to baseline*. Eliminate all incorrect options that are associated with decelerations that develop and resolve more slowly, mirroring the shape of contractions. **Reference:** Ladewig, P. A., London, M. L., & Davidson, M. R. (2010). *Contemporary maternal-newborn nursing care* (7th ed.). Upper Saddle River, NJ: Pearson Education, pp. 423–424.

4 **Answer: 3** **Rationale:** Meconium passage prior to birth occurs in response to a stressful event for the fetus. Moderate bloody show often occurs late in labor. Pink-tinged amniotic fluid occurs because of a small amount of blood usually from the cervix. Accelerations of FHR are considered a normal response and do not indicate fetal distress. **Cognitive Level:** Analyzing **Client Need:** Physiological Adaptation **Integrated Process:** Nursing Process: Assessment **Content Area:** Maternal-Newborn **Strategy:** Critical words are *fetal distress*, indicating the focus of this question is abnormal assessment data. Eliminate incorrect options as they represent common and normal findings during labor. **Reference:** Ladewig, P. A., London, M. L., & Davidson, M. R. (2010). *Contemporary maternal-newborn nursing care* (7th ed.). Upper Saddle River, NJ: Pearson Education, p. 401.

5 **Answer: 3** **Rationale:** Findings on palpation are consistent with shoulder presentation or transverse lie. Vaginal delivery is not possible, so the nurse should anticipate cesarean section. Since the client is in labor, version is contraindicated. **Cognitive Level:** Analyzing **Client Need:** Physiological Adaptation **Integrated Process:** Nursing Process: Planning **Content Area:** Maternal-Newborn

Strategy: The focus of this question is a client in labor with a transverse lie, a presentation that is incompatible with vaginal delivery. The correct answer would be the option that provides a safe alternative to vaginal delivery. **Reference:** Ladewig, P. A., London, M. L., & Davidson, M. R. (2010). *Contemporary maternal-newborn nursing care* (7th ed.). Upper Saddle River, NJ: Pearson Education, pp. 414–415.

6 **Answer: 4 Rationale:** Pressure on the cord must be relieved to save the life of the fetus. Applying upward manual pressure to the presenting part and having the mother assume a knee-chest position are appropriate emergency actions. The physician should be notified after relieving pressure on the cord and starting oxygen. Preventing the cord from drying is not the concern, as it is cord compression that presents the threat to the fetus. Turning the client onto her side and listening to the fetal heart rate will not relieve cord compression. **Cognitive Level:** Applying **Client Need:** Physiological Adaptation **Integrated Process:** Nursing Process: Implementation **Content Area:** Maternal-Newborn **Strategy:** The focus of this question is maintaining the safety of the fetus. The correct option would contain an action to prevent cord compression and promote adequate oxygenation to the fetus. **Reference:** Ladewig, P. A., London, M. L., & Davidson, M. R. (2010). *Contemporary maternal-newborn nursing care* (7th ed.). Upper Saddle River, NJ: Pearson Education, pp. 520–521.

7 **Answer: 1 Rationale:** Prolonged latent-phase labor is associated with uncoordinated, hypertonic, and painful contractions that do little to dilate or efface the cervix. Maternal exhaustion and dehydration are concerns. Medical management is directed toward providing rest and hydration and allowing time for contractions to become coordinated. Often clients awaken from sedation in progressive labor. Although true labor contractions will not stop with sedation, this does little to explain the rationale for sedation to the client. There is very little risk to the fetus unless contractions are intense and less than two minutes apart. Sedation is not provided to allow time to anticipate the need for cesarean delivery. **Cognitive Level:** Applying **Client Need:** Physiological Adaptation **Integrated Process:** Communication and Documentation **Content Area:** Maternal-Newborn **Strategy:** The wording of the question indicates that the correct option is also a true statement. Knowledge of the care of the labor client with hypertonic labor will aid in answering the question. **Reference:** Ladewig, P. A., London, M. L., & Davidson, M. R. (2010). *Contemporary maternal-newborn nursing care* (7th ed.). Upper Saddle River, NJ: Pearson Education, pp. 504–507.

8 **Answer: 3 Rationale:** Early signs of magnesium toxicity that may lead to respiratory arrest are loss of patellar reflexes and decreased respiratory rate (<12/min). Since magnesium is excreted from the body through the renal system, hourly urine output should be assessed. Although blood pressure is a standard assessment for most antepartum clients, there is minimal blood pressure change, if any, associated with administration of magnesium sulfate. Other vital signs, uterine activity and level of consciousness are routine assessments not specific to magnesium toxicity. **Cognitive Level:** Applying **Client Need:** Physiological Adaptation **Integrated Process:** Nursing Process: Assessment **Content Area:** Maternal-Newborn **Strategy:** The focus of the question is the adverse effects of magnesium sulfate. Recall that the drug is a central nervous system depressant and recall route of excretion to choose correctly. **Reference:** Ladewig, P. A., London, M. L., & Davidson, M. R. (2010). *Contemporary maternal-newborn nursing care* (7th ed.). Upper Saddle River, NJ: Pearson Education, p. 486.

9 **Answer: 3 Rationale:** Although rupture of the uterus is rare, there is an increased risk for multiparas and clients undergoing induction or augmentation of labor. Early signs include pain and a tearing sensation, signs of shock, and fetal distress. Blood loss is usually severe but may not be visible. Amniotic fluid embolus is frequently associated with cardiac and respiratory distress. Symptoms of precipitate labor and uterine prolapse do not include pallor, diaphoresis, or fetal distress. **Cognitive Level:** Analyzing **Client Need:** Physiological Adaptation **Integrated Process:** Nursing Process: Assessment **Content Area:** Maternal-Newborn **Strategy:** Critical words in this question are *tearing sensation* and *oxytocin administration*. A tearing sensation is the classic symptom of uterine rupture, a risk with oxytocin administration. Eliminate all incorrect options as the symptom presented would not occur in these conditions. **Reference:** Ladewig, P. A., London, M. L., & Davidson, M. R. (2010). *Contemporary maternal-newborn nursing care* (7th ed.). Upper Saddle River, NJ: Pearson Education, pp. 542–543.

10 **Answer: 4 Rationale:** In a brow presentation, the fetal forehead and the large, diamond-shaped, anterior fontanelle is palpated during vaginal exam. In vertex presentation, the back of the fetal head (occiput) and small, triangular fontanelle is palpated. In breech and shoulder presentations, fetal parts would feel soft and irregular. **Cognitive Level:** Analyzing **Client Need:** Physiological Adaptation **Integrated Process:** Nursing Process: Assessment **Content Area:** Maternal-Newborn **Strategy:** Critical words are *fetal head* and *diamond-shaped fontanelle*. The correct answer is an option containing true information about the presentation that permits palpation of the anterior fontanelle. **Reference:** Ladewig, P. A., London, M. L., & Davidson, M. R. (2010). *Contemporary maternal-newborn nursing care* (7th ed.). Upper Saddle River, NJ: Pearson Education, p. 377.

References

American College of Obstetricians and Gynecologists. (2009). *Revision of labor induction guidelines.* Washington, DC: ACOG.

Davidson, M., London, M., & Ladewig, P. (2012). *Olds' maternal newborn nursing & women's health across the lifespan* (9th ed.). Upper Saddle River, NJ: Pearson Education.

Ladewig, P., London, M., & Davidson, M. (2009). *Contemporary maternal-newborn nursing care* (7th ed.). Upper Saddle River, NJ: Pearson Education.

Martin, J. A., Hamilton, B. E., Sutton, P. D., Ventura, S. J., Matthews, T. J., & Osterman, M. (2010). Births: Final data for 2008. National Vital Statistics Reports (Vol. 59, no. 1). Hyattsville, MD: National Center for Health Statistics. Retrieved August 4, 2011 from http://www.cdc.gov/nchs/data/nvsr/nvsr59/nvsr59_01.pdf

Perry, S. E., Hockenberry, M. J., Lowdermilk, D. L., & Wilson, D. (2010). *Maternal child nursing care* (4th ed.). St. Louis, MO: Mosby.

Ricci, S. (2009). *Essentials of maternity, newborn, and women's health nursing* (2nd ed.). Philadelphia: Lippincott Williams & Wilkins.

The Normal Postpartal Experience 10

Chapter Outline

Physical Changes during the Postpartal Period (Puerperium)

Psychosocial Changes during the Postpartal Period

Nursing Care of the Postpartal Client

Objectives

- ➤ Describe the physical changes that occur in a woman during the postpartal period.
- ➤ Discuss the psychological changes that occur in the new mother.
- ➤ Describe nursing care designed to promote safety and self-care during the postpartal experience of the maternity client.

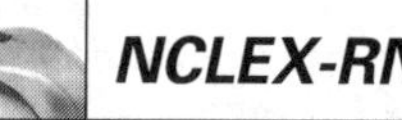

NCLEX-RN® Test Prep

Use the accompanying online resource, NursingReviewsandRationales, to test yourself with hundreds of NCLEX®-style practice questions.

Review at a Glance

afterpains uncomfortable uterine cramps that occur intermittently during first two to three days postpartum; more common in multiparous woman

boggy uterus uterus that is not well-contracted and feels soft when palpated

bonding a process by which parents form an emotional relationship with their infant over time

colostrum fluid in breasts during pregnancy and into early postpartal period; rich in antibodies, high in protein, and acts as a laxative for newborn

diastasis recti separation of two rectus muscles along median line of abdominal wall

en face face-to-face position in which parent's and infant's faces are approximately 20 centimeters apart and on same plane

engorgement swelling of breast tissue; primary engorgement typically lasts 48 hours and reaches a peak between 3rd and 5th days postpartum

engrossment a father's absorption, preoccupation, and interest in his infant

fundus dome-shaped upper portion of uterus between points of insertion of fallopian tubes

Homan's sign client complaint of sharp calf pain when leg is extended and client moves foot in a direction of dorsiflexion, such as walking or stretching legs; can be an early sign of thrombophlebitis

involution reduction in size of uterus after delivery to its pre-pregnant state

let-down reflex release of breast milk caused by contraction of milk glands in response to natural release of oxytocin; also known as milk ejection reflex

lochia alba thin, clear, yellow-to-white vaginal discharge that follows lochia serosa, from approximately 11 days to 3–6 weeks postpartum

lochia rubra red, menstrual-like vaginal discharge, from birth to three days postpartum

lochia serosa serous, pinkish-brown vaginal discharge that follows lochia rubra until approximately 10 days postpartum

postpartum blues a maternal adjustment reaction accompanied by irritability, anxiety, and a mild let-down feeling usually occurring between 2nd and 3rd postpartum day through 1st to 2nd week postpartum

puerperium period starting after third stage of labor and ending with return of uterus to pre-pregnant state at six weeks postpartum

PRETEST

1 The nurse is assessing a client 24 hours after delivery and finds the fundus to be slightly boggy and two centimeters above the umbilicus. What should be the nurse's priority nursing intervention?

1. Document this expected finding and check lochia.
2. Assess the mother's vital signs.
3. After having the mother void, gently massage the fundus until firm.
4. Notify the physician and document.

2 A new mother complains of "afterpains." The nurse's first action should be to do which of the following?

1. Administer an analgesic.
2. Advise her to stop breastfeeding until the pain stops.
3. Encourage her to empty her bladder.
4. Assess her vital signs.

3 The nurse is caring for a woman who gave birth to a daughter yesterday, but greatly desired a son. Today she seems withdrawn, staying in bed and staring at the wall. What is the most appropriate intervention?

1. Monitor this normal response after delivery.
2. Refer the client for a psychiatric consultation.
3. Tell the client she should be thankful her baby is healthy.
4. Encourage the mother to verbalize her disappointment.

4 The nurse is preparing to instruct a new mother on resuming sexual intercourse postpartum. The nurse should include which of the following in the teaching plan? Select all that apply.

1. Pregnancy is not possible prior to the first menses postpartum.
2. An IUD is an appropriate method of birth control in the early postpartum period.
3. Wait until the episiotomy has healed and the lochia has stopped before resuming intercourse.
4. Refrain from intercourse until the first menstrual period after delivery is completed.
5. A water-soluble lubricant may be used if necessary.

5 The nurse is caring for a client who has decided not to breastfeed. What should the nurse include in client teaching to promote lactation suppression? Select all that apply.

1. Applying warm compresses
2. Pumping the breasts
3. Applying ice bags
4. Using medication to suppress lactation
5. Binding the breasts, either with a snug bra or binder

6 A client has a temperature of 100.2°F four hours after delivery. What is the appropriate action for the nurse to take?

1. Encourage increased fluid intake.
2. Do nothing since this is an expected finding at this time.
3. Check the physician's orders for an antibiotic to treat the client's infection.
4. Medicate the client for pain.

7 A client delivered 90 minutes ago. She is alert and physically active in bed. She states that she needs to go to the bathroom. What is the nurse's most appropriate response?

1. "I'll walk you to the bathroom and stay with you."
2. "I'll get a bedpan for you."
3. "It's important that you wipe yourself from front to back after urinating."
4. "Wipe the stitches back and forth to increase circulation."

8 Which laboratory finding should the nurse assess further on a client 24 hours after delivery?

1. Hemoglobin 7.2 grams/dL
2. White blood cell count 20,000/mm^3
3. Trace to 1+ proteinuria
4. Hematocrit 35%

9 The nurse would assess for which common causative factor in a client who shows signs of retarded uterine involution? Select all that apply.

1. The use of general anesthesia
2. Overdistended urinary bladder
3. Mother is a primigravida
4. Uterine infection
5. Prolonged labor

10 A client who had a vaginal delivery had an episiotomy prior to birth. The maternal newborn nurse would evaluate the client's perineum following delivery is using which method?

1. REDA-redness, edema, discharge, approximation
2. REEDA-redness, edema, ecchymosis, discharge, approximation
3. REAA-redness, edema, approximation, assessment
4. RED-redness, edema, discoloration

➤ *See pages 211–213 for Answers and Rationales.*

PRETEST

I. PHYSICAL CHANGES DURING THE POSTPARTAL PERIOD (*PUERPERIUM*)

A. Reproductive

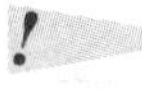

1. **Involution**: a reduction in uterine size after delivery to pre-pregnant state, caused by uterine contractions that constrict and occlude underlying blood vessels at placental site; Table 10-1 presents factors that slow or hasten this process during **puerperium**, the six-week period after delivery

2. **Fundus**: top portion of uterus; a palpable indicator of involution, as shown in Figure 10-1; if contractions of uterine muscle are interrupted, a **boggy uterus**, one that is soft, relaxed, and likely to cause hemorrhage results
3. Lochia: discharge of blood and debris following delivery; types include **lochia rubra**, **lochia serosa**, and **lochia alba**; characteristics of lochia are shown in Table 10-2
   a. Should not contain large clots
   b. Total volume is 240 to 270 mL, and daily volume gradually decreases
   c. Amount may be increased by exertion or breastfeeding
   d. Pooling in uterus or vagina may occur while reclining with increased bleeding upon arising
   e. Unexplained increase in amount or reappearance of lochia rubra is abnormal

Table 10-1 Factors That Influence Involution

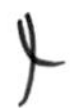

Factors That Enhance Involution	Factors That Slow Involution
Uncomplicated labor and delivery	Prolonged labor and difficult delivery
Breastfeeding	Anesthesia
Early ambulation	Grand multiparity
Complete expulsion of placenta and membranes	Retained placental fragments or membranes
	Full urinary bladder
	Infection
	Overdistention of the uterus

Figure 10-1

Involution of the uterus

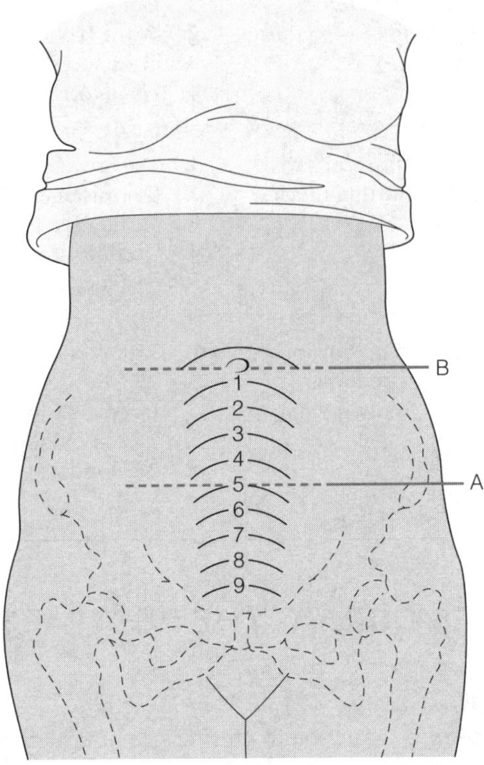

Table 10-2 Characteristics of Lochia

Type	Occurrence	Appearance	Composition
Lochia rubra	1–3 days	Dark red, bloody; fleshy, musty, stale odor that is nonoffensive; may have clots smaller than a nickel	Blood with small amounts of mucus, shreds of decidua, epithelial cells, leukocytes; may contain fetal meconium, lanugo, or vernix caseosa
Lochia serosa	4–10 days	Pink or brownish; watery; odorless	Serum, erythrocytes, shreds of degenerating decidua, leukocytes, cervical mucus, numerous bacteria
Lochia alba	11–21 days, may persist to 6 weeks in lactating women	Yellow to white; may have slightly stale odor	Leukocytes, decidual cells, epithelial cells, fat, cervical mucus, cholesterol, bacteria

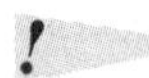

4. **Afterpains**
   a. Caused by intermittent uterine contractions following delivery
   b. Occur in all women but are more painful in multiparous and breastfeeding women
5. Cervix
   a. Soft, irregular, and edematous; may appear bruised with multiple, small lacerations
   b. Closes to 2 to 3 cm after several days, admits a fingertip after one week
   c. Shape permanently changes after first delivery from a round, dimplelike os of nullipara to a lateral, slitlike os of multiparous woman

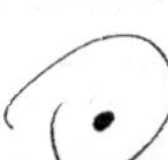

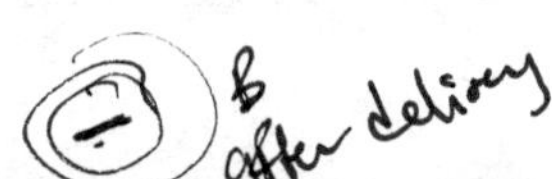

6. Vagina
   a. Smooth walls, edematous with multiple, small lacerations
   b. Client should be free from perineal pain within two weeks
   c. Low estrogen levels postpartum lead to decreased vaginal lubrication and vasocongestion for 6 to 10 weeks, which can result in painful intercourse

B. Abdominal wall

1. Soft and flabby with decreased muscle tone
2. Striae, or stretch marks, that were red during pregnancy will fade to silver or white in Caucasian women; darker-skinned women will have darker striae that remain darker
3. **Diastasis recti**, separation of rectus muscles of abdomen, may improve postpartally depending on woman's physical condition, number of pregnancies, and type and amount of exercise

C. Cardiovascular

1. Returns to pre-pregnant state within two weeks
2. Blood volume that has increased by 40% during pregnancy is eliminated primarily by diuresis
3. First 48 hours postpartum are a time of greatest risk of complications for clients with heart disease
4. Blood pressure should remain consistent with pregnancy baseline
5. Bradycardia of 50 to 70 beats per minute is common during the first 6–10 days; tachycardia is related to increased blood loss, temperature elevation, or difficult, prolonged labor and birth
6. Increased fibrinogen continues for one week resulting in increased erythrocyte sedimentation rate (ESR) and risk for thrombophlebitis
7. Increased white blood cells up to 30,000/mm^3 does not necessarily mean infection or may mask signs of infection; an increase of >30% in six hours indicates pathology
8. Decreased hemoglobin is related to amount of blood loss during delivery; should return to prelabor value in two to six weeks depending on degree of decrease
9. Hematocrit increases by 3rd to 5th day postpartum related to diuresis; a drop indicates abnormal blood loss

Practice to Pass

A client's white blood cell count is 21,000/mm^3 on the first day postpartum. What should you do?

D. Urinary

1. Postpartal diuresis of 2000 to 3000 mL increases urine output in first 12–24 hours after delivery and accounts for a five-pound weight loss
2. Increased glomerular filtration rate assists in diuresis
3. Fluids are also lost through diaphoresis with increased perspiration most commonly occurring at night
4. A full bladder displaces uterus, increasing risk of uterine atony and postpartal hemorrhage
5. Increased bladder capacity and decreased bladder tone lead to decreased sensation and increased risk of urinary retention and infection

E. Gastrointestinal

1. Hunger and thirst are common following birth
2. Risk for constipation increases because of decreased peristalsis, use of opioid analgesics, dehydration and decreased mobility during labor, and fear of pain from having a bowel movement
3. Risk for hemorrhoids increases because of pressure from pushing during second stage of labor

Practice to Pass

A client states she has heard that a woman cannot get pregnant again as long as she is breastfeeding. What should you tell her?

F. Endocrine

1. Estrogen and progesterone levels drop rapidly after delivery of placenta
2. Menstruation usually resumes at 7–9 weeks for nonlactating women with 90% experiencing a menstrual period by 12 weeks; first cycle is usually anovulatory

3. Ovulation and menstruation return time is prolonged in lactating women and affected by length of time woman breast-feeds and whether formula supplements are used; may vary from 2–18 months
4. Lactation
   a. Nipple stimulation leads to release of oxytocin from pituitary gland; this stimulates release of prolactin from pituitary gland, which causes production of milk and **let-down reflex**, release of milk by contractions of alveoli of breasts
   b. **Colostrum** is first milk secreted and is rich in protein and immunoglobulins (for immune protection of newborn)
   c. Primary **engorgement** occurs on second or third day as blood and lymph supply in breasts increases and transitional milk is produced
   d. Mature milk is produced after two weeks; it appears watery and slightly bluish in color, similar to skim milk

II. PSYCHOSOCIAL CHANGES DURING THE POSTPARTAL PERIOD

A. Phases of maternal adjustment

1. Taking-in phase
   a. First one to two days postpartum
   b. Preoccupied with own needs
   c. Passive and dependent
   d. Touches and explores infant
   e. Needs to discuss labor and delivery
2. Taking-hold phase
   a. Begins by 2nd to 3rd day postpartum
   b. Obsessed with body functions
   c. Rapid mood swings
   d. Anticipatory guidance most effective now
3. Letting-go phase
   a. Lasts from 10 days to 6 weeks postpartum
   b. Mothering functions established
   c. Sees infant as a unique person

B. *Bonding* (also known as attachment): process by which parents form an emotional relationship with their infant over time

1. Mother explores infant first with fingertips, then palms, and finally enfolding newborn with whole hands and arms
2. Holds infant in **en face** position, face-to-face position about 20 centimeters apart and on same plane
3. Uses a soft, high-pitched tone of voice
4. **Engrossment** is father's absorption, preoccupation, and interest in infant shortly after birth, which can be stimulated by witnessing birth

C. *Postpartum blues*: a maternal adjustment reaction

1. Transient depression usually occurs between 2nd and 3rd postpartum days and/or within first two weeks postpartum
2. Probably related to changes in hormone levels, fatigue, and psychological stress related to infant dependency
3. Experienced to some degree by a majority of women
4. Characterized by mood swings, anger, tearfulness, feeling let down, anorexia, and insomnia
5. Usually resolves spontaneously, may need evaluation for postpartum depression if symptoms persist or are severe (see also Chapter 11)

III. NURSING CARE OF THE POSTPARTAL CLIENT

A. General considerations with postpartal assessment

1. Evaluate prenatal and intrapartal history for risk factors
2. Provide privacy and encourage client to void prior to assessment
3. Position client in bed with head flat for most accurate findings
4. Proceed in a head-to-toe direction
5. Vital signs are more accurate with woman at rest, will determine need or priority for other assessments
   a. Temperature
      1) Above 100.4°F after first 24 hours may indicate an infection
      2) May be elevated initially after delivery related to dehydration
   b. Pulse
      1) Normal range postpartum is 50–80 beats per minute
      2) Report a pulse greater than 100 beats per minute to health care provider
   c. Respirations: normal range is 16–24 breaths per minute
   d. Blood pressure
      1) Assess for orthostatic hypotension
      2) Monitor more closely for hypertension if client has a history of preeclampsia
6. Women who experience operative procedures, cesarean delivery, or tubal ligation have postpartal needs similar to those of women who gave birth vaginally and those of postoperative clients; monitor breath sounds and have client cough and take deep breaths

Practice to Pass

How should standard precautions be followed during a postpartum assessment?

B. Postpartum assessment: mnemonic BUBBLE-HEB aids in remembering components of assessment

1. **B**reasts
   a. Determine if mother is breast- or bottle-feeding
   b. Palpate for engorgement or tenderness
   c. Inspect nipples for redness, cracks, and erectility, if nursing
2. **U**terus (see Figure 10-2)
   a. Gently place nondominant hand on lower uterine segment just above symphysis pubis; dominant hand palpates top of fundus
   b. Determine uterine firmness and position of fundus midline of abdomen; fundus is 5 cm below umbilicus post-delivery and rises to umbilicus in 6–12 hours
   c. Correlate fundal location with expected descent of 1 centimeter from umbilicus each postpartal day
   d. Inspect any abdominal incisions, cesarean delivery, or tubal ligation, for REEDA: redness, edema, ecchymosis, discharge, and approximation of skin edges
3. **B**ladder
   a. Client should void within 6–8 hours after delivery
   b. Assess frequency, burning, or urgency, which could indicate a urinary tract infection

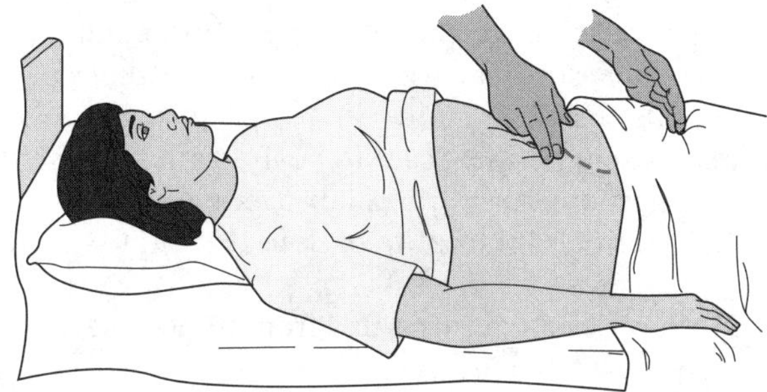

Figure 10-2
Measuring the descent of the fundus

c. Evaluate ability to completely empty bladder

d. Palpate for bladder distention, or use a portable bladder scanner, if unable to void or complete emptying is in question

4. Bowel
   a. Assess for passage of flatus
   b. Inspect for signs of distention
   c. Auscultate bowel sounds in all four quadrants for postoperative clients

Practice to Pass

How should the client be positioned to permit assessment of the perineum?

5. Lochia
   a. Inspect type, quantity, amount, and odor
   b. Correlate findings with expected characteristics of bleeding
   c. Cesarean-delivered women may have less lochia
6. Episiotomy or perineal lacerations
   a. Inspect perineum for REEDA
   b. Inspect for hemorrhoids
7. **Homan's sign**
   a. Pain in calf upon client-initiated movement consistent with dorsiflexion of foot, such as stretching legs or walking; is recorded as a positive sign and may indicate thrombophlebitis
   b. Inspect for pedal edema, redness, or warmth; if abnormal changes are present, assess pedal pulse
8. Emotional status
   a. Assess if client's emotions are appropriate for situation
   b. Determine client's phase of postpartal psychological adjustment
   c. Assess for signs of postpartum blues
9. Bonding: describe how parents interact with infant

C. Priority nursing diagnoses

1. Deficient Fluid Volume
2. Impaired Urinary Elimination
3. Risk for Infection
4. Pain
5. Risk for Constipation
6. Interrupted Family Processes
7. Deficient Knowledge

D. Implementation

1. Prevent hemorrhage
   a. Assess for risk factors
   b. Have client empty bladder frequently
   c. Gently massage fundus, if boggy; teach self-massage of uterus
   d. Administer oxytocic medications, if ordered: oxytocin (Pitocin), methylergonovine maleate (Methergine), ergonovine maleate (Ergotrate)
   e. Monitor for side effects of oxytocics, if administered; hypotension with rapid IV bolus of oxytocin, hypertension with methylergonovine and ergonovine
2. Promote comfort
   a. Apply ice to perineum 20 minutes on/10 minutes off for first 24 hours
   b. Encourage sitz bath, warm or cool, three times per day and prn after first 12–24 hours
   c. Teach client perineal care to be used after every elimination
      1) Squirt or pour warm water over perineum
      2) Blot dry from front to back to prevent tissue trauma and contamination from anal area
      3) Apply clean perineal pad from front to back without touching surface that will be next to client

d. Teach client to tighten buttocks, then sit and relax muscles
e. Apply topical anesthetics (Dermaplast or Americaine spray) or witch hazel compresses (Tucks)
f. Administer analgesics; acetaminophen (Tylenol), non-steroidal anti-inflammatory agents such as ibuprofen (Advil), opioids such as codeine, hydrocodone, or oxycodone (often in a combined tablet with acetaminophen)
g. Utilize patient-controlled analgesia (PCA pump) or morphine epidural if client had cesarean delivery, if appropriate
h. Monitor for side effects of morphine epidural, if administered: late-onset respiratory depression (8–12 hours), nausea and vomiting (4–7 hours), itching (within 3 and up to 10 hours), urinary retention, and drowsiness/sedation

3. Promote bowel elimination
a. Encourage early and frequent ambulation
b. Encourage increased fluids and fiber
c. Administer stool softeners, as ordered; suppositories are contraindicated if client has a third- or fourth-degree perineal laceration involving rectum
d. Teach client to avoid straining; normal bowel pattern returns in two to three weeks

4. Promote urinary elimination
a. Encourage voiding every two to three hours even if no urge is felt
b. Catheterize, as ordered, for urinary retention; indwelling urinary catheter may be placed for 12–24 hours after cesarean delivery

5. Promote successful infant feeding patterns
a. Suppression of lactation and successful bottle-feeding
1) Utilize snug bra or breast binder continuously for five to seven days to prevent engorgement
2) Avoid heat and stimulation of breasts
3) Apply ice packs for 20 minutes four times per day, if engorgement occurs

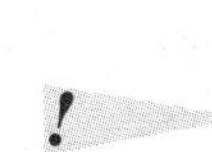

4) Encourage demand feedings every three to four hours, awakening infant during day and allowing to sleep at night
b. Establishment of lactation and successful breastfeeding
1) Utilize a well-fitting bra for continuous support of breasts
2) Teach breast care including avoidance of soap and air drying nipples after feedings

3) Encourage nursing on demand every two to four hours, awakening infant during day and allowing to sleep at night
4) Advise mother to nurse 10 to 15 minutes on first breast and until infant lets go of second; alternate breast used first and rotate positions

5) Suggest football hold or side-lying position with cesarean delivery or tubal ligation to avoid discomfort caused by infant's weight on abdominal incision
6) Provide help with positioning, latching on, and breaking suction when nursing is completed for women who are breastfeeding multiple births
c. Explore impact of culture on feeding practices and support family choices as illustrated in Table 10-3
1) Amount of contact and degree of closeness between mother and newborn is often culturally determined
2) Culture may influence how long breastfeeding continues
3) Feeding practices vary across cultures

6. Promote rest and gradual return to activity
a. Organize nursing care to avoid frequent interruptions
b. Plan maternal rest periods when infant is expected to sleep

Practice to Pass

How would client teaching be modified for a Hmong (Southeast Asian) mother who is breastfeeding twins?

Table 10-3 Cultural Influences on Infant Feeding

Cultural Group	Infant Feeding Practice
North American and European	Exposing the breast is indecent; weaning is a sign of infant development
Hmong (Southeast Asian)	Breast- and bottle-feeding may be combined; expressing or pumping breast milk is unacceptable
Mexican American, Filipino, Navajo, Vietnamese	Colostrum is not offered to the newborn
African American	Plentiful feeding is emphasized; solids are introduced early
Muslim	Breastfeeding is encouraged to 2 years of age

c. Teach woman to resume activity gradually over four to five weeks; avoid lifting, stair-climbing, and strenuous activity
d. Simple postpartal exercises should be started, per orders; encourage client to strengthen muscles affected by childbearing; Kegel exercises tighten perineum by repeatedly attempting to stop flow of urine and then relaxing; raising chin to chest, knee rolls, and buttocks lifts strengthen abdomen
e. Increased lochia or pain indicates overexertion; modify exercise plan

7. Promote adequate nutritional intake
   a. Encourage lactating mothers to add 500 kcal/day to pre-pregnancy diet; bottle-feeding mothers should return to pre-pregnancy diet; diet should be nutrient-dense and balanced for optimal nutrition
   b. Encourage fluid intake of 2000 mL/day
   c. Continue administration of prenatal vitamins and iron, as ordered; iron is best absorbed in presence of vitamin C and may increase constipation
8. Promote psychological well-being
   a. Plan nursing care based on client's phase of psychological adjustment and degree of dependence/independence; provide choices whenever possible
   b. Encourage and support expression of feelings, positive and negative, without guilt
   c. Encourage client to tell story of her labor and birth to integrate expectations and fantasies with reality
   d. Provide recognition and praise for self- and infant-care activities
9. Promote family well-being
   a. Provide an environment that supports family unity and promotes attachment to newborn
   b. Encourage rooming-in, presence of family members
   c. Assist parents in preparing siblings with realistic expectations of newborn, involve siblings in infant care
   d. Teach parents that sibling regression is common
   e. Advise couple to resume sexual activity after episiotomy has healed and lochia has stopped, about three weeks after delivery; level of sexual interest and activity may vary, additional water-soluble lubrication may be needed and breast milk may be released with orgasm
   f. Counsel couples regarding contraception before discharge, assist couple to select a method compatible with health needs and individual preferences; a diaphragm or cervical cap will need to be refitted following delivery; oral contraceptives containing estrogen may interfere with lactation

10. Promote maternal safety
    a. Give Rho (D) gamma globulin (Rhogam, RhIG, Gamulin) if needed to prevent Rh sensitization and future hemolytic disease of newborn (considered safe in breastfeeding mothers under guidance of the health care provider)
        1) Confirm woman is a candidate: Rh-negative mother not sensitized (negative indirect Coombs' test), Rh-positive newborn not sensitized (negative direct Coombs' test), and no known maternal allergy to globulin preparations
        2) Administer 300 micrograms IM within 72 hours of delivery
    b. Give rubella vaccine to provide activity immunity for mother and avoid fetal malformations during a future pregnancy
        1) Confirm woman is a candidate: titer of <1:8 (not immune); no known allergy to neomycin
        2) Administer 0.5 mL subcutaneously prior to discharge
        3) If mother is a candidate for both Rhogam and rubella vaccine, delay rubella vaccine at least six weeks, and preferably three months, to avoid drug interaction and reduced rubella immunity
        4) Teach client to avoid pregnancy for at least three months following vaccination; vaccine contains live virus and can adversely affect fetus; side effects include burning and stinging at injection site, warmth and redness, mild symptoms of disease
    c. Teach client postpartum warning signs to be reported
        1) Bright red bleeding saturating more than one pad/hour or passing large clots
        2) Temperature greater than 100.4°F
        3) Chills
        4) Excessive pain
        5) Reddened or warm areas of breast
        6) Reddened or gaping episiotomy, foul-smelling lochia
        7) Inability to urinate; burning, frequency, or urgency with urination
        8) Calf pain, tenderness, redness, or swelling

E. Evaluation

1. Assessment findings remain normal
2. Maternal physical and psychological well-being is maintained
3. Client verbalizes/demonstrates techniques of self- and infant-care
4. Parents demonstrate positive signs of attachment with their infant

Case Study

A client delivered an infant three hours ago. The nurse assesses the client and finds the following: fundus firm at 1 centimeter below the umbilicus, small amount of lochia rubra, midline episiotomy well approximated. The client states she is "cramping really bad" when she nurses. She has not ambulated since delivery.

1. What else would be important to know about this client?
2. The client states she would like to go to the bathroom. What should the nurse do?
3. The client is unable to void. What should the nurse do next?
4. The client's vital signs are: T 100.8°F, P 56, R 16, BP 110/56. How should the nurse interpret these findings, and what interventions are indicated?
5. What behaviors would the nurse expect to see if this client is bonding positively with her newborn?

For suggested responses, see page 305.

POSTTEST

1 This is the first postoperative day for a client who had a cesarean delivery. The client asks the nurse why she has to get up and walk when it hurts her incision so much. What would the nurse include in a response?

1. Walking decreases the risk of blood clots after surgery.
2. Walking encourages deep breaths to blow off the anesthetic from surgery.
3. Early ambulation is important to stimulate milk production.
4. Walking will decrease the occurrence of afterpains.

2 While assessing the incision of a client two days after cesarean delivery, the nurse notes the skin edges around the incision are red, edematous, and tender to the touch. A scant amount of purulent drainage is noted. What is the most appropriate initial action by the nurse?

1. Cleanse the wound with povidone iodine (Betadine).
2. Notify the physician.
3. Document this expected response.
4. Observe the incision closely for the next 24 to 48 hours.

3 Which interventions should be included when caring for a client with a midline episiotomy with a third-degree laceration? Select all that apply.

1. Increase fiber in diet.
2. Administer bisacodyl (Dulcolax) suppository.
3. Increase fluid intake.
4. Administer an oral stool softener.
5. Administer an enema.

4 The infant of a breastfeeding client was transferred to the neonatal intensive care unit because of respiratory distress. The nurse interprets that follow-up teaching has been effective when the client states which reason to pump the breasts?

1. Prevent breast engorgement
2. Stimulate the milk supply
3. Remove the infected milk
4. Keep the uterus contracted

5 The nurse palpates the uterus of a client immediately after delivery. Where does the nurse expect to feel the fundus?

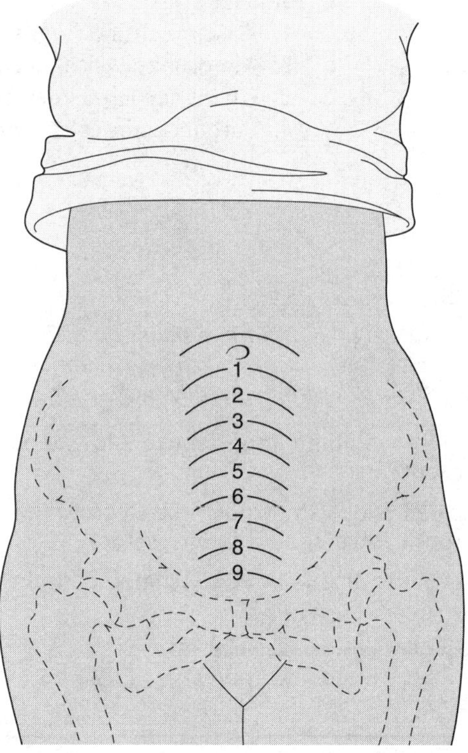

POSTTEST

6 The nurse is assessing a client's fundus and finds it firm, two centimeters above the umbilicus and displaced to the right. What is the most appropriate intervention at this time?

1. Massage the fundus until firm.
2. Have the client void and reassess the fundus.
3. Notify the physician.
4. Start a pad count.

7 A client's prenatal laboratory findings reveal that she is not immune to rubella. The health care provider prescribes rubella vaccine prior to discharge. The nurse concludes that teaching about this medication is effective when the client makes which statement?

1. "I'll need another shot in one month and again in six months."
2. "This shot may cause a fever and make me vomit."
3. "I'll need another shot after each baby I have with Rh-positive blood."
4. "I should not get pregnant for at least three months after the vaccine."

8 A client's vital signs following delivery are: (Day 1) BP 116/72, T 98.6, P 68; (Day 2) BP 114/80, T 100.6, P 76; (Day 3) BP 114/80, T 101.6, P 80. The nurse should suspect which of the following about the client's status?

1. Is dehydrated
2. May have an infection
3. Has normal vital signs
4. Is going into shock

9 The nurse is reviewing infection control policies with a nursing student. The nurse knows that the teaching has been effective when the student states, "The best way to prevent postpartum infection starts

1. in the recovery room with strict use of sterile technique when palpating the fundus."
2. on the postpartum unit by teaching the client the principles of perineal care."
3. by limiting the number of sterile vaginal exams during labor."
4. when the client goes home by avoiding tub baths until the lochia stops."

10 Which assessment should alert the nurse to withhold the scheduled dose of methylergonovine maleate (Methergine) for a postpartum client and notify the health care provider?

1. Blood pressure 142/86
2. Apical pulse 56
3. Blood type O positive
4. Mother is planning to breastfeed

➤ *See pages 213–214 for Answers and Rationales.*

ANSWERS & RATIONALES

Pretest

1 **Answer: 3** **Rationale:** The fundus should remain firm after delivery to decrease the risk of postpartum hemorrhage and decrease one centimeter below the umbilicus each day. All nursing interventions presented are appropriate, but massaging the fundus until firm is the most important to prevent hemorrhage. Full urinary bladders can interfere with uterine contraction. **Cognitive Level:** Applying **Client Need:** Physiological Adaptation **Integrated Process:** Nursing Process: Implementation **Content Area:** Maternal-Newborn **Strategy:** The focus of the question is the priority action to promote maternal safety and prevent hemorrhage related to a boggy uterus. The correct answer would be the option that contains a nursing action to prevent hemorrhage. **Reference:** Ladewig, P. A., London, M. L., & Davidson, M. R. (2010). *Contemporary maternal-newborn nursing care* (7th ed.). Upper Saddle River, NJ: Pearson Education, p. 801.

2 **Answer: 1** **Rationale:** Afterpains are anticipated in the postpartum client and are effectively treated with analgesics. It is unnecessary to stop breastfeeding, empty the bladder, or assess vital signs. **Cognitive Level:** Applying **Client Need:** Physiological Adaptation **Integrated Process:** Nursing Process: Implementation **Content Area:** Maternal-Newborn **Strategy:** The focus of the question is afterpains, a common occurrence that can increase pain. The correct answer would be the option that contains a nursing action to effectively manage pain. **Reference:** Ladewig, P. A., London, M. L., & Davidson, M. R. (2010). *Contemporary maternal-newborn nursing care* (7th ed.). Upper Saddle River, NJ: Pearson Education, p. 807.

3 **Answer: 4** **Rationale:** This client should be encouraged to verbalize her disappointment as the first step in resolving her negative feelings. The other responses are incorrect. This is not a normal response nor is it one that requires a psychiatric referral. **Cognitive Level:** Applying **Client Need:** Psychosocial Integrity **Integrated Process:** Nursing Process: Implementation **Content Area:** Maternal-Newborn

Strategy: Recognize that the data given in the question may be related to disappointment with the sex of the infant. The best response would be the option that facilitates therapeutic communication to encourage the client to express her feelings. **Reference:** Ladewig, P. A., London, M. L., & Davidson, M. R. (2010). *Contemporary maternal-newborn nursing care* (7th ed.). Upper Saddle River, NJ: Pearson Education, p. 808.

4 **Answer: 3, 5 Rationale:** Having sexual intercourse before the episiotomy is healed or the lochia has stopped increases the risk of infection. Water-soluble lubricants can be used, if necessary. An IUD is contraindicated during the early postpartum period. **Cognitive Level:** Applying **Client Need:** Health Promotion and Maintenance **Integrated Process:** Teaching and Learning **Content Area:** Maternal-Newborn **Strategy:** Use the process of elimination and look for statements that are true. Knowledge of client teaching for resumption of sexual activity after delivery will help to answer the question correctly. **Reference:** Ladewig, P. A., London, M. L., & Davidson, M. R. (2010). *Contemporary maternal-newborn nursing care* (7th ed.). Upper Saddle River, NJ: Pearson Education, pp. 803–804.

5 **Answer: 3, 5 Rationale:** Binding the breasts, either with a snug bra or binder, and applying cold to the breasts will help suppress lactation. Milk supply is stimulated by expressing milk and applying heat to the breasts. Medications to suppress lactation are not recommended. **Cognitive Level:** Applying **Client Need:** Health Promotion and Maintenance **Integrated Process:** Teaching and Learning **Content Area:** Maternal-Newborn **Strategy:** Knowledge of the ways to suppress lactation in the nonbreastfeeding mother will help to answer the question correctly. The correct answers are options that include a true statement about a point of client education. **Reference:** Ladewig, P. A., London, M. L., & Davidson, M. R. (2010). *Contemporary maternal-newborn nursing care* (7th ed.). Upper Saddle River, NJ: Pearson Education, pp. 816, 839–840.

6 **Answer: 1 Rationale:** Temperature elevation immediately after delivery is often caused by dehydration during labor. Increasing the client's fluid intake will usually decrease the temperature to within normal limits. There is no indication for analgesia or antibiotics at this time. If the fever persists beyond 24 hours or the client has clinical signs of infection, then further investigation and perhaps treatment is warranted. **Cognitive Level:** Applying **Client Need:** Physiological Adaptation **Integrated Process:** Nursing Process: Implementation **Content Area:** Maternal-Newborn **Strategy:** Recognize that the focus of the question is dehydration fever after delivery. The correct answer would be the option that contains a nursing action to correct this minor and typically temporary finding. **Reference:** Ladewig, P. A., London, M. L., & Davidson, M. R. (2010). *Contemporary maternal-newborn nursing care* (7th ed.). Upper Saddle River, NJ: Pearson Education, pp. 811–816.

ANSWERS & RATIONALES

7 **Answer: 1 Rationale:** Clients are at risk for orthostatic hypotension, especially right after delivery. The nurse should stay with the client the first time she ambulates after delivery to promote safety. Early ambulation prevents circulatory stasis in the lower extremities and should be encouraged. The perineum should be patted (not wiped) dry from front to back to avoid trauma, discomfort, and contamination with bacteria from the anal region. It is unnecessary to use a bedpan. **Cognitive Level:** Analyzing **Client Need:** Physiological Adaptation **Integrated Process:** Nursing Process: Implementation **Content Area:** Maternal-Newborn **Strategy:** The most therapeutic response would be the option that promotes client safety in the immediate postpartal period. Eliminate options that contain false statements as points of client education. Eliminate another as early ambulation is encouraged, not bedrest, to prevent circulatory stasis. **Reference:** Ladewig, P. A., London, M. L., & Davidson, M. R. (2010). *Contemporary maternal-newborn nursing care* (7th ed.). Upper Saddle River, NJ: Pearson Education, pp. 830–831.

8 **Answer: 1 Rationale:** A client with a hemoglobin of 7.2 grams/dL would most likely have significant signs and symptoms of anemia, and this could be life-threatening. It would be important to determine if the client had a large estimated blood loss during delivery or if she is currently bleeding excessively. The hematocrit is within normal limits, and mild proteinuria or leukocytosis up to 30,000/mm^3 are common in early postpartum. **Cognitive Level:** Analyzing **Client Need:** Reduction of Risk Potential **Integrated Process:** Nursing Process: Assessment **Content Area:** Maternal-Newborn **Strategy:** The focus of the question is an abnormal laboratory finding warranting further investigation. Eliminate the option that presents normal data. Eliminate two others because they contain data commonly found in the postpartum. **Reference:** Ladewig, P. A., London, M. L., & Davidson, M. R. (2010). *Contemporary maternal-newborn nursing care* (7th ed.). Upper Saddle River, NJ: Pearson Education, pp. 805–806.

9 **Answer: 1, 2, 4, 5 Rationale:** Among the factors contributing to uterine subinvolution are prolonged labor (frequent contractions), general anesthesia (muscle relaxant), overdistended urinary bladder and uterine infection, among others. Being a primigravida is not necessarily associated with subinvolution. **Cognitive Level:** Analyzing **Client Need:** Physiological Adaptation **Integrated Process:** Nursing Process: Implementation **Content Area:** Maternal-Newborn **Strategy:** The wording of the question indicates that more than one option is correct. Recall common factors that contribute to retarded uterine involution to choose correctly. **Reference:** Ladewig, P. A., London, M. L., & Davidson, M. R. (2010). *Contemporary maternal-newborn nursing care* (7th ed.). Upper Saddle River, NJ: Pearson Education, p. 801.

10 **Answer: 2 Rationale:** Nursing assessment of the perineum includes the following observations, which are abbreviated

as REEDA: redness, edema, ecchymosis, discharge, and approximation. **Cognitive Level:** Analyzing **Client Need:** Physiological Adaptation **Integrated Process:** Nursing Process: Diagnosis **Content Area:** Maternal-Newborn **Strategy:** Critical words are *episiotomy* and *evaluation of perineum*. Recall the mnemonic for perineal assessment to choose correctly. **Reference:** Ladewig, P. A., London, M. L., & Davidson, M. R. (2010). *Contemporary maternal-newborn nursing care* (7th ed.). Upper Saddle River, NJ: Pearson Education, p. 820.

Posttest

1. **Answer: 1 Rationale:** Clients who have had a cesarean delivery are at risk for complications of surgery, including thrombophlebitis. Early ambulation can significantly decrease the risk of blood clots and other postoperative complications. **Cognitive Level:** Applying **Client Need:** Reduction of Risk Potential **Integrated Process:** Nursing Process: Implementation **Content Area:** Maternal-Newborn **Strategy:** The positive wording of the question indicates that the correct answer is also a true statement. Use knowledge of the factors associated with increased risk of thromboembolic disease such as cesarean section and immobility to answer the question. **Reference:** Ladewig, P. A., London, M. L., & Davidson, M. R. (2010). *Contemporary maternal-newborn nursing care* (7th ed.). Upper Saddle River, NJ: Pearson Education, pp. 846–848.

2. **Answer: 2 Rationale:** This client has signs of an incisional infection. The physician needs to be notified first so that treatment can be started as soon as possible. Betadine has not yet been ordered. Documentation should follow reporting. Continued observation would be an ongoing intervention. **Cognitive Level:** Analyzing **Client Need:** Physiological Adaptation **Integrated Process:** Nursing Process: Implementation **Content Area:** Maternal-Newborn **Strategy:** The focus of this question is the collection of assessment data indicating a change in the client's condition: development of infection. The correct answer would be the option that best provides for the safety of the client, reporting the abnormal findings so treatment can be instituted. **Reference:** Ladewig, P. A., London, M. L., & Davidson, M. R. (2010). *Contemporary maternal-newborn nursing care* (7th ed.). Upper Saddle River, NJ: Pearson Education, p. 848.

3. **Answer: 1, 3, 4 Rationale:** A third- or fourth-degree perineal laceration involves the rectal sphincter, therefore suppositories, enemas, and rectal exams are contraindicated until the rectum heals. Increased fiber and fluids or use of stool softeners are appropriate to promote bowel elimination in all postpartum clients. **Cognitive Level:** Applying **Client Need:** Physiological Adaptation **Integrated Process:** Nursing Process: Implementation **Content Area:** Maternal-Newborn **Strategy:** The wording of the question indicates that more than one option is correct Use knowledge of interventions and contraindications for a third- or fourth-degree laceration to make your selections. **Reference:** Ladewig, P. A., London, M. L., & Davidson, M. R. (2010). *Contemporary maternal-newborn nursing care* (7th ed.). Upper Saddle River, NJ: Pearson Education, pp. 820–823.

4. **Answer: 2 Rationale:** Breast-milk production is based on supply and demand. The more the breasts are stimulated to produce milk, by nursing the baby or pumping the breasts, the more milk will be produced. **Cognitive Level:** Analyzing **Client Need:** Health Promotion and Maintenance **Integrated Process:** Nursing Process: Evaluation **Content Area:** Maternal-Newborn **Strategy:** The critical word in the stem of the question is *effective*, which tells you the correct option is also a true statement. Use knowledge of breastfeeding and how to stimulate milk production to aid your selection. **Reference:** Ladewig, P. A., London, M. L., & Davidson, M. R. (2010). *Contemporary maternal-newborn nursing care* (7th ed.). Upper Saddle River, NJ: Pearson Education, pp. 712–713.

5. **Answer:**

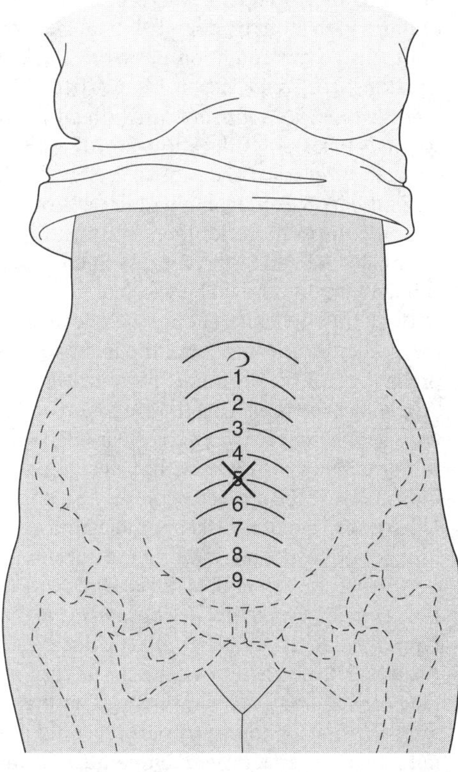

Rationale: Immediately after expulsion of the placenta, the uterus is firmly contracted, about the size of a grapefruit. The fundus is located in the midline of the abdomen and halfway between the symphysis pubis and umbilicus. Within 6–12 hours after delivery, the fundus rises to a level of the umbilicus. The top of the fundus then descends the width of a fingerbreadth each day until it descends into the pelvis by about two weeks, when it is no longer palpable. **Cognitive Level:** Applying **Client Need:** Physiological Adaptation **Integrated Process:** Nursing Process: Implementation **Content Area:** Maternal-Newborn

Strategy: Recall the physiologic process of uterine involution and the changes in fundal position after delivery. **Reference:** Ladewig, P. A., London, M. L., & Davidson, M. R. (2010). *Contemporary maternal-newborn nursing care* (7th ed.). Upper Saddle River, NJ: Pearson Education, pp. 816–818.

6 **Answer: 2** **Rationale:** This client's fundus is already firm, so it is not appropriate to massage the fundus. It is also higher in the abdomen than expected, and it is displaced to the right, which is probably caused by a distended bladder. Having the client void may return the uterus to the expected position; palpating the fundus after voiding will confirm this finding. A pad count would be appropriate if bleeding is increasing; no information given implies that this action is indicated. **Cognitive Level:** Applying **Client Need:** Physiological Adaptation **Integrated Process:** Nursing Process: Implementation **Content Area:** Maternal-Newborn **Strategy:** The critical words in the question are *firm* but *displaced* uterine fundus, common findings with a full bladder. Eliminate options that do not focus on this condition. **Reference:** Ladewig, P. A., London, M. L., & Davidson, M. R. (2010). *Contemporary maternal-newborn nursing care* (7th ed.). Upper Saddle River, NJ: Pearson Education, pp. 817–818.

7 **Answer: 4** **Rationale:** The rubella vaccine is a live virus. If a client becomes pregnant within the first three months after administration, her fetus is at risk for congenital anomalies related to the virus. Women who are not rubella immune should be vaccinated postpartum, prior to discharge. Teaching should include an effective method of birth control and the importance of avoiding pregnancy for the next three months. **Cognitive Level:** Applying **Client Need:** Health Promotion and Maintenance **Integrated Process:** Teaching and Learning **Content Area:** Maternal-Newborn **Strategy:** The wording of the question indicates that the correct answer is also a true statement. Use knowledge of rubella immunizations in the postpartum period to aid in answering the question. **Reference:** Ladewig, P. A., London, M. L., & Davidson, M. R. (2010). *Contemporary maternal-newborn nursing care* (7th ed.). Upper Saddle River, NJ: Pearson Education, p. 839.

8 **Answer: 2** **Rationale:** The vital signs are not normal. An elevation in body temperature greater than 100.4°F after the first 24 hours postpartum could indicate maternal infection. An elevated temperature within the first 24 hours is usually related to dehydration, although the possibility of infection still exists. Rising pulse and falling blood pressure rather than rising temperature is an indicator of hypovolemic shock. **Cognitive Level:** Analyzing **Client Need:** Physiological Adaptation **Integrated Process:** Nursing Process: Diagnosis **Content Area:** Maternal-Newborn **Strategy:** The assessment data includes an abnormal and increasing temperature, a sign of infection. Eliminate options that suggest other complications. **Reference:** Ladewig, P. A., London, M. L., & Davidson, M. R. (2010). *Contemporary maternal-newborn nursing care* (7th ed.). Upper Saddle River, NJ: Pearson Education, pp. 830–832.

9 **Answer: 3** **Rationale:** Even when perfect sterile technique is used when doing a vaginal exam, organisms present on the perineum are transported into the vagina and close to the cervix. By limiting the number of vaginal exams, the risk is decreased. The option discussing technique is incorrect because clean technique, not sterile technique, is used when palpating the fundus. Teaching the client the principles of perineal care and avoiding tub baths until the lochia stops are correct answers, but not the earliest intervention a nurse could perform. **Cognitive Level:** Applying **Client Need:** Safety and Infection Control **Integrated Process:** Nursing Process: Evaluation **Content Area:** Maternal-Newborn **Strategy:** Critical words are *best way to prevent postpartum infection*. Knowledge of medical and surgical asepsis and preventing postpartum complications will aid in choosing the correct answer. **Reference:** Ladewig, P. A., London, M. L., & Davidson, M. R. (2010). *Contemporary maternal-newborn nursing care* (7th ed.). Upper Saddle River, NJ: Pearson Education, pp. 431–435.

10 **Answer: 1** **Rationale:** A potential side effect of Methergine is hypertension. If a client's blood pressure is elevated, the nurse should withhold the scheduled dose and notify the physician. An apical heart rate of 56 is within normal limits postpartum. Blood type and Rh factor are not related to the use of Methergine. The chosen method of feeding method is not impacted by the use of Methergine. **Cognitive Level:** Analyzing **Client Need:** Pharmacological and Parenteral Therapies **Integrated Process:** Nursing Process: Implementation **Content Area:** Maternal-Newborn **Strategy:** The focus of the question is an adverse effect of Methergine, an oxytocic drug. The correct answer is the option that contains a true statement about a side effect. Eliminate incorrect options because they include normal findings or data not related to Methergine use. **Reference:** Ladewig, P. A., London, M. L., & Davidson, M. R. (2010). *Contemporary maternal-newborn nursing care* (7th ed.). Upper Saddle River, NJ: Pearson Education, p. 834.

References

Davidson, M., London, M., & Ladewig, P. (2012). *Olds' maternal newborn nursing & women's health across the lifespan* (9th ed.). Upper Saddle River, NJ: Pearson Education.

Ladewig, P., London, M., & Davidson, M. (2009). *Contemporary maternal-newborn nursing care* (7th ed.). Upper Saddle River, NJ: Pearson Education.

Perry, S.E., Hockenberry, M.J., Lowdermilk, D.L., & Wilson, D. (2010). *Maternal child nursing care* (4th ed.). St. Louis, MO: Mosby.

Ricci, S. (2009). *Essentials of maternity, newborn, and women's health nursing* (2nd ed.). Philadelphia: Lippincott Williams & Wilkins.

The Complicated Postpartal Experience 11

Chapter Outline

Objectives

- Describe nursing assessments that identify the high-risk postpartal client.
- Discuss nursing interventions for the client with postpartal complications related to hemorrhage.
- Describe the nursing care of a client experiencing a puerperal infection.
- Identify the symptoms and management of thromboembolic disorders.
- List the symptoms exhibited in a client experiencing a postpartal psychiatric disorder.

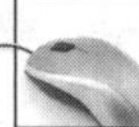

NCLEX-RN® Test Prep

Use the accompanying online resource, NursingReviewsandRationales, to test yourself with hundreds of NCLEX®-style practice questions.

Review at a Glance

disseminated intravascular coagulopathy a pathological form of coagulation that is diffuse rather than localized; several clotting factors are consumed to such extent that generalized bleeding may occur

early-postpartal hemorrhage a loss of blood greater than 500 mL within first 24 hours following birth

endometritis (metritis) infection of endometrium

hematoma a collection of blood resulting from injury to a blood vessel

late-postpartal hemorrhage a loss of blood greater than 500 mL after first 24 hours following birth

mastitis inflammation of breast connective tissue

pelvic cellulitis (parametritis) inflammation involving connective tissue of broad ligament or all pelvic tissue

peritonitis inflammation of peritoneum

postpartal psychiatric disorders according to *DSM-IV-TR*, it is one diagnosable syndrome with three subclasses: adjustment reaction with depressed mood, postpartum major mood disorder, and postpartum psychosis

postpartal (puerperal) infection an infection of reproductive tract within 6-week postpartum period

subinvolution failure of uterus to return to its normal size after pregnancy

thrombophlebitis inflammation of a vein wall resulting in a thrombus

urinary tract infection an infection in urinary tract; cystitis affects lower urinary tract including bladder and urethra; pyelonephritis affects upper urinary tract including ureters and kidneys

uterine atony relaxation of uterine muscle following birth

PRETEST

1 The client is a 36-year-old woman, gravida 6 and para 6, who delivered a 7 pound, 14 ounce baby girl at term after an eight-hour labor. The client's vital signs are stable, and her lochia is bright red, heavy, and contains various clots; some are half dollar size. The nurse would consider the client to be at high risk for uterine atony for which reason?

1. Grandmultiparity
2. Large for gestational age baby
3. Labor of long duration
4. Advancing maternal age

2 Despite the nurse's attempt to massage a boggy fundus, a postpartum client continues to pass several large clots in the presence of bright red lochia. The uterine fundus remains boggy and fundal massage and oxytocin (Pitocin) are not successful. What medication does the nurse expected to be prescribed next?

1. Dinoprostone (Cervidil)
2. Terbutaline sulfate (Brethine)
3. Magnesium sulfate
4. Carboprost (Prostin 15-M or Hemabate)

3 A new mother with mastitis is concerned about breastfeeding while she has an active infection. How should the nurse respond to the client's concern?

1. The infant is protected from infection by immunoglobulins in the breast milk.
2. The infant is not susceptible to the organisms that cause mastitis.
3. The organisms that cause mastitis are not passed in the milk.
4. The organisms will be inactivated by gastric acid.

4 If the nurse suspects a uterine infection in the postpartum client, the nurse should make which priority assessment?

1. Pulse and blood pressure
2. Odor of the lochia
3. Episiotomy site
4. The abdomen for distention

5 A postpartum client develops a temperature during her postpartum course. Which temperature measurement indicates to the nurse the presence of postpartum infection?

1. 99.0°F at 12 hours postdelivery that decreases after 18 hours
2. 100.2°F at 24 hours postdelivery that decreases the second postpartum day
3. 100.4°F at 24 hours postdelivery that remains until the second postpartum day
4. 100.6°F at 48 hours postdelivery that continues into the third postpartum day

6 Which sign of thrombophlebitis should the nurse instruct the postpartal client to look for when at home after discharge from the hospital?

1. Muscle soreness in her legs after exercise
2. Enlarging varicose veins in her legs
3. Localized posterior leg tenderness, heat, and swelling
4. New areas of ecchymosis

7 Which instruction should the nurse include in the discharge teaching plan to assist the postpartal client to recognize early signs of complications?

1. Expect to pass clots, which occasionally can be the size of a golf ball.
2. Report a decrease in the amount of brownish-red lochia.
3. Palpate the fundus daily to make sure it is soft.
4. Notify the health care provider of increased lochia or bright red bleeding.

8 A client delivered a 9 pound, 10 ounce infant assisted by forceps. When the nurse performs the second 15-minute assessment, the client reports increasing perineal pain and a lot of pressure. What action should the nurse take?

1. Apply ice to the client's perineum, reassuring the client that this is normal.
2. Call for assistance from another nurse.
3. Assess the fundus for firmness.
4. Check the perineum for a hematoma.

9 On the client's third postpartum day, the nurse enters the room and finds the client crying. The client states that she does not know why she is crying and she cannot stop. What is the most appropriate reply by the nurse?

1. "There is no need to cry, you have a healthy baby."
2. "Are you dissatisfied with your care? I will see that any issues are addressed."
3. "Many new mothers have shared with us their same confusion of feelings, would you like to talk about them?"
4. "This happens to lots of mothers, and be reassured that it will pass with time."

10 Because postpartum depression occurs in 3 to 30% of postpartal women, the prenatal nurse assesses clients for risk factors for postpartum depression during the prenatal period. Which clients would the nurse consider to be at risk for postpartum depression? Select all that apply.

1. A client who is an unmarried primipara with family support
2. A client who has previously had postpartum blues
3. A client who is a primipara with documented ambivalence about her pregnancy in the first trimester
4. A client who is a primipara with a history of depression and lack of a supportive relationship
5. A client who is a primipara living alone and was consistently ambivalent about pregnancy

➤ *See pages 232–233 for Answers and Rationales.*

I. NURSING CARE OF THE HIGH-RISK POSTPARTAL CLIENT

A. Assessment

1. Degree of homeostasis: amount of intrapartum blood loss, hematocrit, hemoglobin, and CBC results
2. Vital signs: elevated temperature, blood pressure, heart rate; low blood pressure, symptoms of shock
3. Fundus: height, tone, and position
4. ! Lochia: amount, color, consistency, odor, and presence/size of clots (greater than quarter-size of concern)
5. Perineum: edema, ecchymosis, pain, hemorrhoids
6. Bladder: distention and displacement, ability to void
7. Bowel: constipation, distended abdomen, decreased or no bowel sounds (risk of ileus)
8. Breasts: cracked, bleeding, or blistered nipples; engorgement, red streaks, lumps, clogged milk ducts
9. Homan's sign, redness, tenderness, areas of heat in calves; severe abdominal or flank pain
10. Rest, activity tolerance
11. Bonding or attachment behaviors, maternal–infant interaction

B. Priority nursing diagnoses

1. Physiological Integrity: Interrupted Breastfeeding, Deficient Fluid Volume, Impaired Gas Exchange, Fatigue, Pain (perineal), Ineffective Thermoregulation, Ineffective Tissue Perfusion (if blood clot)
2. Safe and Effective Care: Risk for Injury, Risk for Infection, Deficient Knowledge

3. Psychosocial Integrity: Fear, Disturbed Body Image, Ineffective Coping, Impaired Adjustment, Risk for Impaired Parent–Infant Attachment
4. Health Promotion/Maintenance: Deficient Self-Care, Interrupted Family Processes

C. **Planning**

1. Develop a nursing care plan that reflects knowledge of etiology, pathophysiology, and current clinical management for woman experiencing a postpartal complication
2. Goal of nursing care is that client will be free from undetected problems and will maintain physiological and psychosocial integrity

Practice to Pass

You have received a client on the postpartum unit who delivered a large-for-gestational-age infant via low-outlet forceps. What types of problems would you anticipate this client might experience?

D. **Implementation**

1. Teach client normal adaptation
2. Observe for actual or potential problems in immediate postpartal period (first two hours after delivery) and continue into later postpartal period
3. Administer treatment or medication as ordered
4. Educate client about signs of complications prior to discharge
5. Reinforce importance of keeping appointment for postpartal checkup
6. Provide client with telephone numbers that can be used to ask questions

E. **Evaluation**

1. Abnormal findings are identified early
2. Treatment is effective
3. Client is confident in ability to monitor self and access necessary follow-up care upon discharge from hospital

II. POSTPARTAL HEMORRHAGE

! A. ***Early-postpartal hemorrhage***

1. Definition: a blood loss greater than 500 mL in first 24 hours after vaginal delivery or greater than 1000 mL with cesarean delivery; a 10-point drop in hematocrit from admission to postpartum, or requiring need to transfuse following childbirth
2. Predisposing factors: early postpartal hemorrhage occurs within first 24 hours of birth; at term, 600 mL/minute of blood perfuses pregnant uterus; most common causes of postpartal hemorrhage are uterine atony and lacerations

! a. **Uterine atony**

1) Description: lack of uterine muscle tone; normal mechanism for hemostasis after birth of placenta is contraction of interlacing uterine muscles to occlude open areas at site of placental attachment; over 75% of all postpartal hemorrhages are caused by uterine atony; absence of uterine contraction can cause significant blood loss

2) Predisposing factors

a) Conditions that overdistend uterus: delivery of a large infant, multiple gestation, and hydramnios/polyhydramnios

b) Conditions that affect uterine contractility: multiparity, precipitous labor, dysfunctional or prolonged labor, prolonged third stage of labor, and retained placental fragments

c) Medication use: general anesthesia, magnesium sulfate ($MgSO_4$), oxytocin induction or augmentation of labor, and tocolytics

d) Low platelet count secondary to HELLP syndrome of preeclampsia

! b. Lacerations

1) Description: more common after operative obstetrics, a firm uterus with bright red blood or a steady stream or trickle of unclotted blood

2) Types/locations: perineal, vaginal, and cervical

3) Predisposing factors: primiparous state, epidural anesthesia, precipitous childbirth, macrosomia, forceps or vacuum-assisted birth, and mediolateral episiotomy

c. **Hematoma**
   1) Description: a collection of blood, often vulvar or vaginal (Figure 11-1), that occurs because of injury to a blood vessel during spontaneous delivery; in an assisted vaginal delivery, most common site is lateral wall in area of ischial spine
   2) Predisposing factors: prolonged pressure of fetal head on vaginal mucosa, operative delivery (forceps or vacuum extraction), prolonged second stage of labor, precipitous labor, macrosomia, and pudendal anesthesia

d. **Disseminated intravascular coagulopathy** (DIC)
   1) Description: complex disorder caused by overstimulation of clotting and anticlotting mechanisms; leads to overwhelming and diffuse hemorrhage; oozing from puncture sites or development of petechiae may be initial clues of coagulopathy
   2) Predisposing factors: preeclampsia or eclampsia, amniotic fluid embolism, sepsis, abruptio placentae, prolonged intrauterine fetal demise, and excessive blood loss

e. Other causes of early postpartal hemorrhage: uterine rupture or uterine inversion, retained fetal and or placental fragments

B. ***Late-postpartal hemorrhage***
   1. **Subinvolution**: failure of uterus to return to normal size after pregnancy; late-postpartal hemorrhage occurs most often within one to two weeks after childbirth because of retained placental tissue
   2. Blood loss at this time may be excessive but usually poses less risk than immediate postpartal hemorrhage
      a. Lochia often fails to progress from rubra to serosa to alba normally
      b. Lochia rubra that exists longer than two weeks is suggestive of subinvolution
   3. Subinvolution is most commonly diagnosed at postpartal exam at four to six weeks

C. **Nursing assessment**
   1. Assess client's history and labor and delivery record for factors that might predispose client to postpartal hemorrhage
   2. Assess vaginal bleeding after delivery every 15 minutes for one hour, then every 30 minutes for one hour or until stable; more frequent assessments may be necessary depending upon client's condition
      a. Bleeding may be slow and continuous or rapid and profuse
      b. Blood may escape from the vagina or pool in uterus and vagina, becoming evident as clots
      c. Bleeding from a laceration occurs in presence of a firm uterus

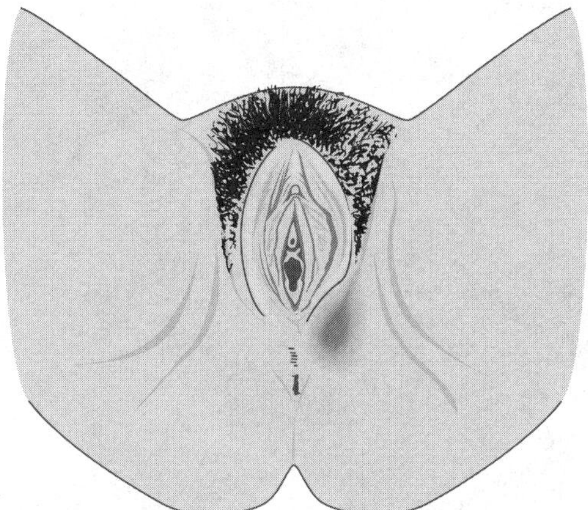

Figure 11-1
Postpartum vulvar hematoma

d. Large and numerous clots may occur

! e. Assist client to a side-lying position and check pad underneath frequently; blood may accumulate under client

f. Weigh peri-pads to estimate blood loss if careful measurement is deemed necessary

3. Palpate fundus for firmness, assess for height in relation to umbilicus and position
4. Assess for signs of shock
5. Assess bladder for fullness and distention
6. Assess for pelvic pain or backache

D. **Priority nursing diagnoses**: Deficient Fluid Volume, Decreased Cardiac Output, Ineffective Tissue Perfusion: Peripheral, Fear

E. **Planning/goal setting**: client will be free from undetected hemorrhage and shock, will have blood volume restored, and will regain homeostasis

F. **Implementation**

1. Remain with client
2. ! Massage boggy uterus gently but firmly, cupping uterus between two hands and avoiding over-massage (see Figure 11-2)
3. ! Administer uterine stimulants as prescribed by health care provider; see Table 11-1 for commonly prescribed uterine stimulants used to prevent and manage uterine atony and hemorrhage
4. If bleeding is excessive, health care provider may elect to perform a bimanual massage
5. ! Monitor vital signs, intake and output, level of consciousness, fundal tone and placement, and amount of bleeding during episode of acute hemorrhage
6. ! Elevate legs 15 to 30 degrees

Figure 11-2

Uterine palpation and massage

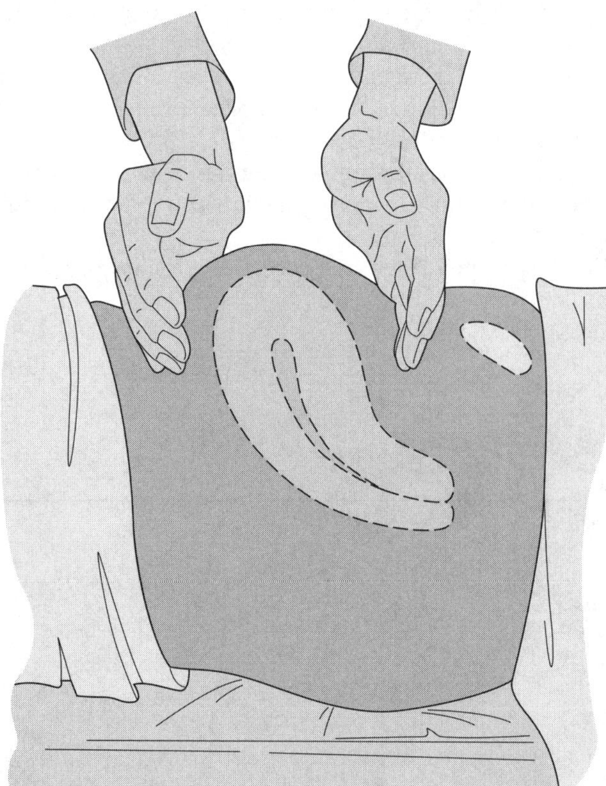

Table 11-1 Uterine Stimulants Used to Prevent and Manage Uterine Atony

Drug	Dosing Information	Contraindications	Expected Effects	Side Effects
Oxytocin (Pitocin, Syntocinon)	IV use: 10–40 units in 500–1000 mL crystalloid fluid @ 50 mU/min administration rate. Onset: immediate. Duration: 1 h. **IV bolus administration not recommended.** IM use: 10 units. Onset: 3–5 min. Duration: 2–3 h.	None for use in postpartum hemorrhage. Avoid undiluted rapid IV infusion, which causes hypotension.	Rhythmic uterine contractions that help to prevent or reverse postpartal hemorrhage caused by uterine atony.	Uterine hyperstimulation, mild transient hypertension, water intoxication rare in postpartum use.
Methylergonovine Maleate (Methergine)	IM use: 0.2 mg q2–4h (5 dose maximum). Onset: 2–5 min. Duration: 3 h. PO use: 0.2 mg q4h (for 6 doses). Onset: 7–15 min. Duration: 3 h (for 1 week). **IV administration not recommended (can cause dangerous hypertension and stroke).**	Women with labile or high blood pressure or known sensitivity to drug, cardiac disease, and Raynaud's disease. Use with caution during lactation.	Sustained uterine contractions that help to prevent or reverse postpartal hemorrhage caused by uterine atony; management of postpartal subinvolution.	Hypertension, dizziness, headache, flushing/hot flashes, tinnitus, nausea and vomiting, palpitations, chest pain. Overdose or hypersensitivity is recognized by seizures; tingling and numbness of fingers and toes.
Prostaglandin (PGF_{2a}, Carboprost tromethamine [Hemabate], Prostin/15M)	IM use: 0.25 mg repeated q15–90 min up to 8 doses maximum. Physician may elect to administer by direct intramyometrial injection.	Women with active cardiovascular, renal, liver disease, or asthma or with known hypersensitivity to drug.	Control of refractory cases of postpartal hemorrhage caused by uterine atony; generally used after failed attempts at control of hemorrhage with oxytocic agents.	N/V, diarrhea, headache, flushing, bradycardia, bronchospasm, wheezing, cough, chills, fever.
Dinoprostone Prostin E2	Vaginal or rectal suppository 20 mcg q2h. Stored in frozen form—must be thawed to room temperature.	Avoid if woman is hypotensive, or has asthma or acute inflammatory disease.	Stimulate uterine contractions.	Fever is common and occurs within 15–45 min of insertion; bleeding, abdominal cramps, N/V.
Misoprostol (Cytotec)	800–1000 mcg rectally. Rapid effects, contractions within minutes.	History of allergy to prostaglandins.	Used to prevent and treat uterine atony after failed attempts to control bleeding with oxytocics.	Diarrhea, abdominal pain, headache.

Source: Davidson, Michele; London, Marcia L.; Ladewig, Patricia W., *Olds' maternal-newborn nursing & women's health across the lifespan*, 9th Ed., ©2012. Reprinted and Electronically reproduced by permission of Pearson Education, Inc., Upper Saddle River, New Jersey.

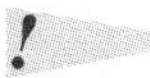

7. Encourage frequent voiding to prevent bladder distention that contributes to uterine atony; an indwelling urinary catheter may need to be inserted or a bed pan may be used during postpartal hemorrhage
8. Replace fluids and administer blood products as ordered
9. Assist with preoperative preparation if needed for surgical removal of placental fragments, ligation of a bleeding vessel, or suturing of a laceration
10. Ensure that surgical consent form is signed, if necessary
11. Support significant other

Practice to Pass

A postpartal client is going home from the hospital. What symptoms of subinvolution will you include in your discharge teaching?

G. Evaluation

1. Client is free from excessive blood loss
2. Lochia is red, moderate in amount, and without clots greater than size of a quarter
3. Fundus is firm, midline, and at level of umbilicus or below
4. Client regains homeostasis according to lab results (hemoglobin and hematocrit)
5. Vital signs are normal
6. Intake and output is adequate
7. Client has positive support during postpartum recovery
8. Client's family is informed of client's status and progress

III. POSTPARTAL (PUERPERAL) INFECTIONS

A. Reproductive tract infections (Table 11-2)

1. Definition: a postpartal (puerperal) infection is any infection in reproductive system within six weeks of delivery
2. Predisposing factors
   a. Cesarean delivery is single most significant risk
   b. Others include anemia, prolonged rupture of membranes, soft tissue trauma or hemorrhage, invasive procedures including use of internal fetal monitoring, multiple vaginal examinations, retention of placental fragments, chorioamnionitis, preexisting bacterial vaginosis, manual removal of placenta, lapses in aseptic technique by staff, use of forceps or vacuum-extraction, diabetic mother, and obesity
3. Types of infection
   a. Localized lesions of perineum, vulva, and vagina

!

      1) Classic signs are pain, redness, warmth, edema, and purulent drainage
      2) Local infection may extend through venous circulation resulting in infectious thrombophlebitis or septicemia
      3) Local infection may extend through lymphatic vessels of uterine wall resulting in the following:
         a) **Pelvic cellulitis (parametritis)**: infection involving connective tissue of broad ligament or connective tissue of all pelvic structures
         b) **Peritonitis**: infection involving peritoneal cavity

Table 11-2 Common Postpartal Infections

Type of Infection	Description	Assessment Findings
Metritis (also called endometritis); extension to parametritis (pelvic cellulitis) possible	Involves endometrium, decidua and uterine myometrium	Temp. usually 101–102°F (38.3–38.9°C); can reach 104°F (40°C) Uterine tenderness on palpation or bimanual exam Subinvolution of uterus Grimacing, guarding, and reports of pain Excessive after pains Positive bacterial culture of lochia
Parametritis (pelvic cellulitis)	Involves connective tissue of broad ligament or of all pelvic structures	Temp. as high as 102–104°F (38.9–40°C) Subinvolution of uterus Abdominal pain extending laterally with possible rebound tenderness
General wound infections	Result from surgical incisions, episiotomy, and lacerations from the birth process	Fever, redness, tenderness, warmth at site, edema, purulent drainage
Urinary tract infection	Result usually from *E-coli* contamination: frequent vaginal exams during labor, urinary catheterization and trauma	Urgency, pressure upon voiding, hematuria, frequency

b. **Endometritis (metritis)**: localized infection of uterine lining usually beginning at placental site; is a common complication after cesarean delivery and has an approximate incidence of 27%; antibiotic prophylaxis at time of cord-clamping has reduced incidence of postpartum endometritis in both elective and emergent cesarean sections
c. Bacterial causative agents are many and include Group B *Streptococcus* (more common at 24–36 hrs or 1–2 days postpartum), genital mycoplasmas (later-onset infections), *Chlamydia trachomatis* (later-onset infections), *Escherichia coli*, *Staphylococcus aureus*, Group A *β-hemolytic streptococcus*, *Clostridium* species, *Klebsiella pneumoniae*, enterococcus, anaerobic streptococcus

4. Nursing assessment
   a. Temperature greater than 100.4°F on any 2 of first 10 days postpartum excluding first 24 hours; possible chills
   b. Abnormal lochia: remains rubra longer, has foul odor, and may be either scant or profuse in amount
   c. Tachycardia
   d. Delayed involution
      1) Fundal height does not descend as expected
      2) Uterus may feel larger and softer
      3) Client may have pain or tenderness over uterus
   e. Pain, tenderness, or inflammation of perineum
   f. Backache
   g. Malaise, fatigue
   h. Abnormal laboratory results: increased erythrocyte sedimentation rate (ESR); leukocytosis—WBC level of 14,000 to 16,000/mm^3 is not unusual during postpartum period; an increase in WBC level of more than 30% in a 6-hour period indicates infection
5. Priority nursing diagnoses: Hyperthermia; Ineffective Protection; Risk for Impaired Parenting; Risk for Impaired Parent/Infant Attachment
6. Planning/goal-setting: client will be free from infection, will participate in prescribed treatment, will develop own maternal role while attaching to newborn, and will exhibit restored homeostasis
7. Implementation
   a. Administer antibiotics as ordered
   b. Use pain rating scale to assess pain before and after administering analgesics
   c. Promote adequate nutrition and hydration (3000 to 4000 mL/day); monitor and record intake and output
   d. Use aseptic technique and good hand hygiene; provide frequent perineal care and educate client in correct technique
   e. Assess vital signs (including temperature, before and after administering antipyretics) monitor laboratory results
   f. Assess fundus for involution and lochia; encourage semi-Fowler's position to facilitate drainage
   g. Promote adequate rest and sleep
   h. Teach family and friends proper hand hygiene when entering and leaving room
   i. Encourage client to care for self first before taking care of baby; allow client to care for and feed infant per client's condition; provide client positive reinforcement
8. Evaluation
   a. Client is comfortable and free of pain
   b. Client obtains adequate nutrition, fluids, and rest
   c. Body temperature decreases and remains normal; infection does not result in more serious complications

d. Client has support and maintains family contact; client and family state they feel informed of client's condition
e. Client has minimal delay in bonding with baby; expresses positive feelings toward baby; shows comfort and competence in caring for baby; and has support and assistance in caring for infant when discharged

B. Wound infections

1. Description: an infection of abdominal incision for cesarean delivery or episiotomy (perineal incision to facilitate vaginal delivery); culture of wound drainage frequently reveals mixed pathogens
2. Predisposing factors
   a. Obesity
   b. Diabetes mellitus
   c. Prolonged postpartal hospitalization
   d. Steroid therapy
   e. Immunosuppression
3. ! Nursing assessment
   a. REEDA assessment
      1) Redness: erythema around wound
      2) Edema: swelling of tissues
      3) Ecchymosis: bruised appearance to skin from bleeding beneath skin surface
      4) Discharge: purulent drainage from incision site
      5) Approximation of skin edges: gaping of wound edges
   b. Generalized fever, localized tissue warmth
   c. Tenderness
4. Priority nursing diagnoses: Risk for Infection; Impaired Skin Integrity; Hyperthermia; Deficient Knowledge; Pain
5. Planning/goal-setting: client will be free from infection, participate in prescribed treatment, express increased comfort, and exhibit restored homeostasis
6. Implementation
   a. Administer antibiotics and antipyretics as ordered
   b. Use pain rating scale before and after administering analgesics
   c. Promote adequate nutrition and hydration (3000 to 4000 mL/day); monitor and record intake and output
   d. Use aseptic technique and good hand hygiene; provide frequent perineal care and educate client in correct technique
   e. Assess vital signs; monitor temperature before and after giving antipyretics; monitor laboratory results
   f. Assess incision or episiotomy site every 8–12 hours for signs of infection
   g. Promote adequate rest and sleep; allow family and friends to visit per client's wishes
   h. Encourage client to care for self first before taking care of infant; allow client to care for and feed infant per client's condition; provide client positive reinforcement
7. Evaluation
   a. Client is comfortable and free of pain
   b. Client obtains adequate nutrition, fluids, and rest
   c. Body temperature decreases and remains normal; infection does not result in more serious complications
   d. Client has support and maintains family contact; client and family state they feel informed of client's condition
   e. Client has minimal delay in bonding with baby; expresses positive feelings toward baby; shows comfort and competence in caring for baby; and has support and assistance in caring for infant when discharged

C. Breast infection (mastitis)

1. Description: **mastitis** is an infection of breast connective tissue, primarily in women who are lactating; usual causative organisms are *Staphylococcus aureus*, *Escherichia coli*, *Haemophilus parainfluenzae*, *Haemophilus influenzae*, and *Streptococcus* species; *Candida albicans* can also cause mastitis
2. Predisposing factors
   a. Traumatized tissue, fissured or cracked nipples
   b. Engorgement, milk stasis or poor drainage of milk, missed feedings
   c. Lowered maternal defenses caused by fatigue or stress
   d. Poor hand hygiene technique
   e. Tight clothing or poor support of pendulous breasts
3. Nursing assessment
   a. Breast consistency, nipple condition
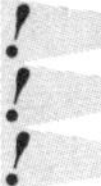
   b. Warm, reddened, painful area
   c. Axillary lymph nodes enlarged or tender
   d. Flu-like symptoms
   e. Generalized fever
4. Priority nursing diagnoses: Hyperthermia; Pain; Ineffective Breastfeeding; Interrupted Breastfeeding
5. Planning/goal-setting: client will be free from infection, have infection treated as soon as possible, participate in prescribed treatment, and maintain successful breastfeeding
6. Implementation
   a. Culture and sensitivity of breast milk may be ordered; note that infection usually is not transmitted to breast milk
   b. Administer antibiotics, analgesics, and antipyretics as ordered
   c. Promote comfort: a well-fitting, supportive bra is needed 24 hours a day
   d. Promote adequate nutrition, hydration, rest, and sleep
   e. Remind mother and staff to use good hand hygiene technique before handling breasts or assisting with breastfeeding; continue breastfeeding as advised by health care provider
   f. Assess vital signs as ordered; monitor temperature before and after administering antipyretic
   g. Educate client regarding breast care, proper latch on, let-down reflex, necessity for frequent breastfeeding, signs of complications, and telephone numbers where client can have questions answered; provide client positive reinforcement
   h. Change position of infant for feeding to relieve pressure on same area of nipple; breastfeed frequently to prevent stasis of milk
7. Evaluation
   a. Client is comfortable and free of pain
   b. Client is adequately hydrated, nourished, and rested
   c. Body temperature decreases and remains normal; infection does not result in breast abscess
   d. Client has support from family in breastfeeding, shows comfort and competence in feeding baby, expresses satisfaction with breastfeeding
   e. Client and family feel informed of client's condition

D. Urinary tract infections

1. Description: **urinary tract infection** (UTI) can occur as *cystitis* (lower urinary tract infection) and often appears two to three days after birth, or as *pyelonephritis* (upper urinary tract infection including ureter and pelvis of kidney); postdelivery UTIs are more likely to occur with bladder overdistention or urinary catheterization, are usually caused by *E. coli* bacteria, and generally occur soon after vaginal delivery

2. Predisposing factors
   a. Normal postpartal diuresis
   b. Increased bladder capacity

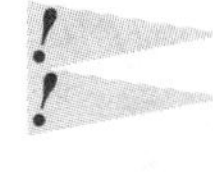

   c. Decreased bladder sensitivity from stretching or trauma
   d. Possible inhibited neural control of bladder following use of general or regional anesthesia

   e. Contamination from catheterization
   f. Obesity
3. Nursing assessment

   a. Overdistention of bladder in early postpartal period as noted by physical exam or results of bladder ultrasound scanner
   b. Frequent urination of small amounts, burning, dysuria, urgency

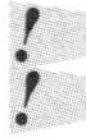

   c. Hematuria
   d. Elevated temperature; low-grade temperature occurs with cystitis, higher fever occurs with pyelonephritis

   e. Flank pain (pyelonephritis)
   f. Costovertebral angle tenderness (pyelonephritis) on palpation
   g. Chills, nausea, vomiting (pyelonephritis)
4. Priority nursing diagnoses: Hyperthermia; Pain; Deficient Knowledge; Urinary Retention
5. Planning/goal-setting: client will be free from infection, have infection treated as soon as possible, participate in prescribed treatment and learn measures to prevent urinary tract infections; lower tract infections will not ascend to become upper urinary tract infections
6. Implementation
   a. Monitor bladder frequently during recovery period to institute preventative measures
   b. Culture and sensitivity of urine may be ordered prior to administration of antibiotics
   c. Administer antibiotics as ordered; commonly sulfamethoxazole/trimethoprim (Bactrim, Septra) or nitrofurantoin (Macrodantin)
   d. Promote comfort: administer as prescribed an analgesic, antispasmodic, and/or antipyretic
   e. Promote nutrition and hydration; increase oral fluids to 3000 to 4000 mL/day
   f. Assess vital signs as ordered; monitor temperature before and after administration of antipyretics
   g. Promote rest and sleep
7. Evaluation
   a. Client voids every two to four hours without urgency or burning
   b. Client is adequately nourished, hydrated, and rested
   c. Lower tract infection does not ascend to become an upper urinary tract infection
   d. Body temperature decreases and remains normal
   e. Client and family feel informed of client's condition

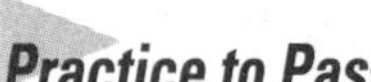

Practice to Pass

A lactating client telephones the nursing unit 24 hours after discharge. She is complaining of breast engorgement and a temperature of 99.9°F. What tips would you give her to relieve the engorgement, and what symptoms would you tell her to look for concerning mastitis?

IV. THROMBOEMBOLIC DISORDERS

A. Description: thromboembolic disorders may occur antepartally but are usually considered a postpartal complication; when a thrombus occurs in response to inflammation in vein wall it is called ***thrombophlebitis***; in this type of thrombosis, the clot is more firmly attached and is less likely to result in an embolism; thromboembolic disorders are more likely to occur after a cesarean birth

B. Contributing factors

1. Increased amounts of blood clotting factors in postpartal period
2. Postpartal thrombocytosis (increased quantity of circulating platelets and increased adhesiveness)
3. Release of thromboplastin substances from tissue of placenta and fetal membranes
4. Increased amounts of fibrinolysis inhibitors

C. Predisposing factors

1. Obesity
2. Increased maternal age
3. High parity
4. Anesthesia or surgery resulting in vessel trauma or venous stasis, prolonged bed-rest; cesarean birth
5. Maternal anemia or diabetes mellitus
6. Hypothermia
7. Heart disease
8. Endometritis
9. Varicosities, injury or trauma to leg
10. History of deep vein thrombosis (DVT)
11. Cigarette smoking

D. Types of thromboembolic disorders

1. ! Superficial thrombophlebitis (more common in postpartum period)
2. Deep vein thrombosis (DVT)
   a. More frequently seen in women with a history of thrombosis
   b. Increased incidence in women with obstetric complications such as hydramnios, preeclampsia, and operative birth
3. Septic pelvic thrombophlebitis
   a. A complication that develops in conjunction with infections of reproductive tract
   b. More common in women with a cesarean birth, incidence is 1 in 800 deliveries
   c. ! DVT and septic pelvic thromboemboli predispose clients to pulmonary embolism
4. Pulmonary embolism
   a. A catastrophic event with high mortality rate; most fatalities occur within 30 minutes
   b. Increased risk with proximal DVT and recurrent thromboembolic disease
   c. Occurs most commonly in postpartum

E. Assessment

1. Superficial thrombophlebitis
   a. Symptoms become apparent about 3rd or 4th postpartal day
   b. Tenderness is apparent in a portion of vein
   c. Local heat and redness is present, may have low-grade fever
   d. Pulmonary embolism is extremely rare
2. Deep vein thrombosis
   a. Frequently occurs in women with a history of thrombosis
   b. ! Characterized by edema of ankle and leg
   c. Initial low-grade fever followed by chills and high fever
   d. Pain located in lower leg or lower abdomen
   e. ! Homan's sign may or may not be positive, but pain results from calf pressure
   f. Peripheral pulses may be decreased
   g. ! May result in pulmonary embolism; signs include dyspnea and chest pain, diagnosis may be verified by ventilation perfusion (V/Q) scan, blood gases, x-ray
3. Septic pelvic thrombophlebitis
   a. Infection ascends upward along venous system, and thrombophlebitis develops in uterine, ovarian, or hypogastric veins

b. Usually unresponsive to antibiotics
c. Characterized by abdominal or flank pain present with guarding
d. Occurs on 2nd to 3rd postpartal day with fever and tachycardia
e. Intermittent fever and chills may persist

4. Pulmonary embolism: dyspnea and chest pain, diagnosis may be verified by V/Q scan, arterial blood gas studies, or x-ray

F. **Priority nursing diagnoses**: Pain; Impaired Gas Exchange; Ineffective Peripheral Tissue Perfusion; Impaired Physical Mobility; Risk for Impaired Parenting

G. **Planning/goal-setting**: thrombosis will be resolved without further complication and client will participate in prescribed treatment

H. **Implementation**

1. Women with varicosities should be evaluated for need for support hose during labor and postpartal period
2. ! Encourage early ambulation following birth; women who have had a cesarean birth should be encouraged to perform regular leg exercises to promote venous return
3. ! If diagnosis of DVT is made, monitor client for signs of pulmonary embolism
4. ! Monitor for signs of bleeding related to heparin or Coumadin therapy, and keep protamine sulfate (heparin antidote) available; keep vitamin K available as antidote if client is receiving oral warfarin (Coumadin)
5. Provide warm, moist soaks keeping legs elevated, if ordered
6. Obtain clotting times as ordered in client who is on anticoagulant therapy
7. Maintain bedrest as ordered; if client may get up, educate client to avoid standing or sitting for long periods of time; advise client against crossing legs or ankles
8. Review need for client to wear support stockings, if ordered, and to plan for rest periods with legs elevated
9. Promote increased fluid intake
10. Promote comfort
    a. Administer non-aspirin analgesic for pain
    b. Elevate extremities on pillow to decrease venous aching
    c. Promote adequate rest and sleep
11. Measure bilateral calf circumference daily and compare measurements for any increase in swelling on affected limb
12. ! Report to health care provider any heavy vaginal bleeding, generalized petechiae, bleeding from mucous membranes, hematuria, or oozing from venipuncture sites when client is medicated with anticoagulant

I. **Evaluation**

1. Client is comfortable, free of pain, and adequately rested
2. Thromboembolic disorder does not result in more serious complications
3. Client and family state they feel informed of client's condition
4. Client has minimal delay in interaction with baby, support and assistance in caring for infant when discharged
5. Client feels comfortable with self-administration of heparin or oral medication upon discharge

Practice to Pass

A newly delivered postpartal client complains of pain in her thighs and lower legs. How would you assess this client for a potential thromboembolic complication?

V. POSTPARTAL PSYCHIATRIC DISORDERS

A. **Description**

1. Many types of psychiatric problems may occur in postpartum period
2. The *Diagnostic and Statistical Manual of Mental Disorders, 4th edition text revision* (*DSM-IV-TR*) classifies postpartum onset mood disorders and proposes that **postpartal psychiatric disorders** be considered one diagnostic syndrome with

three subclasses; a fourth area, postpartum onset of panic disorder, has also been described

a. Adjustment reaction with depressed mood is also known as postpartum, maternal, or baby blues

! **1)** Baby blues typically occur within a few days after infant's birth and are self-limiting, lasting 10 days or longer, more severe in primiparas

2) Is thought to be related to rapid alteration in estrogen, progesterone, and prolactin levels after birth

3) New mothers feel overwhelmed, unable to cope, fatigued, anxious, irritable, and oversensitive; episodic tearfulness occurs without any reason

b. Postpartum major mood disorder, also known as postpartum depression

1) May occur anytime in first postpartum year, most often occurs around fourth week

2) Symptoms: sadness, frequent crying, insomnia, appetite change, difficulty concentrating and making decisions, feelings of worthlessness, obsessive thoughts of inadequacy as a person/parent, lack of interest in usual activities, lack of concern about personal appearance; irritability and hostility toward new baby may be seen

! **3)** Risk factors: primiparity, ambivalence about maintaining pregnancy throughout the pregnancy, history of postpartum depression or bipolar illness, lack of social support, lack of a stable relationship with parents or partner, body image and eating disorders, and lack of a supportive relationship with parents, especially client's father, as a child

4) Treatment: medication, primarily selective serotonin reuptake inhibitors such as sertraline (Zoloft), paroxetine (Paxil) and fluoxetine (Prozac), individual or group psychotherapy, and practical assistance with child care and other demands of daily life; in lactating women, very small amounts of these drugs were found in breast milk and in their infants' serum samples

c. Postpartum psychosis

1) Evident within the first three months postpartum

2) Symptoms: agitation, hyperactivity, insomnia, mood lability, confusion, irrationality, difficulty remembering or concentrating, poor judgment, delusions, and hallucinations

3) Risk factors: previous postpartum psychosis, history of bipolar disorder, prenatal stressors such as lack of support, obsessive personality, and a family history of mood disorder

4) 10 to 25% reoccurrence rate in subsequent pregnancies

5) Treatment: hospitalization, antipsychotic medications, sedatives, electroconvulsive therapy, removal of the infant, social support, and psychotherapy

d. Postpartum onset panic disorder: characterized by frightening panic attacks that includes acute onset of anxiety, fear, rapid breathing, palpitation, and a sense of doom

B. Assessment

1. History of previous psychological problems

2. Adequacy of coping skills

3. Degree of self-esteem

! **4.** Presence of mood swings, emotional distress, restlessness, irritability, guilt, extreme anxiety about the baby, anorexia, inability to complete activities of daily living, or trouble concentrating or expressing self

C. Priority nursing diagnoses: Risk for Impaired Parenting; Compromised Family Coping; Ineffective Coping; Risk for Impaired Parent–Infant Attachment

D. Planning/goal-setting: client and family will recognize common postpartum psychological changes; client will be free from psychological maladaptation; client and family will recognize signs of psychological impairment and will contact appropriate resources identified at time of discharge; and client will function adequately as a parent

E. Implementation

1. Observe client with baby, by herself, and with family and friends
2. Recognize early signs of problems
3. Seek client referral to psychiatrist for evaluation of psychological status
4. Support positive parenting behaviors
5. Discuss client's plans for her infant and herself
6. Refer client to social services, if indicated

F. Evaluation

1. Client uses appropriate coping strategies to care for self and baby
2. Client has realistic expectations for self and baby
3. Client perceives that she is receiving support she needs
4. Client has support for depressive episodes
5. Client and family share feelings and concerns openly
6. Appropriate bonding is observed and baby is safe
7. Home is a safe environment

Practice to Pass

You are assessing a client's interaction with her newborn infant. What types of behavior would you see if the client was suffering from a postpartal psychiatric disorder?

Case Study

The client is a 16-year-old gravida 1, para 1 who delivered her infant by cesarean at 37 weeks' gestation following prolonged rupture of membranes and failure to progress during labor.

1. What factors increase the client's risk for a postpartal infection?
2. What ongoing nursing assessments are necessary to identify an infection?
3. What signs and symptoms are used to diagnose an infection?
4. What is the first step in treating an infection?
5. What nursing diagnoses are pertinent to a client with a postpartal infection?

For suggested responses, see pages 305–306.

POSTTEST

POSTTEST

1 The nurse should monitor which postpartum clients who are at high risk for thrombophlebitis? Select all that apply.

1. A client who had a cesarean delivery
2. A client of normal pre-pregnant weight
3. A client who has five children
4. A client who smokes cigarettes
5. A client who kept active during pregnancy

2 Which of the following actions by a lactating client would the nurse support to help the client prevent mastitis? Select all that apply.

1. Apply vitamin E cream to soften the nipples.
2. Wear a tight, supportive bra.
3. When the client's nipples are sore, offer the infant a bottle.
4. Encourage the client to breastfeed her infant frequently.
5. Teach breastfeeding techniques soon after birth and reinforce as needed.

3 The home health nurse is making a home visit to a postpartal client. The nurse would document and report which of the following as a symptom of infection?

1. Lochia that is pink tinged
2. Apical pulse of 68
3. Generalized abdominal tenderness
4. Oral temperature of 99.2°F

4 Which intervention, if medically prescribed and then carried out by the nurse, would have the most direct effect on reducing postpartum hemorrhage?

1. Continuous fundal massage to decrease bleeding and contract the uterus
2. Trendelenburg position to facilitate cardiac function
3. Bladder catheterization to maintain uterine contraction
4. Administration of a tocolytic drug

5 The nurse interprets that which factor in a client's history places the woman at greatest risk for postpartal endometritis?

1. Cesarean delivery after 24 hours of labor and failure to progress
2. Use of external fetal monitoring during labor
3. Ruptured membranes for four hours prior to delivery
4. Spontaneous vaginal delivery after eight hours of labor

6 After delivery of a large-for-gestational-age infant, the nurse notes bright red blood continuously trickling from the client's vagina. Her fundus is firm and midline. The nurse suspects which of the following as the most likely cause of bleeding?

1. Lacerations
2. Hematoma
3. Uterine atony
4. Retained fragments of conception

7 A client is in the immediate postpartal period after delivery of a 9-pound, 14-ounce baby. The client is a gravida 6, para 5. The nurse notices some new blood stains on the top sheet and discovers the client lying in a pool of blood. The fundus is located above the umbilicus and is boggy. What would be the nurse's priority action?

1. Take the client's blood pressure
2. Have the client empty her bladder
3. Start an IV
4. Massage the uterus

8 A woman who delivered three weeks ago calls the postpartum unit with breastfeeding questions. She wants to know if she can continue to breastfeed while she has the flu. She states that she feels achy all over and has chills and a fever of 103°F. What other question is important for the nurse to ask?

1. "Have you been sleeping well?"
2. "Are you still experiencing vaginal flow?"
3. "Do you have any reddened areas or tenderness on your breasts, or unusual breast discharge?"
4. "Do you have any swelling in your legs or visual disturbances?"

9 It is most important for the nurse to have which drug readily available when the client is being treated with heparin therapy for thrombophlebitis?

1. Calcium gluconate
2. Vitamin K
3. Protamine sulfate
4. Ferrous sulfate

10 The home-care nurse is caring for a postpartal client and suspects the development of postpartum psychosis. Which client findings support the nurse's judgment? Select all that apply.

1. Has a history of a bipolar (manic-depressive) disorder
2. Reports voices telling her the baby is evil and must die
3. Can't remember details of delivery or when the infant fed last
4. Is tearful without an identifiable reason
5. Is calm and remains seated during the home visit

➤ *See pages 233–235 for Answers and Rationales.*

POSTTEST

ANSWERS & RATIONALES

Pretest

1 **Answer: 1** **Rationale:** Women that are parity of six or above (grandmultiparity) are at the greatest risk of uterine atony because of repeated distention of uterine musculature during pregnancy. Labor leads to muscle stretching, diminished tone, and muscle relaxation. The client's age is not a factor in uterine atony, the length of labor is not considered to be prolonged or precipitous, and the size of the baby is considered appropriate for gestational age, and is not considered to be macrosomic. **Cognitive Level:** Analyzing **Client Need:** Physiological Adaptation **Integrated Process:** Nursing Process: Diagnosis **Content Area:** Maternal-Newborn **Strategy:** The focus of the question is risk identification for uterine atony. Eliminate two options as this client's infant is of normal size and labor was of average duration. Eliminate maternal age, which is not a risk factor for hemorrhage. **Reference:** Ladewig, P. A., London, M. L., & Davidson, M. R. (2010). *Contemporary maternal-newborn nursing care* (7th ed.).Upper Saddle River, NJ: Pearson Education, pp. 888–892.

2 **Answer: 4** **Rationale:** Cervidil is used to ripen the cervix before labor; terbutaline sulfate is a tocolytic, and could cause further muscle relaxation; magnesium sulfate is used to decrease contractions or prevent seizures; and Hemabate is a prostaglandin, used to manage uterine atony. Oxytocin remains the first-line drug, the prostaglandins now are more commonly used as the second-line drug, and carboprost (Prostin 15-M or Hemabate) is the most commonly used uterotonin. As many as 68% of clients respond to a single carboprost injection, with 86% responding by the second dose. **Cognitive Level:** Applying **Client Need:** Physiological Adaptation **Integrated Process:** Nursing Process: Planning **Content Area:** Maternal-Newborn **Strategy:** The focus of the question is a second-line agent to stimulate uterine contraction. Eliminate the three options that identify drugs that do not possess this action. **Reference:** Ladewig, P. A., London, M. L., & Davidson, M. R. (2010). *Contemporary maternal-newborn nursing care* (7th ed.).Upper Saddle River, NJ: Pearson Education, p. 457.

3 **Answer: 3** **Rationale:** The organisms are localized in breast tissue and are not excreted in the breast milk. The other answers are factually incorrect. **Cognitive Level:** Applying **Client Need:** Physiological Adaptation **Integrated Process:** Nursing Process: Implementation **Content Area:** Maternal-Newborn **Strategy:** The wording of the question indicates that the correct option is also a true statement. Knowledge of the care of the woman with mastitis and the pathophysiology will aid in choosing correctly. **Reference:** Ladewig, P. A., London, M. L., & Davidson, M. R. (2010). *Contemporary maternal-newborn nursing care* (7th ed.).Upper Saddle River, NJ: Pearson Education, pp. 899–901.

4 **Answer: 2** **Rationale:** An abnormal odor of the lochia indicates infection in the uterus. The vital signs may be affected by an infection, but that is not definitive enough to suspect a uterine infection. A distended abdomen usually indicates a problem with gas, perhaps a paralytic ileus. Inspection of the episiotomy site would not provide information regarding a uterine infection. **Cognitive Level:** Applying **Client Need:** Physiological Adaptation **Integrated Process:** Nursing Process: Assessment **Content Area:** Maternal-Newborn **Strategy:** The critical words in the question are *uterine infection*. The correct answer would be the option that includes an assessment specific to uterine infection. The three incorrect options should be eliminated because they are not specific assessments for uterine infection. **Reference:** Ladewig, P. A., London, M. L., & Davidson, M. R. (2010). *Contemporary maternal-newborn nursing care* (7th ed.).Upper Saddle River, NJ: Pearson Education, pp. 892–893.

5 **Answer: 4** **Rationale:** A temperature elevation greater than 100.4°F on two postpartum days not including the first 24 hours meets the criteria for infection. This criterion is the most common standard in the United States. It is not abnormal for a postpartum client to run a low-grade fever in the first 24 hours. This can be caused by the body's reaction to labor, dehydration, or a reaction to epidural anesthesia. Postpartum nurses should assess other signs and symptoms of infection in addition to fever and WBCs when evaluating the possibility of infection in mothers who had epidural analgesia. **Cognitive Level:** Applying **Client Need:** Physiological Adaptation **Integrated Process:** Nursing Process: Assessment **Content Area:** Maternal-Newborn **Strategy:** The focus of the question is assessment data that defines puerperal morbidity. This definition includes a time element (after 24 hours) and a threshold for elevated temperature (greater than 100.4°F). Eliminate incorrect options because they do not meet the definition for postpartal infection. **Reference:** Ladewig, P. A., London, M. L., & Davidson, M. R. (2010). *Contemporary maternal-newborn nursing care* (7th ed.).Upper Saddle River, NJ: Pearson Education, p. 892.

6 **Answer: 3** **Rationale:** These are classic signs of thrombophlebitis that appear at the site of inflammation; the other signs listed are not. **Cognitive Level:** Applying **Client Need:** Physiological Adaptation **Integrated Process:** Teaching and Learning **Content Area:** Maternal-Newborn **Strategy:** The wording of the question indicates the correct option is also a true statement. Knowledge of the signs and symptoms of thrombophlebitis will help to choose the correct answer. **Reference:** Ladewig, P. A., London, M. L., & Davidson, M. R. (2010). *Contemporary maternal-newborn nursing care* (7th ed.).Upper Saddle River, NJ: Pearson Education, pp. 902–907.

7 **Answer:** 4 **Rationale:** An increase in lochia or a return to bright red bleeding after the lochia has changed to pink indicates a complication. The other statements are false. **Cognitive Level:** Applying **Client Need:** Physiological Adaptation **Integrated Process:** Nursing Process: Planning **Content Area:** Maternal-Newborn **Strategy:** The wording of the question indicates the correct option is also a true statement. Knowledge of complications for the postpartal client will aid in choosing the correct answer. **Reference:** Ladewig, P. A., London, M. L., & Davidson, M. R. (2010). *Contemporary maternal-newborn nursing care* (7th ed.).Upper Saddle River, NJ: Pearson Education, pp. 850–854.

8 **Answer:** 4 **Rationale:** Bleeding into the connective tissue beneath the vulvar skin may cause the formation of vulvar hematomas, which develop as a result of injury to tissues with spontaneous as well as operative deliveries (use of forceps). One of the first signs of a hematoma may be complaint of pressure, pain, or an inability to void. An ice pack to the perineum can be used to reduce swelling, but a hematoma is abnormal and should be reported to the physician. The fundus should be assessed, but the client's complaints warrant perineal or vaginal assessment. **Cognitive Level:** Applying **Client Need:** Physiological Adaptation **Integrated Process:** Nursing Process: Assessment **Content Area:** Maternal-Newborn **Strategy:** The question presents abnormal assessment data that warrants further assessment. The correct answer would be the option that includes an action for the nurse to take to obtain additional assessment findings related to perineal pain and pressure. **Reference:** Ladewig, P. A., London, M. L., & Davidson, M. R. (2010). *Contemporary maternal-newborn nursing care* (7th ed.).Upper Saddle River, NJ: Pearson Education, pp. 887–889.

9 **Answer:** 3 **Rationale:** Creating an environment where a client and her family can discuss emotional concerns is essential. Sharing time with the new mother to discuss thoughts and feelings is important to clients. Responding with patronizing answers does nothing to assist the mother to talk about her thoughts and feelings and may increase her sense of isolation and feelings of inadequacy and despair. **Cognitive Level:** Applying **Client Need:** Psychosocial Integrity **Integrated Process:** Communication and Documentation **Content Area:** Maternal-Newborn **Strategy:** The focus of the question is therapeutic communication. The correct answer would be the option that validates and explores the client's feelings. **Reference:** Ladewig, P. A., London, M. L., & Davidson, M. R. (2010). *Contemporary maternal-newborn nursing care* (7th ed.).Upper Saddle River, NJ: Pearson Education, pp. 808, 907–908.

10 **Answer:** 4, 5 **Rationale:** Risk factors for postpartum depression include primiparity, ambivalence about maintaining the pregnancy throughout the pregnancy, history of previous depression or bipolar illness, lack of a stable support system, lack of a stable relationship with parents or partner, poor body image, and lack of a supportive relationship with parents, especially her father as a child. Ambivalence regarding pregnancy is a normal response in the first and into the second trimester, but should be resolved by the third trimester. Postpartum blues occurs in approximately 50 to 80% of postpartum women; the blues does not particularly indicate that a woman will develop postpartum depression. **Cognitive Level:** Analyzing **Client Need:** Psychosocial Integrity **Integrated Process:** Nursing Process: Assessment **Content Area:** Maternal-Newborn **Strategy:** The focus of the question is risk factors for postpartum depression. Eliminate two options that contain findings common in a normal pregnancy and a third because the presence of support can reduce the risk of psychological complications. **Reference:** Ladewig, P. A., London, M. L., & Davidson, M.R. (2010). *Contemporary maternal-newborn nursing care* (7th ed.).Upper Saddle River, NJ: Pearson Education, p. 908.

Posttest

1 **Answer:** 1, 3, 4 **Rationale:** The postpartal woman is prone to develop superficial thrombophlebitis from increased clotting factors, increased number and adhesiveness of platelets during the postpartal period. Numerous factors place clients at risk. Among the most common are cesarean deliveries, lack of mobility, obesity, cigarette smoking, previous history, trauma such as leg stirrups during birth, varicosities, diabetic mothers, multiparas, and anemia. **Cognitive Level:** Analyzing **Client Need:** Physiological Adaptation **Integrated Process:** Nursing Process: Assessment **Content Area:** Maternal-Newborn **Strategy:** The wording of the question indicates that more than one option is correct. Use knowledge of risk factors for thrombophlebitis to make your selections. **Reference:** Ladewig, P. A., London, M. L., & Davidson, M. R. (2010). *Contemporary maternal-newborn nursing care* (7th ed.). Upper Saddle River, NJ: Pearson Education, pp. 902–903.

2 **Answer:** 4, 5 **Rationale:** Preventing stasis of the milk and emptying the breast frequently will help prevent mastitis. Vitamin E cream will not help to prevent mastitis. A supportive bra is helpful, but a bra that is tight will not be comfortable. Offering a bottle will reduce the milk supply if it occurs frequently and will not help mastitis. **Cognitive Level:** Applying **Client Need:** Health Promotion and Maintenance **Integrated Process:** Nursing Process: Implementation **Content Area:** Maternal-Newborn **Strategy:** The question is worded in a positive manner, indicating that the correct options are items that will prevent mastitis. Eliminate one option immediately because of the word *tight*. Use knowledge about the prevention of mastitis to choose the correct answers. **Reference:** Ladewig, P. A., London, M. L., & Davidson, M. R. (2010). *Contemporary maternal-newborn nursing care* (7th ed.). Upper Saddle River, NJ: Pearson Education, pp. 675–679.

3 **Answer:** 3 **Rationale:** The signs of a postpartal infection would include a temperature of greater than 100.4°F on

two successive days after the first 24 postpartal hours, tachycardia, foul-smelling lochia, and pain and tenderness of the abdomen. The pinkish lochia is normal, and the temperature might indicate a cold or breast milk coming in. Bradycardia would be an unrelated finding. **Cognitive Level:** Analyzing **Client Need:** Physiological Adaptation **Integrated Process:** Nursing Process: Assessment **Content Area:** Maternal-Newborn **Strategy:** The focus of the question is an infection, an abnormal finding in the postpartum. Postpartal infections are usually located in the uterus. The correct answer would be the option that contains abnormal assessment data associated with uterine infection. **Reference:** Ladewig, P. A., London, M. L., & Davidson, M. R. (2010). *Contemporary maternal-newborn nursing care* (7th ed.). Upper Saddle River, NJ: Pearson Education, pp. 892–893.

4 **Answer: 3 Rationale:** A full bladder may cause uterine atony and contribute to bleeding. If a client has hemorrhaged, a Foley catheter may also be needed to allow accurate measurement of urine output, which is an indicator for kidney function. Overly aggressive stimulation of the fundus may cause decreased uterine tone; this is detrimental because overstimulation of the uterine muscle fibers can contribute to uterine atony. Avoid the Trendelenburg position because it has been reported to interfere with cardiac and respiratory function by increasing pressure on chemoreceptors and decreasing the area for lung expansion. A tocolytic agent relaxes the uterus; in this case, an oxytocic drug to contract the uterus would be indicated. **Cognitive Level:** Analyzing **Client Need:** Physiological Adaptation **Integrated Process:** Nursing Process: Implementation **Content Area:** Maternal-Newborn **Strategy:** First, eliminate factors that cause uterine relaxation, which would increase bleeding. Next, recall that Trendelenburg position has harmful effects to eliminate it. **Reference:** Ladewig, P. A., London, M. L., & Davidson, M. R. (2010). *Contemporary maternal-newborn nursing care* (7th ed.). Upper Saddle River, NJ: Pearson Education, pp. 885–892.

5 **Answer: 1 Rationale:** Factors contributing to postpartum endometritis include the introduction of pathogens with invasive procedures, prolonged labor, and prolonged rupture of membranes. The risk of endometritis is greatest after a cesarean delivery, especially after a long labor and prolonged rupture of membranes. The other options are neither invasive nor do they increase the client's risk for infection. **Cognitive Level:** Analyzing **Client Need:** Physiological Adaptation **Integrated Process:** Nursing Process: Assessment **Content Area:** Maternal-Newborn **Strategy:** The focus of the question is risk for uterine infection. Eliminate the incorrect options because they include common noninvasive actions or data that represent normal birth experiences. **Reference:** Ladewig, P. A., London, M. L., & Davidson, M. R. (2010). *Contemporary maternal-newborn nursing care* (7th ed.). Upper Saddle River, NJ: Pearson Education, pp. 892–893.

6 **Answer: 1 Rationale:** Suspect lacerations if the client is bleeding and the fundus is firm. If the cause were uterine atony, the fundus would not be firm. When there are fragments of the placenta or the membranes, the uterus will not contract effectively. **Cognitive Level:** Analyzing **Client Need:** Physiological Adaptation **Integrated Process:** Nursing Process: Diagnosis **Content Area:** Maternal-Newborn **Strategy:** The critical words in the question are *continuous bleeding with a firm uterine fundus*, a classic symptom of a laceration. Eliminate hematoma because bleeding would be concealed and two other options that would be associated with uterine atony. **Reference:** Ladewig, P. A., London, M. L., & Davidson, M. R. (2010). *Contemporary maternal-newborn nursing care* (7th ed.). Upper Saddle River, NJ: Pearson Education, p. 887.

7 **Answer: 4 Rationale:** Of the options given the only one that immediately affects the bleeding is uterine massage. It might be important to start an IV with oxytocin at a rapid rate, and to allow the client to empty her bladder; however, the first action is to massage the uterus to stop or slow down the blood flow. **Cognitive Level:** Analyzing **Client Need:** Physiological Adaptation **Integrated Process:** Nursing Process: Implementation **Content Area:** Maternal-Newborn **Strategy:** The focus of the question is hemorrhage in the presence of uterine relaxation. The correct answer would be the option that contains a nursing action to contract the uterus and prevent further hemorrhage. **Reference:** Ladewig, P. A., London, M. L., & Davidson, M. R. (2010). *Contemporary maternal-newborn nursing care* (7th ed.). Upper Saddle River, NJ: Pearson Education, pp. 886–887.

8 **Answer: 3 Rationale:** Mastitis most frequently occurs at two to four weeks after delivery with initial flu-like symptoms plus breast tenderness and redness. The client may be describing symptoms of a breast infection. Sleep, lochia, and edema with visual disturbances are not associated with breast problems. **Cognitive Level:** Analyzing **Client Need:** Physiological Adaptation **Integrated Process:** Nursing Process: Assessment **Content Area:** Maternal-Newborn **Strategy:** The focus of the question is breastfeeding and the potential complication of mastitis. The correct answer would be the option that obtains further assessment data related to the breasts. **Reference:** Ladewig, P. A., London, M. L., & Davidson, M. R. (2010). *Contemporary maternal-newborn nursing care* (7th ed.). Upper Saddle River, NJ: Pearson Education, pp. 899–900.

9 **Answer: 3 Rationale:** Protamine sulfate is the drug used to combat bleeding problems related to heparin overdose. One option raises serum calcium levels; another is the antidote for warfarin, and the other option is an iron supplement. **Cognitive Level:** Applying **Client Need:** Pharmacological and Parenteral Therapies **Integrated Process:** Nursing Process: Implementation **Content Area:** Maternal-Newborn **Strategy:** The focus of the question is anticoagulation related to heparin use. The correct answer would be the option

that contains a drug with an action to combat bleeding. **Reference:** Wilson, B., Shannon, M., & Shields, K. (2011). *Pearson Nurse's drug guide 2011.* Upper Saddle River, NJ: Pearson Education, p. 740.

10 **Answer: 1, 2, 3 Rationale:** Postpartum psychosis usually becomes evident within three months of delivery. Delusions and hallucinations are common. The risk for suicide or infanticide is increased by the psychotic woman's distorted thoughts about herself or the baby. The psychotic woman would typically display agitation, hyperactivity, and confusion. Adjustment reaction with depressed mood, commonly known as maternal or baby blues, occurs in 50–70% of women and is characterized by feelings of fatigue, anxiety, or being overwhelmed by the new maternal role. A key feature is episodic tearfulness without reason that typically occurs within a few days of birth and resolves spontaneously about the 10th postpartal day. **Cognitive Level:** Analyzing **Client Need:** Psychosocial Integrity **Integrated Process:** Nursing Process: Assessment **Content Area:** Maternal-Newborn **Strategy:** The question is worded as a positive statement. The correct answer would be the options that contain true statements of assessment findings for postpartal psychosis. **Reference:** Ladewig, P. A., London, M. L., & Davidson, M. R. (2010). *Contemporary maternal-newborn nursing care* (7th ed.). Upper Saddle River, NJ: Pearson Education, p. 908.

References

Davidson, M., London, M., & Ladewig, P. (2012). *Olds' maternal newborn nursing & women's health across the lifespan* (9th ed.). Upper Saddle River, NJ: Pearson Education.

Ladewig, P., London, M., & Davidson, M. (2009). *Contemporary maternal-newborn nursing care* (7th ed.). Upper Saddle River, NJ: Pearson Education.

Perry, S.E., Hockenberry, M. J., Lowdermilk, D. L., & Wilson, D. (2010). *Maternal child nursing care* (4th ed.). St. Louis, MO: Mosby.

Ricci, S. (2009). *Essentials of maternity, newborn, and women's health nursing* (2nd ed.). Philadelphia: Lippincott Williams & Wilkins.

12 The Normal Newborn Experience

Chapter Outline

Nursing Care of the Normal Newborn

Physiologic Changes at Birth

Newborn Nutrition

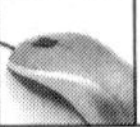

NCLEX-RN® Test Prep

Use the accompanying online resource, NursingReviewsandRationales, to test yourself with hundreds of NCLEX®-style practice questions.

Objectives

- Identify nursing assessments to be performed on the newborn on admission to the nursery.
- Describe the changes required in each body system for successful transition from intrauterine to extrauterine life.
- Identify client teaching for the new mother related to infant nutrition.

Review at a Glance

acrocyanosis peripheral cyanosis; blue color of hands and feet

Babinski reflex a neurological reflex where newborn toes will hyperextend and fan apart with dorsiflexion of big toe when foot is stroked upward from heel and across ball of foot

Barlow's maneuver when infant's thigh is adducted and gently pressed downward; dislocation is felt if femoral head slips out of acetabulum

caput succedaneum swelling of tissue over presenting part of fetal head caused by pressure during labor; crosses suture lines

cephalohematoma blood from ruptured vessels between skull bone and external covering (periosteum); does not cross suture line

ductus arteriosus in fetal circulation, an anatomic shunt between pulmonary artery and arch of aorta

ductus venosus in fetal circulation, a structure that shunts arterial blood into inferior vena cava

Epstein's pearls small white specks on gum lines of newborns

Erb-Duchenne paralysis (Erb's palsy) paralysis of arm and chest wall from a birth injury to brachial plexus or 5th to 6th cervical nerves

foramen ovale in fetal circulation, a shunt that connects right and left atria

grasp reflex elicited by placing an object in newborn's hand, resulting in a firm hold of that object

lanugo fine, downy hair found on all body parts of fetus (except palms of hands and soles of feet), from 20 weeks' gestation to birth; begins to decrease at 36 to 40 weeks

latch-on proper position of infant on nipple/aerola to allow the transfer of milk, tongue down with lactiferous sinuses covered

meconium dark green or black material present in large intestine of a full-term infant; the first stool passed

milia tiny, white pustules on face and chin resulting from unopened sebaceous glands

Mongolian spots dark or bluish, flat pigmented areas on skin of lower back and buttocks in some infants of African-American, Hispanic, or Asian heritage

Moro reflex elicited by startling the newborn; thighs and knees flex and fingers fan and then clench as arms are thrown out, then brought together

Ortolani's maneuver a manual procedure performed to rule out possibility of congential hip dysplasia; hip joint is abducted and lifted, and a click is felt as femur enters acetabulum

pilonidal dimple dimple located on skin surface at base of spine not connected to the spine

plantar grasp pressure applied with a finger against ball of infant's foot causes the toes to flex

rooting reflex an infant's tendency to turn head and open lips to suck when one side of mouth is touched

sucking reflex elicited by inserting a finger or nipple in newborn's mouth

tonic neck reflex elicited when infant's head is turned to one side, the arm and leg of that side extend while extremities on opposite side flex; fencing position

trunk incurvature reflex (Galant reflex) stroking one side of spine while infant lies prone causes pelvis to flex toward stimulated side

vernix caseosa a protective cheese-like, whitish substance present on fetal skin; decreases with increased gestational age

PRETEST

1 A newborn's head circumference is 34 cm (13.6 inches) and chest circumference is 32 cm (12.5 inches). Which nursing action would be appropriate?

1. Refer the newborn for evaluation for psychomotor retardation.
2. Prepare the mother for the probability that the physician will want to transilluminate the cranial vault.
3. Measure the occipitofrontal circumference daily.
4. Record the findings and take no further action.

2 The nurse tests the newborn's Babinski reflex by doing which of the following?

1. Touching the corner of the newborn's mouth or cheek
2. Changing the newborn's equilibrium
3. Placing a finger in the palm of the newborn's hand
4. Stroking the lateral sole from the heel upward and across the ball of the foot

3 A new mother questions the nurse about the "lump" on her baby's head. The nurse explains that is a "collection of blood between the skull bone and its covering (periosteum)" and is called which of the following?

1. Caput succedaneum
2. Molding
3. Cephalohematoma
4. Subdural hematoma

4 The maternal newborn nurse who assesses a newborn should find that the heart rate is within which range within three minutes of birth?

1. 100–130 beats per minute
2. 110–180 beats per minute
3. 110–160 beats per minute
4. 130–170 beats per minute

5 The nurse understands that the results of which assessment of gestational age must be determined within 12 hours of birth for valid results?

1. Breast tissue enlargement in female infants
2. The usual posture the infant assumes
3. Assessment of the creases on the soles of feet
4. The angle of the Scarf sign

6 A newborn admitted to the nursery 15 minutes after birth is moderately cyanotic, has a mottled trunk, active movement of the extremities, and is wrapped in a cotton blanket. With this information, what is the primary assessment by the nurse at this time?

1. Evaluate the umbilical stump for bleeding.
2. Assess the infant's temperature.
3. Perform a visual scan for visible abnormalities.
4. Assess the infant for a patent airway.

7 The nurse observes that a one-day postpartum client who is breastfeeding her first child appears frightened. The client says, "The baby has been breathing funny, fast and slow, off and on." What is an appropriate response by the nurse?

1. "That's normal when the baby breastfeeds."
2. "There's nothing to worry about. I'll go take the baby back to the nursery now."
3. "I'll watch the baby for a while to see if there is something wrong."
4. "Be reassured; it's a normal breathing pattern. I'll sit here while you finish feeding him."

8 Which behavior by a new mother observed by the nurse indicates good bottle-feeding technique? Select all that apply.

1. Keeps the nipple full of formula throughout the feeding
2. Props the bottle on a rolled receiving blanket
3. Points the bottle at the infant's tongue
4. Enlarges the nipple hole to allow for a steady stream of formula to flow
5. Keeps the infant close with head elevated

9 A mother is beginning to experience nipple discomfort while breastfeeding. What would be the nurse's first priority in the plan of care?

1. Have the mother pump until the nipples heal and give breast milk from the bottle.
2. Remove the baby from the breast and reposition.
3. Give the mother a nipple shield to wear.
4. Have the mother breastfeed only from the nipple that is not injured.

---

10 A mother asks, "Is it true that breast milk will prevent my baby from catching colds and other infections?" The nurse should make which reply based on current research findings?

1. "Your baby will have increased resistance to illness caused by bacteria and viruses, but may still contract infections."
2. "You shouldn't have to worry about your baby's exposure to contagious diseases until the breastfeeding period of time is over."
3. "Breast milk offers no greater protection to your baby than formula feedings."
4. "Breast milk will give your baby protection from all illnesses to which you are immune."

➤ *See pages 248–249 for Answers and Rationales.*

I. NURSING CARE OF THE NORMAL NEWBORN

A. Physical assessment

1. Vital signs

   a. Heart rate is 110–160 beats/min, irregular, especially when crying, and perhaps a functional murmur; may be as high as 180 briefly when crying; count apical pulse for one full minute
   b. Respirations are 30–60 breaths/min with short periods of apnea, irregular; cry is vigorous and loud; may be slightly elevated during crying, but over 60/min (tachypnea) two hours after delivery or less than 30/min (bradypnea) may indicate a problem; count for one full minute
   c. Temperature is 36.5–37°C (97.7–98.6°F) axillary; stabilizes about 8 to 10 hours after birth; poor thermostability is related to heat loss via *convection* (loss to cooler air currents), *radiation* (indirect heat transfer from body to cooler surfaces), *evaporation* (from wet skin) and *conduction* (direct heat loss to cooler objects)
   d. Blood pressure is 80/46; varies with changes in newborn's activity and blood volume; more accurate when newborn is resting
2. Pain assessment: intermittent crying not lasting more than 60 seconds, not high-pitched, quiets easily, and no tears noted
3. Priority nursing diagnosis: Ineffective Thermoregulation; Ineffective Breathing Pattern; Decreased Cardiac Output
4. Planning and implementation
   a. Maintain newborn on radiant warmer or in isolette with servocontrol to maintain skin temperature 36.5 to 37°C (97.5 to 98.6°F)
   b. Allow infant to assume a flexed position to decrease surface area of skin exposed to environment, thereby reducing heat loss; assure that infant remains dry
   c. Monitor axillary and skin probe temperature per institution's protocol

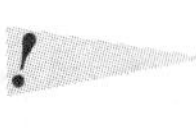

   d. Monitor respirations for tachypnea and skin color changes for mottling
5. Evaluation: at two hours of age the newborn maintains an axillary temperature of 97.7–98.6°F, a heart rate of 120–160/min, respirations 30–60/min with no signs of distress, skin color pink, and remains in flexed position

B. General assessment (performed in cephalocaudal or head to toe/tail manner)

1. Head
    - **a.** One-fourth of body size, molding of fontanels and suture spaces, round, and moves easily from left to right and up to down
    - **b.** Frontal occipital circumference (FOC), measured around forehead and occipital area, is 32 to 37 cm (12.5 to 14.5 in.) or 2 cm greater than chest circumference
    - **c.** Symmetric exception may be caused by birth trauma, i.e., **caput succedaneum** (swelling of soft tissue under scalp), or **cephalohematoma** (collection of blood beneath cranial bone and periosteum)
    - **d.** Anterior and posterior fontanels should be open, with posterior fontanel closing sooner (8 to 12 weeks) than anterior fontanel (18 months)
2. Hair: silky smooth, grows toward face, high above eyebrow, variations in texture depend on ethnic background
3. Face: symmetric movement
4. Eyes
    - **a.** Clear blue/slate-gray or brown in color
    - **b.** Pupils equal and reactive to light, blink reflex present, sclera is bluish white
    - **c.** May have subconjunctival hemmorrhage (small broken tiny capillaries on sclera; will disappear in few weeks)
    - **d.** Edematous eyelids
    - **e.** Lacrimal structures (tearing) functions at about 2 months
5. Nose: patent nares bilaterally, no discharge, may have flat bridge, sneezing done to clear nostrils
6. Mouth
    - **a.** Symmetrical when cries, hard palate intact, uvula midline, reflexes present
    - **b.** **Rooting reflex** (infant turns to side stimulated and opens mouth to suck), **sucking reflex** (exhibits sucking when object placed in mouth or touches lips)
    - **c.** May have **Epstein's pearls** (small white specks, inclusion cysts, on gum ridges), tongue not protruding
7. Ears: well-formed notch of ear on straight line with outer canthus of eye
8. Neck: short, freely movable, has **tonic neck reflex** or fencer position (when head is turned to one side, extremities on same side extend and extremities on opposite side flex)
9. Chest
    - **a.** Clavicles straight and intact, barrel-shaped chest with bilateral expansion with inspirations
    - **b.** Breath sounds clear
    - **c.** Heart rate ausculated at border of left sternum extending left to midclavicle; regular rate and rhythm
    - **d.** Point of maximum impulse (PMI) lateral to midclavicular line at 3rd to 4th intercostal space
10. Breasts: nipples symmetric, may have whitish discharge or supernumerary (extra, small) nipples on chest surface
11. Abdomen
    - **a.** Soft, dome-shaped, round, some laxness of muscles, moves with respirations
    - **b.** Bowel sounds when relaxed
    - **c.** Umbilical cord is white, gelatinous with two arteries and one vein, clamped with no foul odor
    - **d.** Femoral pulses palpable and equal, no bulges or nodes along bilateral inguinal areas
12. Genitalia
    - **a.** Male: pendulous scrotum with rugae, testes descended into scrotum, penis with urinary meatus at tip of glans on ventral surface of penile shaft

b. Female: labia minora may have **vernix caseosa** (white, cheesy protective covering that decreases as gestational age increases) and smegma in creases, labia majora normally covers labia minora and clitoris, discharge (blood-tinged mucus or pseudomenstruation) may be present because of maternal hormones

13. Extremities and trunk
    a. Trunk: short, flexed synchronized movement
    b. **Trunk incurvature reflex (Galant reflex)**: newborn lies prone and when one side of spine is stroked, it causes pelvis to flex toward stimulated side
    c. Hips: stable with no clicks or snaps upon movement
    d. To rule out hip dislocation, **Barlow's maneuver** adducts legs over hips and a snap is felt as femur leaves acetabulum; with **Ortolani's maneuver**, hip joint is abducted and lifted, and a click is felt as femur enters acetabulum
    e. Arms: equal in length with symmetrical movement; **grasp reflex** present (newborn grasps when object is placed in hand); lack of movement may indicate **Erb-Duchenne paralysis** or Erb's palsy, when newborn is unable to move upper arms; an asymmetric Moro response may be caused by damage to 5th and 6th cervical roots of the brachial plexus; five digits on each hand with normal palmar creases, nails present
    f. Legs: equal length, bowed, well-flexed, symmetric skin folds, peripheral pulses present
    g. Feet: creases on soles, may have "positional" clubfoot caused by intrauterine position but should be able to turn toward midline; **plantar grasp** present (pressure on soles of feet elicits curling of toe); **Babinski reflex** present (stroking sole upward and across ball of foot elicits fanning and extension of toes); disappears at 12 months
    h. Back: spine straight and flexible, may have small **pilonidal dimple**, a small dimple at base of spine but without connection to spinal cord
    i. Anus: patent, well placed, may have meconium stool
14. Skin
    a. Color consistent with ethnic background, pink-tinged
    b. **Acrocyanosis**: bluish discoloration of hands and feet may be present
    c. May have mottling: lacy pattern of dilated blood vessels under skin caused by fluctuation of general circulation
    d. May have **milia**—obstructed secretions of sebaceous glands
    e. May have **Mongolian spots**—dark or bluish pigmented areas on dorsal area of skin of buttocks of Asian, African-American, or Hispanic descent
    f. May have **lanugo**—downy, fine hair of fetus between 20 weeks and birth, noticeably found on shoulders, forehead, and cheeks

C. Gestational age assessment using Ballard tool (Ballard score)

1. An assessment that evaluates six neuromuscular and six physical characteristics; performed during first few hours of birth
2. A score of 1 to 5 is assigned to each characteristic and total score correlates to a gestational age, i.e., a term newborn given a score of 3 for each characteristic scores an 18 for neuromuscular assessment and 18 for physical characteristics; the total of 36 points correlates to 38+ weeks' gestation
3. Numerical rating is then marked on graph along with newborn's birth weight, length, and head circumference to classify newborn based on maturity and intrauterine growth
4. An overall rating below tenth percentile indicates infant is *small for gestational age (SGA)*; between 10th and 90th percentile indicates infant is *appropriate for gestational age (AGA)*; above 90th percentile indicates that infant is *large for gestational age (LGA)*

Practice to Pass

An anxious new mother asks you, "What's wrong with my baby? What are those white spots on her nose and chin?" What is your response?

5. Determining ratings for each subscore
   a. Wear gloves when assessing newborn after birth prior to first bath
   b. First evaluate observable characteristics without disturbing newborn then proceed to characteristics that require more handling of infant
   c. Maternal conditions such as preeclampsia, eclampsia, diabetes mellitus, and maternal analgesia and anesthesia during intrapartal period may affect some gestational age components
   d. Neuromuscular maturity: during first 24 hours, newborn's nervous system is unstable; reflexes and assessments dependent on newborn's brain centers may be unreliable and need to be repeated in 24 hours
      1) Posture: well-flexed with elbow, hip, and knee joints at 90° angle
      2) Square window sign (wrist): elicited by flexing newborn's hand toward ventral forearm until resistance is felt and measuring angle
      3) Arm recoil: in supine position, elbows are flexed and held for five seconds, then extended at newborn's side and released; upon release, a term newborn will form an angle of less than 90° and recoil back to a flexed position
      4) Popliteal angle: in a supine position, thigh is flexed on abdomen and chest with one hand; with index finger of other hand behind ankle, try to extend lower leg until resistance is felt
      5) Scarf sign: in supine position, draw an arm across chest toward opposite shoulder until resistance is felt; note location of elbow in relation to midline of chest
      6) Heel-to-ear extension: in supine position, gently draw foot toward ear on same side until resistance is felt; knee may bend; hold buttocks down to avoid rolling newborn and note proximity of foot to ear and degree of knee extension
   e. Physical maturity: not influenced by labor and birth and do not change significantly within first 24 hours after birth
      1) Skin: opaque texture, few distinct larger veins, dry, some peeling
      2) Lanugo: minimal, decreases as gestational age increases
      3) Plantar surface: a reliable indicator of gestational age in first 12 hours of life; beginning at top of foot, creases should cover at least two-thirds of entire foot surface
      4) Breast: using forefinger and middle finger, gently measure breast tissue between them in millimeters; at term gestation, measurement should be between 5 and 10 mm; nipple should be raised above skin level
      5) Eye/ear: eyes are open and clear; ears—when top and bottom of pinna are folded over each other, pinna will spring back quickly when released; upper two-thirds of pinna incurves
      6) Male genitalia: testes descended, scrotum pendulous and covered with rugae
      7) Female genitalia: labia majora increases as gestation increases and nearly covers clitoris at 36 to 40 weeks; at 40 weeks, labia majora cover labia minora and clitoris

Practice to Pass

Many factors can influence the term newborn's gestational age score. What factors might affect the posture, sole creases, and amount of breast bud tissue?

II. PHYSIOLOGIC CHANGES AT BIRTH

A. **Cardiovascular**: expansion of lungs with first breath increases pulmonary blood flow and decreases pulmonary vascular resistance
   1. Increased aortic pressure and decreased venous pressure: clamping of umbilical cord increases vascular resistance, and aortic blood pressure increases
   2. Increased systemic pressure and decreased pulmonary artery pressure caused by loss of placenta; lung expansion increases pulmonary blood flow and dilates pulmonary vessels; pulmonary vascular beds open and perfuse other body systems
   3. The **foramen ovale** (an opening that previously connected right and left atria), functionally closes in about one to two hours, and anatomically closes in a few weeks to one year, increasing left atrial pressure; some shunting may occur early in transition and with crying

4. The **ductus arteriosus** (in fetal circulation, an anatomic shunt between pulmonary artery and arch of the aorta) closes, reversing blood flow, so now blood flows from aorta to pulmonary artery because of increased left arterial pressure
5. The **ductus venosus** closes (in fetal circulation, shunts arterial blood into inferior vena cava); is thought to be related to severance of umbilical cord, results in redistribution of blood and cardiac output; closure forces perfusion of liver

B. Respiratory: initial respirations are triggered by physical, sensory, and chemical factors

1. Physical: effort required to expand lungs and fill collapsed alveoli, changes in pressure gradient
2. Sensory: temperature, noise, light, sound
3. Chemical: changes in blood (decreased O_2 level, increased CO_2 level, decreased pH) as a result of transitory asphyxia during delivery
4. ! Newborn is an obligatory nose-breather, and any obstruction will cause respiratory distress; ability to maintain respiratory function is influenced by newborn's large heart that reduces lung space; is also influenced by weak intercostal muscles, horizontal ribs and high diaphragm, which restrict space available for lung expansion
5. Priority nursing diagnoses: Impaired Gas Exchange; Ineffective Breathing Pattern
6. Planning and implementation
   a. ! Monitor newborn's respirations for any signs of respiratory distress (increased rate, audible grunting, nasal flaring, retractions) per institutional protocol; normal limits are 30 to 60/min
   b. Monitor color of skin, oral area, and extremities for any signs of hypoxia
   c. Keep newborn on warmer for closer observation; maintain dryness
   d. Keep infant NPO if respirations are above 60/min
   e. Maintain oral area free from mucus or emesis
7. Evaluation: newborn's respirations are within normal limits, color is pink, temperature stable with no signs of respiratory distress

Practice to Pass

What position do most newborns usually assume during transition? Why?

C. Neurologic: newborn's brain is one-fourth the size of an adult's and myelination of nerve fibers is incomplete

1. Newborn exhibits uncoordinated movements, labile temperature regulation, poor control over musculature, easy startling, and tremors of extremities
2. Newborn reflexes are important indicators of normal development; these include **Moro reflex** (elicited by startling newborn; flexion of thighs and knees and fingers that fan, then clench as arms are thrown out, then brought together) and previously discussed Babinski grasp, plantar grasp, sucking, and tonic neck reflexes
3. Periods of reactivity: pattern of behavior during first several hours after birth
   a. ! First period of reactivity: 30 to 60 minutes after birth; awake and alert; may display nursing and attachment behaviors with random diffuse movements
   b. Period of inactivity to sleep phase: activity diminishes, heart and respiratory rates decrease, and newborn enters sleep phase lasting from a few minutes to two to four hours; will be difficult to awaken
   c. Second period of reactivity: awakes from deep sleep, lasting four to six hours; close observation is required for changes in heart rate, respiration, and color

D. Musculoskeletal: newborn should have full range of motion—when extremities are fully extended, they should return to a flexed position; any variations should be further investigated

E. Gastrointestinal changes

1. Digestive enzymes are active at birth and can support extrauterine life by 36 to 38 weeks' gestation
2. Necessary muscular and reflex developments for transporting food are present at birth
3. Digestion of protein and carbohydrates is easily accomplished, but fat digestion and absorption are poor due to absence of pancreatic enzymes

4. Little saliva is manufactured until 3 months
5. An immature lower esophageal sphincter often leads to regurgitation or spitting up
6. **Meconium**, stool that contains bile, epithelial cells, and amniotic cells, is excreted within 24 hours in 90% of normal newborns
7. Wide variations occur among newborns regarding interest in food

F. **Genitourinary changes**

1. Functioning nephrons are complete by 34 to 36 weeks' gestation
2. Glomerular filtration rate (reabsorption and filtration) is low; therefore, newborn may tend to reabsorb sodium and excrete large amounts of water
3. Decreased ability to excrete drugs and excessive fluid loss can lead to acidosis and fluid imbalance; uric acid crystals may cause a pink to reddish stain in diaper (also known as brick deposits or "brick dust spots")

G. **Hepatic**

1. If mother's iron intake has been adequate, iron stores from mother are sufficient to carry newborn through 5th month of extrauterine life; iron supplements may be given after this age
2. Liver controls amount of circulating unconjugated bilirubin, a pigment derived from hemoglobin that is released with breakdown of red blood cells
3. Unconjugated bilirubun can leave vascular system and permeate other extravascular tissues (e.g., skin, sclera, oral mucous membranes), resulting in a yellow coloring termed *jaundice* or *icterus*
4. Because unconjugated bilirubin binds to albumin (protein) and is eliminated in stools, early and increased feeding may be encouraged to promote increased excretion of stool; phototherapy requires eye protection (bili-mask)

H. **Integumentary**

1. As newborn maturity increases, so does maturity of skin; greater skin maturity leads to better protection of newborn from heat loss and infection
2. Skin color depends on activity level, temperature, hematocrit levels, and race
3. Plethora is a ruddy (red) appearance and usually indicates a hematocrit greater than 65% and should be evaluated; a polycythemic infant should be monitored closely for onset of cyanosis, respiratory distress, hypoglycemia, and jaundice
4. When the infant cries, skin becomes bright red because of immature capillary system; acrocyanosis is common

I. **Immune system**

1. Of three major types of immunoglobulins (IgG, IgA, and IgM), only IgG crosses placenta; therefore, infants receive passive immunity from mother in form of IgG near end of gestation (also called passive acquired immunity)
2. Infants eventually produce antibodies (active acquired immunity) beginning at about 3 months, but IgA is missing from respiratory, urinary, and gastrointestinal tracts until approximately 4 to 6 months of age, unless newborn is breastfed or until infant produces own antibodies
3. Infants who are breastfed are provided antibodies from breast milk for as long as mother chooses to breastfeed and are provided protection from many infectious diseases, including influenza, mumps, and chickenpox

III. NEWBORN NUTRITION

A. **Nutrition guidelines**: a well, healthy newborn needs 105 to 108 kcal/kg/24/hr of nutrition and 140 to 160 mL/kg/24 hr of fluid intake; weight gain is 4 to 8 ounces/ week; weight doubles by 5 months of age, and triples by age of 1 year

B. **Priority nursing diagnosis**: Deficient Knowledge; Ineffective Breastfeeding; Imbalanced Nutrition: Less Than Body Requirements; Imbalanced Nutrition: More Than Body Requirements

Practice to Pass

A new mother asks, "How long should I continue to feed my newborn formula? It's so expensive. When can I give him cow's milk?" How should the nurse respond?

C. **Planning and implementation**: teaching guidelines for formula/bottle-feeding
   1. Formula meets energy and nutrient requirements of newborn/infants, but does not have immunologic properties and digestibility of human milk
   2. Standard formulas are available in three types
      a. Concentrated liquid: diluted with water at a 1:1 ratio
      b. Powder: mixed with water, usually one scoop to two ounces of water
      c. Ready-to-feed: can be poured directly into a bottle; must be refrigerated once opened and discarded after 24 hours
      d. The American Academy of Pediatrics (AAP) recommends that infants be given formula or breast milk until 12 months of age
      e. Soy formulas are available for infants who cannot tolerate cow's milk protein and lactose
   3. Preparation of formula
      a. Aseptic sterilization: supplies are sterilized separately from formula by boiling them in water for 20 minutes
      b. Terminal sterilization: formula is poured into unsterilized bottles that are sterilized together for 25 minutes
      c. With sanitary conditions, bottles and formula are not routinely sterilized, but all equipment is cleaned thoroughly, including top of formula can
      ! d. Formula may be warmed to room temperature in a container of warm water; bottles should never be warmed in a microwave; hot spots may develop and burn infant's mouth/throat; heating also changes nutritional composition of formula
   4. Feeding techniques
      a. Hold infant close with head elevated
      b. Keep bottle tipped so that nipple remains full of formula
      ! c. Never prop bottle or put infant to bed with a bottle in his or her mouth; propping can cause aspiration and middle ear infections
      d. Discard any formula left in bottle because of risk of bacterial growth

D. **Planning and implementation**: teaching guidelines for breastfeeding
   1. Influences on supply and demand (infant need)
      a. Maternal supply is related to frequency of feedings until about three to four weeks when milk supply is well established; thereafter, the critical factor for supply to meet demand is breast emptying
      b. Infants self-regulate their intake and control breast milk production by extent to which they "empty" breast; a lactating breast is never "emptied" completely, but infant chooses how much to take
   2. Suckling sequence and proper **latch-on** (see Figure 12-1)
      a. Nipple and areola are drawn into mouth enough for lips to cover 1 to 1.5 inches of areola
      b. Jaw should move up and down in a rhythmic motion during milk transfer; ears may wiggle; cheeks should be full and rounded, not sucked in
      c. Upper and lower lips should be flanged
      d. Tongue should be troughed—cup-shaped, beginning at bottom of mouth and extending over lower alveolar ridge; in this way, tongue draws nipple in and presses it against hard palate, forming a teat; tongue then humps up from back to front of areola in a "rolling-like" movement for milk transfer
   3. Frequency of feedings: increasing frequency will not increase supply unless transfer of milk is successfully occurring; audible swallowing is best indicator of milk transfer; swallowing is more frequent as more milk is transferred
      a. Schedules should not be imposed on breastfeeding newborns as they have a stomach capacity of about 30 mL, and breast milk is more easily digested than artificial milk (formula)

Figure 12-1

Latch-on position

Adapted from Lawrence, R.A. (1994). *Breastfeeding: A guide for the medical profession* (4th ed.). St. Louis, MO: Mosby, p.219.

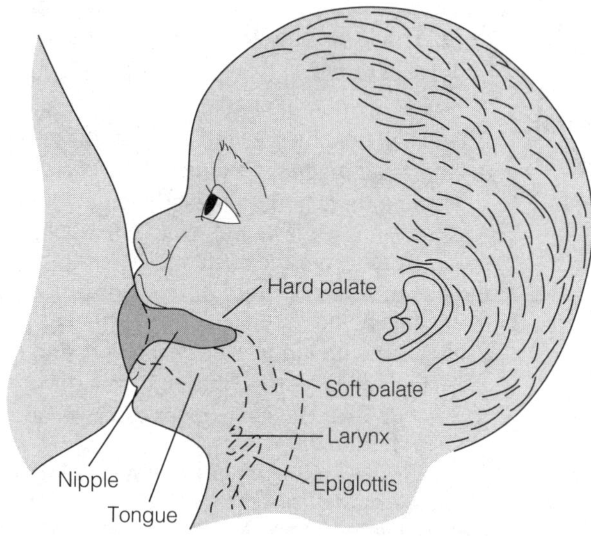

- **b.** Breastfeeding infants should be fed when hunger cues are displayed; rooting, sucking on fists, clenched fists; these cues may be exhibited from 90 minutes to three hours after the last feeding; crying is the last sign of hunger
- **c.** Night feedings will be necessary during first six to eight weeks; fat content of breast milk is high in evening, which may help infant to consume more calories and therefore feel more satiated; infants who consume more calories during day may be able to have longer stretches of sleep at night

4. Duration of feedings

- **a.** Research does not document the common myth that limiting time at breast will minimize or prevent sore nipples; sore nipples are almost always caused by incorrect positioning of infant at breast or poor latch-on
- **b.** Mothers should watch the infant, not the clock; what an infant is doing at breast is a better indicator of milk transfer than amount of time spent there
- **c.** Newborns/infants with different sucking styles take different amounts of time to complete a feeding, anywhere from 10 to 30 minutes; foremilk is milk that is produced and stored between feedings, looks like skimmed milk—bluish in tint and usually has less fat content than hindmilk, which is produced during and released at end of a feeding and looks much richer with a yellowish tint
- **d.** Signs of satiation are slowing of audible swallowing, pauses between sucking bursts, infant takes him- or herself off breast, hunger cues disappear, and infant is relaxed, drowsy, sleeping

5. Positioning for feeding; good positioning is paramount for proper latch-on and effective suckling

- **a.** Body position for mother starts with good posture; straight back, pillows under arms (and under infant), feet touching floor or a footstool beneath her feet
- **b.** Hand position: during early weeks, breast should be supported with a hand; use caution that fingers do not cover lactiferous sinuses or areola that infant needs to take into his or her mouth; later on, infant will be able to support breast after initial latch-on
- **c.** Cradle hold: infant is in chest-to-chest position, facing breast close enough to touch with nose and chin, with shoulder resting slightly lower on mother's forearm and hand supporting infant's buttocks; opposite hand is used to support breast
- **d.** Side-lying position: infant is lying alongside mother with a rolled-up blanket behind infant and a pillow behind mother to help maintain position; this position is suggested for night-time feedings and mothers who had cesarean deliveries

Box 12-1

Ten Steps to Successful Breastfeeding

Every facility providing maternity services and care for newborn infants should do the following:

1. Have a written breastfeeding policy routinely communicated to all healthcare staff.
2. Train all health care staff in the skills necessary to implement this policy.
3. Inform all pregnant women about the benefits and management of breastfeeding.
4. Help mothers initiate breastfeeding within a half-hour of birth.
5. Show mothers how to breastfeed and how to maintain lactation even if they are separated from their infants.
6. Give newborn infants no food or drink other than breast milk unless it is medically indicated.
7. Practice rooming-in—allow mothers and infants to stay together—24 hours a day.
8. Encourage breastfeeding on demand.
9. Give no artificial teats or pacifiers (also called dummies or soothers) to breastfeeding infants.
10. Foster the establishment of breastfeeding support groups and refer mothers to them on discharge from the hospital or clinic.

!

e. Football or clutch position: infant is positioned in mother's arm with his or her head, back, and shoulders in palm of hand; infant is tucked up under mother's arm, lining up infant's lips with nipple

6. Breastfeeding support is necessary for beginning or continuing of breastfeeding (see Box 12-1)

a. Encourage use of breastfeeding support groups or telephone hotlines at hospitals

b. Lactation consultants are trained and certified to provide assistance to breastfeeding mothers who experience problems

c. La Leche League is an international breastfeeding support and information group, with local groups often meeting in neighborhoods

d. Hospitals and birthing centers that subscribe to World Health Organization's (WHO) Baby Friendly Hospital promote "10 steps to successful breastfeeding" and stop distribution of breast milk substitutes

Practice to Pass

A new breastfeeding mother says she is not sure that her newborn is "getting any milk." How do you respond?

E. Evaluation: infant is gaining 0.5 to 1 ounce per day, doubles weight by 5 months of age and triples weight by 1 year of age; infant has six wet or soiled diapers per day and is alert and responsive; skin is elastic; mucous membranes are moist

Case Study

The client delivered her first child by cesarean delivery. She had an uneventful recovery. Her clinical status is within normal limits, and her vital signs are stable but her blood pressure is somewhat elevated one hour after delivery. She emphatically tells you that she does not want to feed the baby, even though before delivery she stated, "I really want to breastfeed immediately after delivery." Now, she wants you to feed her newborn in the nursery. You want to comply with the client's wishes but you are concerned about the conflicting statements made by the mother prior to and after delivery and the benefits of early breastfeeding.

1. What does your assessment data reveal about the mother?
2. What is your first nursing action based on your assessment data?
3. When do you take the newborn to his mother?
4. How much instruction do you give the mother when you take the newborn to her?
5. What are the priorities for helping the newborn and his mother have a positive experience?

For suggested responses, see page 306.

POSTTEST

1 At two days of age, the nurse hears a murmur over the right and left auricles of the newborn's heart. The nurse concludes that this may represent patency of which infant structure?

1. Open umbilical vein
2. Foramen ovale
3. Patent ductus arteriosus
4. Patent ductus venosus

2 The maternal-newborn nurse formulates which nursing goal for a newborn in transition within the first few hours after birth?

1. To facilitate development of a close parent–infant relationship
2. To assist parents in developing healthy attitudes about childrearing practices
3. To identify actual or potential problems that may require immediate or emergency attention
4. To provide the parents of the newborn with information about well-baby programs

3 The nurse conducts a neurological assessment of the newborn. Which findings indicate the need for further evaluation? Select all that apply.

1. Asymmetrical fine jumping movements of the leg and arm muscles
2. Fanning and hyperextension of toes when the sole is stroked upward from the heel
3. Grasping a finger placed in the neonate's palm
4. Muscle flaccidity not relieved by holding the newborn
5. Weak and ineffective sucking movements

4 Most newborns void in the first 24 hours after birth. The nurse interprets that which of the following is responsible for a reddish stain, sometimes called "red brick dust spots," or "brick deposits," on the newborn's diaper?

1. Uric acid crystals in the urine
2. Mucus and urate in the urine
3. Excess bilirubin in the urine
4. Excess iron in the urine

5 A nurse providing care to a newborn would use which concept underlying adaptation of the newborn's immune system when planning nursing care?

1. Iron stores from the mother are sufficient to carry the newborn through the fifth month of extrauterine life.
2. Unconjugated bilirubin can leave the vascular system and permeate the other extravascular tissues.
3. The newborn is unable to limit invading organisms at their point of entry.
4. Most newborns void in the first 24 hours after birth and 5 to 20 times thereafter.

6 The nurse who is trying to prevent heat loss in the newborn recalls that which physical characteristics serve to increase a newborn's loss of heat? Select all that apply.

1. Infant assuming the flexed position
2. Blood vessel dilation and reddened skin
3. Limited subcutaneous fat
4. Larger body surface relative to that of an adult
5. Larger cranial bones relative to that of an adult

7 A postpartal client is bottle-feeding her newborn. The nurse should teach the client to take which actions when the baby regurgitates small amounts of formula? Select all that apply.

1. Measure temperature by tympanic route.
2. Recognize this as a normal occurrence.
3. Discontinue feedings for six to eight hours.
4. Report this immediately to the pediatrician.
5. Understand that this may result from overfeeding.

8 A mother recently gave birth to her second child and began breastfeeding in the LDRP (labor, delivery, recovery, postpartum) suite. What would be an appropriate suggestion for the nurse to make?

1. Bottle-feed the baby between breastfeeding sessions
2. Routinely use plastic-lined nipple shields
3. Impose time limits for breastfeeding sessions
4. Offer both breasts at each feeding

9 A postpartal client has decided to bottle-feed her infant. The nurse would teach the client that which of the following is an acceptable guideline for the use and storage of canned formula?

1. Powdered formulas are the least expensive but must be refrigerated.
2. Tap water in cities is clean and need not be sterilized for preparing infant formula.
3. Refrigerating unused portions of the infant's formula after feeding is a good practice.
4. Unused formula in an opened can should be discarded after 48 hours.

10 The nurse is assisting a new mother in breastfeeding. The mother asks how she will know if her infant is getting anything from her breasts. The nurse responds that which of the following is the best indicator that the infant is getting breast milk?

1. Very loud burping after five minutes at the first breast
2. Finishing both breasts within three to five minutes
3. Audible swallowing
4. Sleeping four hours between feedings

➤ *See pages 250–251 for Answers and Rationales.*

ANSWERS & RATIONALES

Pretest

1 **Answer: 4** **Rationale:** This finding is normal. No further action is required. The newborn head measurement will be greater than or equal to the chest measurement. **Cognitive Level:** Analyzing **Client Need:** Health Promotion and Maintenance **Integrated Process:** Nursing Process: Implementation **Content Area:** Maternal-Newborn **Strategy:** The focus in the question is normal assessment findings. The correct answer would be the option that contains accurate documentation of the information with no additional action. **Reference:** Ladewig, P. A., London, M. L., & Davidson, M. R. (2010). *Contemporary maternal-newborn nursing care* (7th ed.). Upper Saddle River, NJ: Pearson Education, pp. 598–599.

2 **Answer: 4** **Rationale:** A Babinski reflex is elicited by stroking the lateral aspect of the sole of the heel upward and across the ball of the foot. A positive test (in newborns) of fanning the toes and dorsiflexing the big toe is an indicator of fetal well-being. Touching the corner of the mouth or cheeks elicits the rooting reflex. Changing the newborn's equilibrium elicits the Moro reflex. Placing a finger in the palm of the newborn's hand elicits the palmar grasp reflex. **Cognitive Level:** Applying **Client Need:** Health Promotion and Maintenance **Integrated Process:** Nursing Process: Implementation **Content Area:** Maternal-Newborn **Strategy:** Recall that the Babinski reflex involves a response of the newborn's foot. Eliminate the options that do not include assessment of the foot. **Reference:** Ladewig, P. A., London, M. L., & Davidson, M. R. (2010). *Contemporary maternal-newborn nursing care* (7th ed.). Upper Saddle River, NJ: Pearson Education, p. 615.

3 **Answer: 3** **Rationale:** Cephalhematoma is a collection of blood between the skull bone and periosteum. Caput succedaneum is swelling of tissue over the presenting part of the fetal head caused by pressure during labor. Molding is an overlapping of cranial bones or shaping of the fetal head to accommodate the bony and soft parts of the birth canal during labor. Subdural hematoma refers to bleeding between the dural and arachnoid membranes. **Cognitive Level:** Applying **Client Need:** Health Promotion and Maintenance **Integrated Process:** Teaching and Learning **Content Area:** Maternal-Newborn **Strategy:** Recall the definition of cephalohematoma to aid in answering this question. **Reference:** Ladewig, P. A., London, M.L., & Davidson, M.R. (2010). *Contemporary maternal-newborn nursing care* (7th ed.). Upper Saddle River, NJ: Pearson Education, p. 603.

4 **Answer: 3** **Rationale:** The normal range is 110–160 beats/min. The rate varies with activity, increasing to 160 while crying and decreasing to 110 while in deep sleep. Bradycardia—rates below 110, and tachycardia—rates above 160, are not normal and require further evaluation and intervention. **Cognitive Level:** Analyzing **Client Need:** Health Promotion and Maintenance **Integrated Process:**

POSTTEST

ANSWERS & RATIONALES

Nursing Process: Assessment **Content Area:** Maternal-Newborn **Strategy:** The focus of the question is normal assessment findings. Incorrect options can be eliminated because they contain abnormal findings. **Reference:** Ladewig, P. A., London, M. L., & Davidson, M. R. (2010). *Contemporary maternal-newborn nursing care* (7th ed.). Upper Saddle River, NJ: Pearson Education, pp. 566–567.

5 **Answer: 3 Rationale:** After 12 hours, edema of tissues present in most newborns begin to resolve and creases appear; these creases do not have the same predictive value as those assessed before resolution of newborn edema. Breast tissue enlargement, posture, and angle of the Scarf sign remain predictive beyond the first 12 hours after birth. **Cognitive Level:** Applying **Client Need:** Health Promotion and Maintenance **Integrated Process:** Nursing Process: Assessment **Content Area:** Maternal-Newborn **Strategy:** This question is time related. The correct answer would be the option that contains a true statement for this period of time after birth. Knowledge of normal newborn care is essential to answer the question correctly. **Reference:** Ladewig, P. A., London, M. L., & Davidson, M. R. (2010). *Contemporary maternal-newborn nursing care* (7th ed.). Upper Saddle River, NJ: Pearson Education, p. 591.

6 **Answer: 2 Rationale:** These symptoms reflect cold stress and require the temperature to be taken immediately. These symptoms are not associated with bleeding from the umbilical stump, congenital abnormalities, or respiratory distress. **Cognitive Level:** Analyzing **Client Need:** Health Promotion and Maintenance **Integrated Process:** Nursing Process: Assessment **Content Area:** Maternal-Newborn **Strategy:** The focus of the question is abnormal findings related to cold stress. The critical word in the stem is *cyanotic*. The correct answer would be the option that contains a true assessment for cold stress. **Reference:** Ladewig, P. A., London, M. L., & Davidson, M. R. (2010). *Contemporary maternal-newborn nursing care* (7th ed.). Upper Saddle River, NJ: Pearson Education, pp. 765–766.

7 **Answer: 4 Rationale:** Periodic breathing with no color or heart rate changes is normal in the newborn adapting to extrauterine life. The nurse provides verbal reassurance and also physical reassurance by his or her presence. Stating there's nothing to worry about and the nurse will watch the infant does not reassure the mother and confirms the mother's fears. Stating it's normal provides information but does not address the mother's subjective sense of fear. **Cognitive Level:** Analyzing **Client Need:** Health Promotion and Maintenance **Integrated Process:** Communication and Documentation **Content Area:** Maternal-Newborn **Strategy:** Use of therapeutic communication techniques is the key to answering communication questions. The correct answer is the one that provides factual information and also addresses the client's concern or worry. **Reference:** Ladewig, P. A., London, M. L., & Davidson, M. R. (2010). *Contemporary maternal-newborn nursing care* (7th ed.). Upper Saddle River, NJ: Pearson Education, pp. 564–565.

8 **Answer: 1, 5 Rationale:** Keeping the infant close with head elevated is an optimal position for bottle-feeding. Keeping the nipple full of formula prevents the infant from sucking air. Propping the bottle and enlarging the nipple hole can cause aspiration of formula. Pointing the bottle at the infant's tongue could cause the infant to gag and vomit. **Cognitive Level:** Analyzing **Client Need:** Health Promotion and Maintenance **Integrated Process:** Nursing Process: Evaluation **Content Area:** Maternal-Newborn **Strategy:** The question is worded positively, indicating that the correct options are also correct actions. Use principles related to prevention of aspiration to help make your selections. **Reference:** Ladewig, P. A., London, M. L., & Davidson, M. R. (2010). *Contemporary maternal-newborn nursing care* (7th ed.). Upper Saddle River, NJ: Pearson Education, pp. 683–687.

9 **Answer: 2 Rationale:** Discomfort while breastfeeding is almost always caused by improper latch-on. Removing the infant from the breast and repositioning with proper position can reduce the discomfort. Having the mother pump and give the breast milk from a bottle can interfere with the breastfeeding process and may cause nipple confusion. Giving the mother a nipple shield to wear and having the mother breastfeed from the uninjured nipple will not solve poor latch-on, and feeding from one breast will cause engorgement in the other breast. **Cognitive Level:** Applying **Client Need:** Health Promotion and Maintenance **Integrated Process:** Nursing Process: Planning **Content Area:** Maternal-Newborn **Strategy:** The focus of the question is nipple discomfort, commonly caused by poor positioning of the newborn while feeding. The correct answer would be the option that contains a true statement aimed at correct positioning of the infant. **Reference:** Ladewig, P. A., London, M. L., & Davidson, M. R. (2010). *Contemporary maternal-newborn nursing care* (7th ed.). Upper Saddle River, NJ: Pearson Education, pp. 870–876.

10 **Answer: 1 Rationale:** Breast milk will not protect the baby from all illnesses. Lactoferrin (a whey protein in human milk) inhibits the growth of iron-dependent bacteria in the GI tract together with secretory IgA (another whey protein in human milk), which protects against respiratory and GI bacteria, viral organisms, and allergies. Breast milk does have other enzymes and proteins that protect the infant from illness. **Cognitive Level:** Applying **Client Need:** Health Promotion and Maintenance **Integrated Process:** Communication and Documentation **Content Area:** Maternal-Newborn **Strategy:** The wording of the question indicates the correct option is also a true statement of fact. Knowledge of breastfeeding will aid in answering the question correctly. **Reference:** Ladewig, P. A., London, M. L., & Davidson, M. R. (2010). *Contemporary maternal-newborn nursing care* (7th ed.). Upper Saddle River, NJ: Pearson Education, pp. 579–580, 710.

Posttest

1 **Answer: 2 Rationale:** The foramen ovale is an opening between the right and left atria that should close shortly after birth so the newborn will not have a murmur or mixed blood traveling through the vascular system. The open umbilical vein, patent ductus arteriosus, and patent ductus venosus are incorrect as they do not connect the right and left atria. **Cognitive Level:** Analyzing **Client Need:** Physiological Adaptation **Integrated Process:** Nursing Process: Assessment **Content Area:** Maternal-Newborn **Strategy:** The critical words in question are *right and left auricles*. The correct answer is the option that contains a structure located between the right and left atria of the heart. **Reference:** Ladewig, P. A., London, M. L., & Davidson, M. R. (2010). *Contemporary maternal-newborn nursing care* (7th ed.). Upper Saddle River, NJ: Pearson Education, pp. 565, 740–743.

2 **Answer: 3 Rationale:** One of the nursing goals of newborn care during the first few hours after birth is to identify actual and potential problems that might require immediate attention. Facilitating development of relationships, assisting in developing health attitudes about childrearing practices, and providing information about well-baby programs are considered to be continuing care goals. All of these should be the focus after the initial goals are met. **Cognitive Level:** Applying **Client Need:** Health Promotion and Maintenance **Integrated Process:** Nursing Process: Planning **Content Area:** Maternal-Newborn **Strategy:** This question is time related. The transition period occurs in the first four hours after birth when the newborn transition to extrauterine life is most critical. The correct answer would be the option that contains an action to ensure assessment and safety during this critical period of adjustment. **Reference:** Ladewig, P. A., London, M. L., & Davidson, M. R. (2010). *Contemporary maternal-newborn nursing care* (7th ed.). Upper Saddle River, NJ: Pearson Education, p. 567.

3 **Answer: 1, 4, 5 Rationale:** The usual position of the infant is partially flexed and all movements should be symmetrical. Any weak, absent, asymmetrical, or fine jumping movements suggest nervous system disorders and indicate the need for further evaluation. Common reflexes found in the normal newborn include the Babinski (or plantar), which is fanning, and hyperextension of the toes when the sole is stroked upward from the heel toward the ball of the foot and the grasping reflex, elicited by stimulating the newborn to grasp on an object by touching the palm of the hand. **Cognitive Level:** Applying **Client Need:** Health Promotion and Maintenance **Integrated Process:** Nursing Process: Assessment **Content Area:** Maternal-Newborn **Strategy:** This question is worded as a negative statement. The correct answer would be the options that contain abnormal assessment findings that warrant further investigation. **Reference:** Ladewig, P. A., London, M. L., & Davidson, M. R. (2010). *Contemporary maternal-newborn nursing care* (7th ed.). Upper Saddle River, NJ: Pearson Education, pp. 592–596.

4 **Answer: 1 Rationale:** Uric acid crystals in the urine may produce the reddish "brick dust" stain on the diaper. Mucus and urate do not produce a stain. Bilirubin and iron in the urine occur with hepatic adaptation. **Cognitive Level:** Analyzing **Client Need:** Health Promotion and Maintenance **Integrated Process:** Nursing Process: Assessment **Content Area:** Maternal-Newborn **Strategy:** The focus of the question is a colored stain in the diaper. The correct answer would be the option that contains a true statement. Incorrect options can be eliminated because these substances do not leave a red stain in the diaper. **Reference:** Ladewig, P. A., London, M. L., & Davidson, M. R. (2010). *Contemporary maternal-newborn nursing care* (7th ed.). Upper Saddle River, NJ: Pearson Education, pp. 578–579.

5 **Answer: 3 Rationale:** The newborn cannot limit the invading organism at the port of entry. The other options are true adaptations in other body systems. **Cognitive Level:** Applying **Client Need:** Health Promotion and Maintenance **Integrated Process:** Nursing Process: Planning **Content Area:** Maternal-Newborn **Strategy:** Because the question is worded in a positive manner, the correct answer would be the option that contains a true statement about adaptation in the immune system of the newborn. Eliminate incorrect options as they do not contain information related to immune function. **Reference:** Ladewig, P. A., London, M. L., & Davidson, M. R. (2010). *Contemporary maternal-newborn nursing care* (7th ed.). Upper Saddle River, NJ: Pearson Education, pp. 579–580.

6 **Answer: 2, 3, 4 Rationale:** The flexed position of the term infant decreases the surface area exposed to the environment, thereby reducing heat loss. Blood vessels are closer to the skin than in an adult and constrict when exposed to cooler temperatures. Limited subcutaneous fat will increase a newborn's heat loss. Larger body surface than an adult increases the newborn's heat loss. The size of the cranial bones has no effect on heat loss. **Cognitive Level:** Analyzing **Client Need:** Health Promotion and Maintenance **Integrated Process:** Nursing Process: Assessment **Content Area:** Maternal-Newborn **Strategy:** The focus of the question is conservation of heat in the newborn. Eliminate incorrect options that either conserve heat or have no effect on heat loss. **Reference:** Ladewig, P. A., London, M. L., & Davidson, M. R. (2010). *Contemporary maternal-newborn nursing care* (7th ed.). Upper Saddle River, NJ: Pearson Education, pp. 765–766.

7 **Answer: 2, 5 Rationale:** Small amounts of regurgitation of formula are common, often caused by "overfeeding" or an immature cardiac sphincter. Regurgitation of formula is not necessarily a sign of infection, or a reason to take a temperature, or discontinue a feeding. Vomiting, forceful, or persistent expulsion of formula should be further investigated. **Cognitive Level:** Applying **Client Need:** Health Promotion and Maintenance **Integrated Process:** Nursing

Process: Planning **Content Area:** Maternal-Newborn **Strategy:** Because the wording in the stem of the question is positive, the correct options will all be true statements. Knowledge of normal newborn care related to bottle-feeding will aid in answering this question correctly. **Reference:** Ladewig, P. A., London, M. L., & Davidson, M. R. (2010). *Contemporary maternal-newborn nursing care* (7th ed.). Upper Saddle River, NJ: Pearson Education, p. 577.

8 **Answer: 4 Rationale:** Mothers are encouraged to offer both breasts to the infant in the beginning for simultaneous stimulation, but it is not imperative nor harmful if the infant does not feed off of one breast at a session. Giving supplemental feedings can upset the natural supply and demand and can shorten the breastfeeding experience. Prolonged exposure to plastic liners or wet nursing pads may result in skin breakdown. Time limits should not be imposed on breastfeeding infants as they each have different styles of suckling. **Cognitive Level:** Applying **Client Need:** Health Promotion and Maintenance **Integrated Process:** Nursing Process: Implementation **Content Area:** Maternal-Newborn **Strategy:** The question is worded in a positive manner, so the correct option is a true statement. Knowledge of breastfeeding will aid in answering this question correctly. **Reference:** Ladewig, P. A., London, M. L., & Davidson, M. R. (2010). *Contemporary maternal-newborn nursing care* (7th ed.). Upper Saddle River, NJ: Pearson Education, pp. 675–679.

9 **Answer: 1 Rationale:** Opened cans of formula must be used within a 24-hour period. There are no nutrients in whole milk that can enhance formula. The least expensive option is powdered formula but it must be properly prepared and stored. Tap water is not always safe. Any formula not taken by the infant should be disposed of as bacteria from the infant's mouth can enter the bottle and contaminate the remaining formula. **Cognitive Level:** Applying **Client Need:** Health Promotion and Maintenance **Integrated Process:** Teaching and Learning **Content Area:** Maternal-Newborn **Strategy:** The correct answer would be an option that contains a true statement about a point of client education. Recall contraindications for storage of infant formulas to aid in answering the question correctly. **Reference:** Ladewig, P. A., London, M. L., & Davidson, M. R. (2010). *Contemporary maternal-newborn nursing care* (7th ed.). Upper Saddle River, NJ: Pearson Education, pp. 683–687.

10 **Answer: 3 Rationale:** Audible swallowing during a feeding produces sounds heard as a soft "ka" or "ah." Burping is related to how much air the infant swallows during feedings Newborns usually spend 15 to 20 minutes at the breast in the first few weeks. Some older infants may be able to finish a feeding in three to five minutes. Because breast milk is more digestible than formula, and a newborn's stomach is small, feeding is usually needed more frequently than every four hours. Frequent feedings are important in the early days to establish lactation. **Cognitive Level:** Analyzing **Client Need:** Health Promotion and Maintenance **Integrated Process:** Nursing Process: Implementation **Content Area:** Maternal-Newborn **Strategy:** Because the question is worded in a positive manner, the correct option is a true statement. Knowledge of breastfeeding will aid in answering the question correctly. **Reference:** Ladewig, P. A., London, M. L., & Davidson, M. R. (2010). *Contemporary maternal-newborn nursing care* (7th ed.). Upper Saddle River, NJ: Pearson Education, pp. 657–679.

References

Davidson, M., London, M., & Ladewig, P. (2012). *Olds' maternal newborn nursing & women's health across the lifespan* (9th ed.). Upper Saddle River, NJ: Pearson Education.

Ladewig, P., London, M., & Davidson, M. (2009). *Contemporary maternal-newborn nursing care* (7th ed.). Upper Saddle River, NJ: Pearson Education.

Perry, S.E., Hockenberry, M. J., Lowdermilk, D. L., & Wilson, D. (2010). *Maternal child nursing care* (4th ed.). St. Louis, MO: Mosby.

Ricci, S. (2009). *Essentials of maternity, newborn, and women's health nursing* (2nd ed.). Philadelphia: Lippincott Williams & Wilkins.

13 The Complicated Newborn Experience

Chapter Outline

Nursing Care of High-Risk Newborn
Problems Related to Maturity
Problems Related to Size
Problems Related to Birth Trauma
General Care of the Neonate Experiencing Respiratory Distress
Congenital Infections
Cold Stress
Hyperbilirubinemia
Hypoglycemia
Infant of a Diabetic Mother (IDM)
Substance Abuse

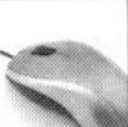

NCLEX-RN® Test Prep

Use the accompanying online resource, NursingReviewsandRationales, to test yourself with hundreds of NCLEX®-style practice questions.

Objectives

- Describe nursing assessments that identify the high-risk newborn.
- Discuss nursing interventions for the newborn with problems related to maturity or size.
- Identify the components of nursing care for the newborn experiencing birth trauma.
- Relate the consequences of maternal infections to the care of the newborn.
- Identify nursing actions to prevent cold stress in the newborn.
- Differentiate between physiologic and pathologic jaundice.
- Identify nursing responsibilities in the care of newborns receiving phototherapy.
- Discuss nursing care of the newborn experiencing respiratory distress.
- Describe the components of care for the infant of a diabetic mother.
- Relate the consequences of maternal substance abuse to the care of the newborn.

Review at a Glance

bronchopulmonary dysplasia (BPD) chronic pulmonary disease occurring in infants whose lungs require supplemental oxygen

continuous positive airway pressure (CPAP) pressurized air delivered to lungs to keep them expanded during exhalation

exchange transfusion replacement of 70 to 80% of circulating blood by withdrawing recipient's blood and injecting donor's blood in equal amounts

extracorporeal membrane oxygenation (ECMO) prolonged heart–lung bypass to allow lungs to heal

intrauterine growth restriction (IUGR) fetal undergrowth from any cause

intraventricular hemorrhage (IVH) bleeding into ventricle in brain, causing increased intracranial pressure

kernicterus damage to brain tissue caused by very high levels of bilirubin in blood

meconium aspiration syndrome (MAS) respiratory disease of term, postterm, and SGA neonates caused by inhalation of meconium into lungs

necrotizing enterocolitis (NEC) acute gastrointestinal disorder in a hypoxic neonate

neutral thermal environment an environment that provides for minimal heat loss or expenditure

oxygen hood method of delivering oxygen through a plastic hood placed over infant's head

phototherapy treatment of infants with hyperbilirubinemia by exposing them to bright lights called *bililights*

retinopathy of prematurity (ROP) formation of fibrotic tissue behind lens of eye causing blindness; associated with preterm infants who require high supplemental oxygen levels

respiratory distress syndrome (RDS) respiratory disease that affects premature babies; caused by lack of surfactant

transient tachypnea of the newborn (TTN) respiratory distress in a term infant related to delayed absorption of fluid in lungs from delivery

umbilical artery line (UAL) catheter threaded through umbilical artery; used to monitor blood pressure, give IV fluids and obtain blood samples

umbilical venous line (UVL) catheter threaded through umbilical vein; used to obtain blood samples and give IV fluids and medications

PRETEST

1 The nurse is admitting a neonate two hours after delivery. Which assessment data should the nurse be concerned about? Select all that apply.

1. Hands and feet blue with otherwise pink color
2. Bilateral nasal flaring
3. Minimal response to verbal stimulation
4. Apical heart rate 140–156
5. Chest retractions

2 Of the following nursing diagnoses for a high-risk newborn, which requires the most immediate intervention by the nurse?

1. Acute Pain related to frequent heel sticks
2. Imbalanced Nutrition: Less Than Body Requirements related to limited oral intake
3. Ineffective Airway Clearance related to pulmonary secretions
4. Deficient Knowledge related to infant care needs

3 On admission to the nursery it is noted that the mother's membranes were ruptured for 48 hours before delivery and her temperature is 102°F (38.9°C). What information from this newborn's assessment should the nurse evaluate further?

1. Temperature instability
2. Irregular respiratory rate
3. Jitteriness
4. Excessive bruising of presenting part

4 The nurse would take which action as part of nursing care of the infant experiencing neonatal abstinence syndrome?

1. Place stuffed animals and mobiles in the crib to provide visual stimulation.
2. Position the baby's crib in a quiet corner of the nursery.
3. Avoid the use of pacifiers.
4. Spend extra time holding and rocking the baby.

5 A mother was diagnosed with gonorrhea immediately after delivery. When providing nursing care for the infant, what is an important goal of the nurse?

1. Prevent the development of ophthalmia neonatorum.
2. Lubricate the eyes.
3. Prevent the development of thrush.
4. Teach the danger of breastfeeding with gonorrhea.

6 A full-term newborn weighed 10 pounds, 5 ounces at birth. What would be a priority nursing diagnosis for this infant?

1. Ineffective Thermoregulation related to lack of subcutaneous fat
2. Risk for Injury related to macrosomia
3. Impaired Gas Exchange related to lack of surfactant
4. Deficient Knowledge related to newborn care

PRETEST

7 The nurse finds the mother of a 28 weeks' gestation infant crying in her room. The mother states, "I just know my baby is going to die." What is the most therapeutic response by the nurse?

1. "I know this seems overly optimistic, but it is likely that everything will be fine."
2. "Why do you think that?"
3. "You seem very worried about what will happen to your baby."
4. "My baby was born at 27 weeks and he is fine now."

8 A nurse is admitting an infant of a diabetic mother (IDM). At 1 hour of age, the nurse notices that the newborn is very jittery. Which action by the nurse is most appropriate?

1. Begin oxygen by nasal cannula.
2. Assess the newborn's blood glucose.
3. Place the newborn under a radiant warmer.
4. Initiate use of a cardiac/apnea monitor.

9 A newborn's temperature is 97.4°F. What is the priority nursing intervention by the nurse?

1. Notify the health care provider immediately.
2. Take the newborn to the nursery and observe for two hours.
3. Reassess the temperature in four hours.
4. Wrap the newborn in two warm blankets and place a cap on the head.

10 A nurse is assessing a neonate born 12 hours ago and notes a yellow tint to the sclera. The nurse should read the medical record for what other assessment that is important to note at this time?

1. Blood glucose level
2. Blood type and Rh factor of both mother and newborn
3. Most recent infant blood pressure
4. Length of time membranes ruptured prior to delivery

➤ *See pages 275–276 for Answers and Rationales.*

I. NURSING CARE OF HIGH-RISK NEWBORN

A. Assessments that identify high-risk newborns

1. Certain prenatal and intrapartal risk factors will increase risk of a neonate experiencing complications after delivery
   a. Maternal preexisting diabetes mellitus or development of gestational diabetes during pregnancy; a primary concern in infants of diabetic mothers (IDM) is hypoglycemia after delivery
   b. Mother received opioid analgesics/anesthetics during labor, especially systemically and immediately before delivery; opioids cross placenta and can cause respiratory depression in neonate after delivery
   c. Fetal asphyxia causes fetus to pass meconium into amniotic fluid, which could be aspirated during delivery; common causes of fetal asphyxia include placental insufficiency, prolapsed cord, placental abruption, and placenta previa
   d. Difficult or prolonged labor, which increases risk of birth trauma
   e. Multiple gestation pregnancy
   f. Preterm or postterm delivery
   g. Life-threatening congenital anomalies
   h. Maternal or neonatal infection
   i. Small for gestational age (SGA) or large for gestational age (LGA)
2. ! Apgar scores: an Apgar score of less than 6 at 1 minute or 7 at 5 minutes indicates neonate is not making a satisfactory transition to extrauterine life and requires careful monitoring
3. ! Changes in physical assessment are often vague, so a thorough assessment is essential (see Box 13-1)

Box 13-1

Critical Neonatal Assessment Indicators

The appearance of any of these signs in a neonate could indicate the presence of a serious complication:

- Respiratory: bradypnea or tachypnea, respiratory distress, weak or absent respiratory effort
- Cardiovascular: bradycardia or tachycardia, murmur
- Neuromuscular: lethargy, temperature instability, tremors, unusual behaviors such as lip-smacking
- Gastrointestinal: poor feeding tolerance, poor suck/swallow reflex
- Skin color: cyanosis (acrocyanosis is normal for the first 24 to 48 hours after delivery), jaundice (especially within the first 24 hours)
- Obvious major anomalies

4. Gestational age
   a. Gestational age less than 37 weeks' gestation based on due date
   b. Perform a quick assessment if due date is unknown; follow up with a thorough gestational age assessment as soon as possible
      1) Eyelids fused until 26 weeks' gestation
      2) Creases cover a third of soles of feet at 36 weeks' gestation
      3) Breast buds are absent until 37 weeks' gestation
      4) Ear cartilage has little recoil until 30 weeks' gestation
      5) Vernix caseosa covers body by 31 to 33 weeks' gestation
      6) Lanugo covers shoulders by 33 to 36 weeks' gestation

B. General planning and implementation for all high-risk newborns

1. Constantly monitor infant for subtle changes in condition and intervene promptly when necessary
   a. Decrease risk of nosocomial infections; each neonate should have his or her own supplies; practicing effective hand hygiene is most important method of preventing infection
   b. Conserve infant's energy and decrease physiologic stress by organizing care and minimizing interruptions; monitor each neonate for signs of stress
   c. Provide appropriate stimulation for infant growth and development; high-risk neonates have same developmental needs as healthy neonates

Practice to Pass

An infant's pulse oximeter alarms with a saturation of 78%. What should the nurse do first?

2. Common procedures/tests/equipment
   a. Pulse oximeter
      1) Estimates arterial oxygen saturation through a sensor placed on skin
         a) Sensor should be placed on palm of hand, sole of foot, or wrapped around finger

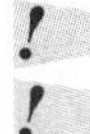

         b) Assess skin integrity at sensor site every 4 hours and rotate site every 12 hours
      2) Pulse oximeter reading of 90% or higher reflects safe clinical range
   b. Arterial blood gas (ABG)
      1) Direct measurement of amount of oxygen, carbon dioxide, and bicarbonate in a sample of arterial blood by arterial puncture or from umbilical artery line (UAL)
      2) Compare oximeter reading at time blood sample obtained to correlate values

      3) Apply pressure to puncture site for three to five minutes if obtained by arterial puncture
   c. Blood glucose monitoring (Dextrostick, Accucheck)

      1) Warm foot prior to obtaining blood sample to increase circulation
      2) Lance heel to obtain blood sample; this test is performed at bedside; heel is preferred site (see Figure 13-1)

Figure 13-1

Newborn heel sticks

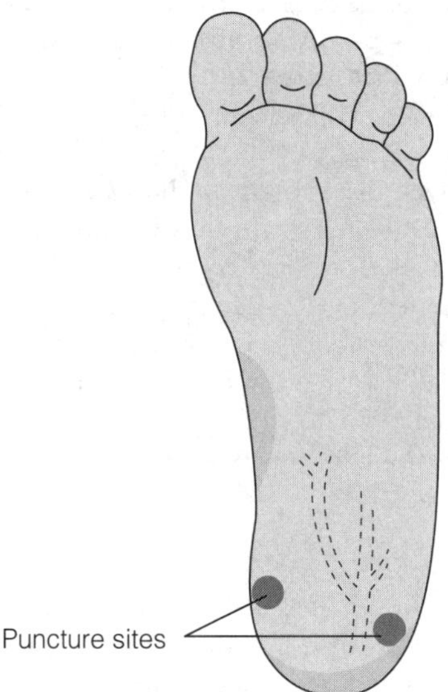

d. Umbilical lines
   1) An **umbilical arterial line (UAL)** is inserted into an umbilical artery and is used primarily to obtain arterial blood gases
   2) An **umbilical venous line (UVL)** is inserted into umbilical vein and can be used for IV fluids, medications and to obtain blood for laboratory tests
   3) All infants with umbilical lines should be closely assessed for blue discoloration or blanching on lower extremities or buttocks, which could indicate an embolus or vasospasm and may necessitate removal of line
   4) Assess closely for line placement, bleeding from umbilicus or disconnected tubing; position infant in a side-lying or prone position for close monitoring

e. Oxygen administration
   1) Oxygen can be administered by **oxygen hood** (hood placed over infant's head), nasal cannula, **continuous positive airway pressure (CPAP)** (pressurized air), or endotracheal tube (ET)
   2) Oxygen should be warmed and humidified prior to administration to decrease insensible fluid loss and heat loss
   3) Monitor amount of oxygen being administered and oxygen saturation and/or ABGs; it is important to administer minimum amount of oxygen to meet infant's oxygen needs to prevent complications

f. Gavage tubes
   1) Used to decompress stomach or to administer formula, breast milk, or oral medications
   2) It is preferred to insert tube orally instead of nasally because infants are obligate nose-breathers
   3) A 5 Fr. or 8 Fr. tube is commonly used; measure tube from earlobe to nose and then to tip of xyphoid process; insert tube and secure placement
   4) Check placement of tube prior to administering any feeding or medication; feedings should be administered over three to five minutes to avoid dumping syndrome; offer a pacifier during feeding

3. Parenting the high-risk newborn
   a. Parents are initially in a state of shock and disbelief and may grieve loss of the "perfect baby" that they fantasized about during pregnancy

b. Priority nursing diagnoses for parents of high-risk infants: Compromised Family Coping; Deficient Knowledge; Anticipatory Grieving; Powerlessness; Social Isolation
c. Planning and intervention
   1) Assess bonding
   2) Explain equipment and infant's condition
   3) Present positive, realistic attitude and establish trust
   4) Encourage parents to touch infant and perform care-taking activities as infant's condition allows
   5) Encourage parents to verbalize feelings
   6) Teach parents care of infant in preparation for discharge
   7) Give instant pictures of infant to parents prior to transfer to neonatal intensive care unit (NICU)—allow parents to utilize own photo equipment with guidance
d. Evaluation: parent(s) demonstrate effective coping with newborn's situation

II. PROBLEMS RELATED TO MATURITY

A. Prematurity

1. Description: infant born before completion of 37th week of pregnancy
   a. Prognosis and severity of complications related to level of maturity: the earlier the infant is born, the greater the chance of complications
   b. Major complications are related to **respiratory distress syndrome (RDS)** (disorder caused by lack of surfactant), difficulty regulating body temperature, infection, and hemorrhage
   c. Are generally ready for discharge near their due date
2. Etiology
   a. Earliest age of viability is 23 to 24 weeks' gestation
   b. Maternal risk factors: age, smoking, poor nutrition, placental problems (placenta previa, placental abruption, preeclampsia/eclampsia), previous preterm delivery, incompetent cervix
   c. Fetal risk factors: multiple gestation pregnancy, infection
   d. Other risk factors: low socioeconomic status, environmental exposure to harmful substance(s)
3. Assessment and pathophysiology
   a. Respiratory
      1) Insufficient surfactant allows alveoli to collapse with each expiration
      2) Inadequate number and maturity of alveoli makes adequate alveolar gas exchange difficult
      3) Skeletal muscles are weak so newborn may not be able to reposition head and body to maintain patent airway
      4) Signs of respiratory distress typically develop within one to two hours after delivery (see Box 13-2)
      5) Respiratory failure is most common cause of death in preterm infants within first 72 hours of life
   b. Cardiovascular
      1) Incomplete muscular coat of pulmonary blood vessels
      2) Lowered pulmonary resistance increases left-to-right shunting
      3) Patent ductus arteriosus causes pulmonary congestion, increased respiratory effort, CO_2 retention, and bounding femoral pulses
   c. Temperature regulation
      1) Lack of subcutaneous fat to insulate body
      2) Large body surface area in proportion to body weight, so more likely to lose heat faster

Box 13-2

Signs of Neonatal Respiratory Distress

- Tachypnea
- Intercostal and/or subcostal retractions
- Nasal flaring
- Expiratory grunting
- Seesaw respiratory movements
- Diminished breath sounds
- PaO_2 less than 50 mm Hg
- PCO_2 above 60 mm Hg
- Increasing exhaustion
- Cyanosis (late finding)

3) Small muscle mass
4) Absent sweat or shiver mechanisms
5) Increased insensible fluid loss
6) Increased risk of hypothermia

d. Low resistance to infection
1) Lack of immunoglobulins from mother (these usually cross placenta during third trimester)
2) Difficulty localizing infection and poor WBC response
3) Increased risk of infection

e. Hematopoietic: bruises easily related to fragile capillaries and prolonged prothrombin time

f. Hepatic
1) Increased risk of hyperbilirubinemia related to immature liver and difficulty eliminating bilirubin released by normal breakdown of red blood cells
2) Decreased liver glycogen stores so infant is prone to hypoglycemia
3) Prolonged drug metabolism related to immature liver
4) Immature production of clotting factors resulting in increased risk of bleeding disorders

g. Gastrointestinal
1) Weak suck/swallow reflex until 33 to 34 weeks' gestation and poor gag/cough reflexes increase risk of aspiration
2) Increased risk of **necrotizing enterocolitis (NEC)**, a serious neonatal inflammation of intestines related to immature GI system and hypoxia

h. Renal
1) Unable to concentrate urine effectively increasing risk of dehydration
2) Prolonged drug excretion time related to immature kidneys

i. Neuromuscular
1) Immature control of vital functions
2) Increased risk of **intraventricular hemorrhage (IVH)**, which is bleeding into ventricles of brain
3) Increased risk of apnea
4) Poor muscle tone
5) Weak or absent reflexes
6) Weak, feeble cry

4. Priority nursing diagnoses: Impaired Gas Exchange; Ineffective Thermoregulation; Imbalanced Nutrition: Less Than Body Requirements

5. Planning and implementation

a. Respiratory
1) Maintain respirations at 30 to 60/min, assess every 1 to 2 h and prn

2) Assess oxygenation and administer O_2 as ordered
  a) Auscultate breath sounds
  b) Monitor for signs of respiratory distress
  c) Suction prn
  d) Monitor oxygen saturation and/or arterial blood gases
3) Position with head slightly elevated in supine position; prone position may also be used to facilitate chest expansion

b. Thermoregulation
1) Maintain **neutral thermal environment** (temperature that prevents heat loss) and prevent cold stress
  a) Place infant under radiant warmer or in double-wall isolette
  b) Warm oxygen, equipment, and linen before contact with infant
  c) Generally, infant can be weaned to an open bassinet when his or her temperature is stable and infant is gaining weight
  d) Ensure infant remains dry
2) Assess infant's temperature q 2 to 3 hours and prn; may use skin probe

c. Monitor for signs of sepsis (changes in behavior, temperature variations, difficulty feeding, tachycardia)

d. Feeding
1) Feed according to abilities
2) Assess tolerance of feedings
  a) Monitor suck/swallow reflex to assess risk of aspiration; if poor, gavage feed as indicated
  b) Use "preemie" nipple if bottle feeding; burp frequently
  c) Assess for abdominal distention and emesis, which could indicate that neonate is not tolerating feedings
3) Monitor intake and output (I&O), daily weight; assess for dehydration

e. Monitor for hypoglycemia
f. Monitor for hyperbilirubinemia
g. Organize care to minimize stress
h. Provide skin care with special attention to cleanliness and careful positioning to prevent skin breakdown
i. Assess apical heart rate for 1 min q 1 to 2 h
j. Monitor potential bleeding sites (umbilicus, injection sites)
k. Monitor overall growth and development; check daily weight, measure length and occipital frontal circumference (OFC) weekly
l. Monitor closely for medication side effects caused by decreased ability to metabolize and excrete medications

6. Evaluation: infant will not develop complications related to preterm birth

7. Potential complications related to prematurity

a. Respiratory distress syndrome (RDS)
1) Also known as hyaline membrane disease; results from deficient or ineffective pulmonary surfactant production
2) Primarily associated with prematurity
3) Usually appears during first 24 to 48 hours after birth and peaks around 72 hours
4) Other predisposing factors include fetal hypoxia and postnatal hypothermia
5) Factors protecting neonate against RDS
  a) Chronic fetal stress, such as maternal hypertension and preeclampsia
  b) Prenatal administration of betamethasone to mother, which accelerates fetal lung maturity
  c) Administration of artificial surfactant (Exosurf, Survanta) in infant's airway after delivery, which helps keep alveoli from collapsing and causing atelectasis

6) At risk for **bronchopulmonary dysplasia (BPD)**, a chronic pulmonary disease in which alveolar epithelium is damaged, requiring mechanical ventilation and oxygen during first weeks of life

b. **Retinopathy of prematurity (ROP)**
   1) Etiology: multifactorial in origin; prolonged exposure to high concentrations of oxygen may cause hemorrhage within retina and lead to retinal detachment and loss of vision; other risk factors include intraventricular hemorrhage, chronic lung disease, apnea, hypoxia, sepsis, acidosis, multiple gestation, exposure to bright lights, blood transfusions; survival of very-low-birth-weight infants may be the most important factor in increased incidence of ROP
   2) All premature infants who received oxygen should be screened prior to discharge by an ophthalmologist
   3) Most cases of ROP regress spontaneously with no long-term visual impairment
   4) Treatment options may include laser photocoagulation, cryotherapy, surgical vitrectomy, or scleral buckling

c. Intraventricular hemorrhage (IVH)
   1) Etiology: rupture of thin, fragile capillaries within ventricles of brain leading to increased intracranial pressure
   2) Prematurity and hypoxia are primary risk factors
   3) Assessment: neurological changes such as hypotonia and lethargy, bulging fontanels, increasing OFC, bradycardia, apnea

d. Necrotizing enterocolitis (NEC)
   1) Etiology: decreased blood flow and perfusion to intestines because of hypoxia and hypoxemia at birth
   2) Assessment: abdominal distention, poor feeding, vomiting, blood in stool
   3) Treatment involves NPO, IV fluids and antibiotics until intestines healed

e. Apnea and bradycardia
   1) Preterm neonates are at risk for apnea related to immature regulation of vital functions; if apnea is prolonged, eventually bradycardia occurs
   2) Infants almost always go into respiratory arrest first, followed by cardiac arrest; by supporting respiratory function, heart rate should return to normal range
   3) ! If apnea occurs, first stimulate respirations with gentle tactile stimulation; if this is unsuccessful, reposition neonate and finally support respirations with a manual resuscitation bag if necessary

B. Postmaturity

1. Definition and etiology
   a. Infant born after completion of 42 weeks of pregnancy
   b. Problems are caused by progressively less efficient actions of placenta that result in decreased oxygen and impaired nutrition transport
   c. Infant is at risk for birth injury related to dystocia
   d. Placental insufficiency may occur with an aging placenta that can no longer meet needs of fetus; increases risk of fetal asphyxia, which can result in passage of meconium in utero and increased risk of **meconium aspiration syndrome (MAS)**, inhalation of meconium into lungs
2. Assessment
   a. Absence of vernix and minimal lanugo
   b. Dry, cracked skin related to metabolism of fat to meet energy needs in utero
   c. Hypoglycemia related to metabolism of glycogen to meet energy needs in utero
   d. Minimal subcutaneous fat
   e. Skin and cord yellow to green caused by meconium staining
   f. Long fingernails and often has scratches on face and trunk

3. Priority nursing diagnoses: Impaired Gas Exchange; Hypothermia; Imbalanced Nutrition: Less Than Body Requirements
4. Interventions
   ! a. Assess for hypoxia
   b. Assess for presence of meconium at delivery
   c. Assess for presence of birth injuries
   ! d. Assess for signs of hypoglycemia; monitor blood glucose
   e. Initiate early feeding
   f. Maintain a neutral thermal environment
5. Evaluation: neonate will make a successful transition to extrauterine life with stable respiratory function, temperature, blood glucose

III. PROBLEMS RELATED TO SIZE

A. Small for gestational age (SGA)

1. Definition: birth weight below 10th percentile; may have proportional or disproportional growth
2. Etiology: placental insufficiency, infections, smoking, hypertension, malnutrition, substance abusing mothers
3. Assessment
   a. Skin: loose and dry, little fat or muscle mass
   b. Little scalp hair
   c. Hypoglycemia
   d. Weak cry
4. Priority nursing diagnoses: Hypothermia; Impaired Gas Exchange; Imbalanced Nutrition: Less Than Body Requirements
5. Interventions
   ! a. Assess for presence of meconium during labor and delivery; thoroughly suction airway immediately after delivery if present
   b. Assess temperature and provide neutral thermal environment
   c. Assess for signs of hypoglycemia
   ! d. Weigh daily and assess changes in weight
6. Evaluation: infant is free of signs of respiratory distress, maintains stable temperature and blood glucose level, and gains weight

B. Large for gestational age (LGA)

1. Definition: birth weight above 90th percentile
2. Etiology
   a. Primary cause: most are unknown but most well-known is infant of diabetic mother (IDM)
   b. If preterm, at risk for respiratory distress syndrome
   c. If postterm, at risk for meconium aspiration
3. Increased risk of the following:
   a. Hyperbilirubinemia related to increased bilirubin released from damaged red blood cells secondary to traumatic delivery
   b. Hypoglycemia present in infants of diabetic mothers
   c. Polycythemia
   d. Birth injury: fractured clavicle, Erb-Duchenne paralysis secondary to shoulder dystocia
4. Assessment
   a. Measure birth weight; assessment depends on whether infant is preterm, postterm, or at term
   b. Signs of birth trauma related to size of infant
   c. Hypoglycemia, especially with an IDM

5. Priority nursing diagnosis: Risk for Injury related to size and gestational age of newborn
6. Interventions
   a. Continued assessment of birth injury; look for shoulder dystocia and fracture of clavicle
   b. Continue monitoring of blood glucose and bilirubin levels
   c. Monitor for polycythemia
   d. Educate and support family when child is bruised and injured
7. Evaluation: infant will transition to extrauterine life without birth trauma or injury

IV. PROBLEMS RELATED TO BIRTH TRAUMA

A. Facial paralysis

1. Etiology: temporary facial paralysis caused by pressure on facial nerve during delivery
2. ! Assessment: face on affected side is unresponsive when neonate cries, eye remains open, forehead will not wrinkle
3. Self-resolves within hours or days of delivery, permanent paralysis is rare
4. ! Assess and support ability to feed orally

B. Erb-Duchenne paralysis

1. Definition: brachial paralysis of upper portion of arm
2. Etiology
   a. Most common type of paralysis associated with difficult delivery
   b. Paralysis is related to stretching or pulling head away from shoulder during difficult delivery
3. Assessment
   a. ! Flaccid arm with elbow extended and hand rotated inward
   b. ! Moro reflex absent on affected side
   c. Grasp reflex intact
4. Interventions
   a. Intermittent immobilization
   b. ! Brace, splint, or pin sleeve to mattress
   c. Reposition q 2 to 3 hours
   d. ! Delay range of motion until 10th day to prevent further damage

C. Fractures

1. Etiology
   a. Clavicle is most frequently fractured bone during delivery
   b. Other bones fractured during delivery are skull, humerus, and femur
   c. Cephalopelvic disproportion (CPD) is often a predisposing factor
2. ! Assessment (fractured clavicle): assess for deformity and bruising, limited range of motion, crepitus over affected bone, and absence of Moro reflex on affected side
3. Priority nursing diagnoses: Impaired Physical Mobility; Pain
4. Interventions (fractured clavicle)
   a. ! Instruct parents to handle affected arm gently
   b. Usually self-resolves
5. Evaluation: infant will not show signs of permanent damage related to birth trauma

D. Asphyxia

1. Definition: inadequate tissue perfusion which fails to meet metabolic needs of tissues
2. Etiology
   a. Nonreassuring fetal heart rate pattern during labor (late or variable decelerations, loss of variability, bradycardia), difficult delivery, prematurity, passage of meconium in utero
   b. Initial goal is to identify neonates at risk so resuscitation can begin immediately if necessary

Figure 13-2

External cardiac massage

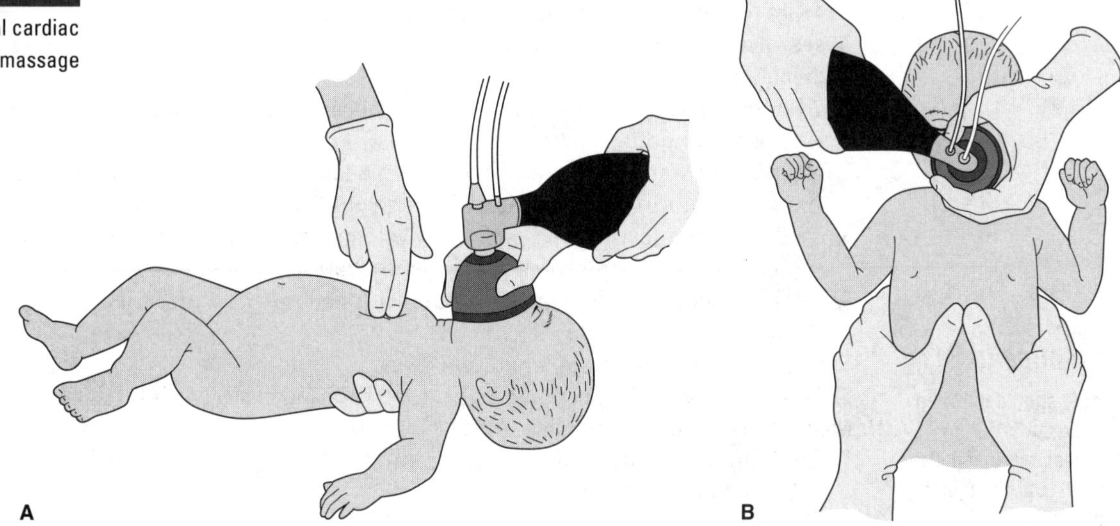

3. Assessment
   a. Fetal scalp pH during labor; 7.20 or less considered ominous sign of fetal asphyxia
   b. Apgar score of 4 to 7 indicates need for stimulation; score less than 4 indicates need for resuscitation; resuscitative efforts should begin immediately if needed
   c. Passage of meconium prior to or during delivery
4. Priority nursing diagnoses: Ineffective Breathing Pattern; Decreased Cardiac Output
5. Interventions
   a. At delivery, hold neonate in a head-down position and thoroughly suction mouth and nares
   b. Place neonate under prewarmed radiant warmer
   c. Stimulate respiratory effort by rubbing back and feet
   d. If respirations inadequate, place neonate in "sniffing" position; inflate neonate's lungs with positive pressure using bag and mask with 100% oxygen at rate of 40 to 60 breaths/min
   e. Once breathing is established, check heart rate; if heart rate is less than 60, or 60 to 80 and not increasing, begin cardiac compressions; lower third of the sternum should be compressed with two fingertips or both thumbs at rate of 100 compressions/min; a 3:1 ratio of compressions to assisted ventilation is used (see Figure 13-2)
   f. Resuscitative medications, primarily epinephrine, should be administered after 30 seconds of assisted ventilation and compressions if neonate's heart rate is not above 80 beats/min
   g. Administer naloxone (Narcan) if mother received opioid analgesics (narcotics) near time of delivery
6. Evaluation: newborn's metabolic and physiologic processes are stabilized, and recovery proceeds without complications

V. GENERAL CARE OF THE NEONATE EXPERIENCING RESPIRATORY DISTRESS

A. Common causes of respiratory distress in neonates

1. Respiratory distress syndrome (RDS); typically preterm infants
2. Meconium aspiration syndrome (MAS); typically term and postterm infants

3. **Transient tachypnea of newborn (TTN)** from delayed absorption of fluid in lungs from delivery; typically affects term and postterm infants

B. Assessment (refer back to Box 13-2)

C. Interventions

1. Maintain neutral thermal environment because of increased oxygen demand if neonate is hypothermic
2. Administer warmed, humidified oxygen as ordered, generally attempting to keep oxygen saturation greater than 90% and PaO_2 between 50 and 70 mm Hg
3. Withhold oral feedings if respiratory rate greater than 60 breaths/min because of increased risk of aspiration; notify health care provider
4. Position neonate side lying or supine with neck slightly extended ("sniffing position"); arms at sides
5. Suction prn to maintain a patent airway
6. Monitor oxygen saturation and/or arterial blood gases (ABGs) as ordered

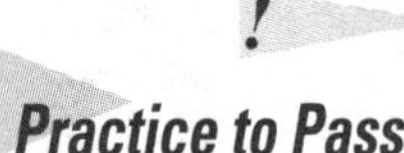

Practice to Pass

How should interventions differ during resuscitation if meconium is present in the amniotic fluid?

D. Meconium aspiration syndrome (MAS)

1. Definition: aspiration of meconium into tracheobronchial tree during first few breaths after delivery in a term neonate
2. Etiology
   a. Prenatal asphyxia causes increased fetal intestinal peristalsis, relaxation of anal sphincter and passage of meconium into amniotic fluid; this fluid may be aspirated into lungs during first few breaths after delivery
   b. Meconium in lungs produces a ball-valve action (air is allowed in but cannot be exhaled) and is irritating to airway; as lungs become hyperinflated, pulmonary perfusion decreases leading to increased hypoxia
   c. Can lead to persistent pulmonary hypertension of newborn (PPHN)
3. Assessment
   a. May demonstrate signs of fetal distress during labor and delivery
   b. Apgar score less than 6 at one and five minutes
   c. Immediate signs of respiratory distress at delivery (cyanosis, tachypnea, retractions)
   d. Overdistended, barrel-shaped chest
   e. Diminished breath sounds
   f. Yellow staining of skin, nails, and umbilical cord
4. Priority nursing diagnosis: Ineffective Gas Exchange
5. Interventions
   a. Suction oropharynx then nasopharynx after neonate's head is born and shoulders and chest are still in birth canal to remove as much meconium as possible before newborn's first breath
   b. If meconium is thick in amniotic fluid, place neonate under radiant warmer, visualize glottis, and suction any meconium from trachea before stimulating respirations
   c. Administer oxygen to maintain adequate PO_2 and oxygen saturation
   d. Anticipate need for mechanical ventilation, high-frequency ventilation or **extracorporeal membrane oxygenation (ECMO)**, which is used for prolonged heart–lung bypass to allow lungs to heal
   e. Perform chest physiotherapy routinely
6. Evaluation
   a. Risk of MAS is promptly identified and early intervention is initiated
   b. Neonate is free of respiratory distress and maintains acid–base balance

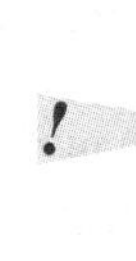

E. Transient tachypnea of newborn (TTN)

1. Etiology
   a. Failure to clear airway of excess lung fluid at delivery
   b. Primarily occurs in term infants, especially if delivered by cesarean because they have not experienced mechanical squeeze that occurs during a vaginal delivery

2. Assessment
   a. Expiratory grunting, nasal flaring, mild cyanosis
   b. Tachypnea by 6 hours of age, respiratory rate may get as high as 100 to 140 breaths/min
3. Priority nursing diagnosis: Ineffective Gas Exchange
4. Interventions
   a. Administer oxygen as needed to maintain PO_2 and oxygen saturation within normal limits
   b. Usually self resolves within 72 hours
5. Evaluation: neonate is free of respiratory distress and maintains acid–base balance

VI. CONGENITAL INFECTIONS

A. TORCH (see also Chapter 6)

1. Toxoplasmosis
   a. Etiology
      1) Caused by protozoan *Toxoplasma gondii*
      2) Contracted by eating raw or undercooked meat or contact with feces of infected cats; can be found in garden soil, maternal–fetal transmission during pregnancy
      3) Often results in spontaneous abortion if contracted during first trimester
      4) Severe neonatal disorders associated with congenital infection include seizures, coma, microcephaly, and hydrocephalus
   b. Interventions: to prevent maternal–fetal transmission, women should:
      1) Use good hand hygiene
      2) Avoid eating raw meat
      3) Avoid exposure to cat litter, garden soil, and uncovered children's sand boxes during pregnancy
      4) Have toxoplasma titer checked prenatally if cats live in household or if client is an avid gardener
2. Other infections, usually Hepatitis B (HBV)
   a. Transmitted from mother to neonate in about 90% of cases
   b. Transmitted transplacentally and by contact with blood and body fluids
   c. Infected neonates may be symptom free or have acute hepatitis, with a 75% mortality rate
   d. Infants of mothers with positive HbsAg should receive hepatitis B immune globulin (HBIG) 0.5 mL IM within first 12 hours of life; they should also receive hepatitis B vaccine, with first dose within first 12 hours of life, the second dose at 1 month and the third dose at 6 months
   e. Centers for Disease Control (CDC) recommends all women be screened prenatally for HbsAg to determine newborns at risk
3. Rubella
   a. Etiology
      1) Also called German measles
      2) Up to 20% of women of childbearing age are not rubella immune; a rubella titer of 1:8 or greater indicates immunity
      3) Eighty to ninety percent of fetuses exposed during first trimester will be affected either by spontaneous abortion or congenital anomalies
   b. Assessment: clinical signs of congenital infections are congenital heart disease, **intrauterine growth restriction (IUGR)** or fetal undergrowth, and hearing loss
   c. Interventions: infants born with congenital rubella syndrome are infectious and should be isolated

4. Cytomegalovirus (CMV)
   a. Respiratory or sexual transmission; neonate can contract during delivery through an infected birth canal
   b. Most common cause of congenital viral infection; most (90 to 95%) of these infants are asymptomatic at birth; remaining 5 to 10% may experience hemolytic anemia and jaundice, hydrocephaly or microcephaly, pneumonitis, deafness, and fetal or neonatal death
   c. Disease is usually progressive through infancy and childhood
5. Herpes (HSV)
   a. Etiology: herpes simplex virus type 1 or type 2
   b. Maternal symptoms include vesicles on genitalia, thighs, and/or buttocks that are usually painful; fetal symptoms include fever or hypothermia, jaundice, seizures, poor feeding; 50% develop vesicular skin lesions
   c. There is no known cure
   ! d. Virus can be lethal to fetus and is transmitted during birth; cesarean delivery is indicated if mother has active lesions at time of delivery
   e. Antiviral medications (famciclovir, acyclovir, valacylovir) are still under investigation for safe use during pregnancy

B. Sexually transmitted infections

1. Syphilis
   a. Etiology
      1) Caused by *treponema palladium*, a spirochete
      2) Organism crosses placenta after 16 weeks' gestation and infects fetus; Langhans' layer in chorion prevents fetal infection early in pregnancy until this layer begins to atrophy between 16 and 18 weeks' gestation
      3) There is no increased risk of anomalies, but spirochete may cause inflammatory and destructive changes in liver, spleen, kidneys, and bone marrow
      ! 4) If syphilis is untreated during pregnancy, 25% of pregnancies will end in stillbirth and 40 to 50% of neonates born to these women will have symptomatic congenital syphilis
   ! b. Assessment: clients with syphilis have a positive serologic test (VDRL)
2. Gonorrhea
   a. Causative organism is *Neisseria gonorrhea*
   b. Neonate can be exposed to organism during birth; this can result in sepsis or ophthalmia neonatorum, which can cause permanent blindness
   c. Penicillin is treatment of choice
   ! d. Eye prophylaxis with erythromycin (Ilotycin) ointment within four hours after birth can decrease risk of ophthalmia neonatorum
3. Chlamydia
   a. Most common sexually transmitted infection
   b. Caused by *Chlamydia trachomatis*
   c. Can be transmitted to neonate during delivery and cause neonatal conjunctivitis and pneumonia
   ! d. Eye prophylaxis with erythromycin ointment shortly after birth can prevent neonatal conjunctivitis; silver nitrate has been used prophylactically in past but is not effective against *Chlamydia trachomatis*
4. Candidiasis
   a. Etiology
      1) Neonatal oral yeast infection is commonly called thrush
      2) Caused by yeast normally found in vagina, most commonly *Candida albicans*

3) Excessive yeast growth occurs more commonly in sick newborns and those receiving antibiotics or steroids
4) Neonate may contract thrush during birth process or from contaminated hands or feeding equipment

b. Assessment
1) Thrush presents as white patches on oral mucosa, gums, and tongue, which cannot be manually removed and may bleed when touched
2) Occasional difficulty in swallowing

c. Priority nursing diagnoses: Pain; Imbalanced Nutrition: Less Than Body Requirements

d. Interventions
1) Antifungal medications are applied to affected area to treat infection; feed sterile water prior to administration to rinse out milk
2) Nystatin (Mycostatin) is applied to newborn's mouth with a medicine dropper or swabbed over mucosa, gums, and tongue after a feeding
3) Gentian violet may also be swabbed over mucosa, gums, and tongue, being careful to guard against staining skin, clothes, and equipment

e. Evaluation
1) Neonate's mouth is intact, lesions are healed, with no evidence of infection
2) Neonate has oral intake and maintains weight or regains weight lost, if any

5. HIV/AIDS

a. Etiology
1) During pregnancy, transmission can occur to fetus across placenta or from contaminated blood and blood products given to mother, or through semen; after delivery, can occur through breast milk
2) Maternal to newborn transmission rates are 15 to 25% without prophylactic medication; transmission rate drops to less than 2% when mothers are given zidovudine (ZDV) prenatally, deliver by elective cesarean at 38 weeks (prior to rupture of membranes) and avoid breastfeeding
3) It may take up to 15 months for infants to form own antibodies against HIV
4) HIV testing should be done at birth, 1 to 2 months of age, and at 4 to 6 months of age

b. Assessment
1) Can show signs and symptoms of disease within days of birth
2) Urinary system infections
3) Failure to thrive with developmental delays
4) Hepatomegaly and/or splenomegaly, swollen glands
5) Recurrent respiratory infections, rhinorrhea, interstitial pneumonia
6) Recurrent or persistent oral and genital candidiasis infections
7) Recurrent diarrhea, weight loss

c. Priority nursing diagnoses: Imbalanced Nutrition: Less Than Body Requirements; Risk for Impaired Skin Integrity; Risk for Infection; Impaired Physical Mobility; Impaired Growth and Development

d. Interventions
1) Use of standard precautions; specific isolation not required
2) Promote comfort
3) Keep well nourished; encourage bottle-feeding as HIV virus has been found in breast milk
4) Thorough cord care to prevent infection, prevent exposure to infections
5) The infant should receive all vaccines except oral poliovirus
6) Skin and mouth care
7) Administer zidovudine (ZDV) as ordered

e. Evaluation: potential opportunistic infections are identified early and treated promptly

C. Sepsis

1. Definition: generalized infection that has spread rapidly through bloodstream
2. Pathophysiology: immature immune system, inability to localize infection, and lack of IgM immunoglobulin, which is necessary to protect against bacteria and does not cross placenta
3. When sepsis is suspected, cultures will be obtained and antibiotics started immediately; after 72 hours of treatment, antibiotics may be discontinued if final culture reports are negative and symptoms have subsided; antibiotics will generally be continued for 10 to 14 days if final culture reports are positive
4. Etiology
   a. Prolonged rupture of membranes
   b. Long, difficult labor
   c. Resuscitation and other invasive procedures
   d. Maternal infection

   e. Beta-hemolytic streptococcal vaginosis is most common cause of neonatal sepsis and meningitis; cervical culture should be obtained prior to delivery; if positive, antibiotics given during intrapartum period decrease risk of transmission
   f. Aspiration of amniotic fluid, formula, or mucus
   g. Nosocomial: caused by infected health care workers or equipment
5. Assessment
   a. Symptoms often vague initially
   b. Temperature instability, especially hypothermia
   c. Feeding intolerance as evidenced by decreased intake, abdominal distention, vomiting, poor sucking
   d. Subtle behavior changes, "the infant just doesn't look right," lethargy, seizure activity, pallor
   e. Progressive respiratory distress
   f. Hyperbilirubinemia
   g. Tachycardia initially, followed by periods of apnea and bradycardia
6. Priority nursing diagnoses: Risk for Infection; Deficient Fluid Volume
7. Interventions

   a. Obtain cultures (blood, urine, cerebral spinal fluid) before antibiotics are initiated
   b. Administer antibiotics as ordered
   c. Observe for changes in vital signs and physical assessment
8. Evaluation
   a. Newborn will remain free from sepsis
   b. Early signs of sepsis will be recognized and appropriate therapy will be initiated
   c. If therapy is necessary, newborn will not suffer negative consequences

Practice to Pass

Your patient is HIV-positive and wants to breastfeed. She's heard that HIV-positive women in underdeveloped countries are encouraged to breastfeed and she does not understand why she is being told to bottle-feed her baby. What should the nurse tell her?

VII. COLD STRESS

A. Overview

1. Neonates produce body heat by nonshivering thermogenesis
2. This process requires increased oxygen and glucose consumption to burn brown fat; subcutaneous fat acts as an insulator and helps conserve body heat
3. A flexed position decreases exposed surface area and conserves body heat

B. Etiology

1. At risk for hypothermia because of large surface-area-to-mass ratio

2. Large amount of heat is lost from head
3. All newborns are at risk for hypothermia, especially preterm and small-for-gestational-age infants

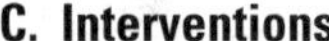

Practice to Pass

An isolette temperature has been steadily increasing over the past 12 hours in order to keep the infant's temperature stable. For what problems should the nurse assess closely?

C. Interventions

1. Maintain neutral thermal environment
   a. Reduce or eliminate heat lost through drafts and contact with cold objects
   b. Postpone initial bath until temperature has stabilized
   c. Dry infant immediately after delivery and when bathing
2. Place newborn under servo-controlled warmer or on mother's abdomen immediately after delivery
3. Assess body temperature; keep axillary temperature 97.6° (36.4°C) to 99.2°F (37.3°C)
4. If axillary temperature is less than 97.6°F (36.4°C)
   a. Put hat on infant's head
   b. Wrap newborn with warm blankets
   c. Assess oxygenation status and assess for hypoglycemia

   d. Rewarm infant slowly to prevent hypotension and apnea
5. Be aware that chronic hypothermia could be an early sign of sepsis

VIII. HYPERBILIRUBINEMIA

A. Etiology

1. Bilirubin is formed by breakdown of hemoglobin from red blood cells (RBCs); there are two types of bilirubin: direct (conjugated), which is water-soluble and easier for body to eliminate, and indirect (unconjugated), which is fat-soluble so it can more easily cross blood–brain barrier but is harder for body to eliminate
2. Before birth, unconjugated bilirubin is eliminated by placenta; after delivery, bilirubin is converted from an unconjugated to a conjugated form in liver and is excreted via bile ducts into intestines; it can be reabsorbed from intestines if peristalsis slows
3. **Kernicterus** is a potential complication of hyperbilirubinemia; direct (unconjugated) bilirubin is deposited in basal ganglia of brain and causes permanent impaired neurological function; bilirubin level, gestational age, condition, and poor fluid–caloric balance increase risk of kernicterus at low serum bilirubin levels

B. Physiologic jaundice/hyperbilirubinemia

1. A normal newborn has two times as much bilirubin as an adult related to a higher concentration of circulating RBCs, an impaired ability of liver to conjugate bilirubin related to immaturity and transition from fetal to neonatal circulation, and a shorter lifespan of the fetal RBC
2. Factors that increase risk of physiologic jaundice
   a. Resolution of enclosed hemorrhage (cephalohematoma, large amount of bruising from difficult delivery)
   b. Infection
   c. Dehydration
   d. Sepsis
3. Physiologic jaundice begins after first 24 hours of life

C. Pathologic jaundice/hyperbilirubinemia

1. Usually related to hemolytic disease of newborn
   a. Rh incompatibility
      1) If mother is Rh-negative and fetus is Rh-positive, fetal Rh-positive RBCs enter maternal bloodstream through breaks in maternal–fetal circulation late in pregnancy and after separation of placenta at delivery, causing maternal antibody formation; in a subsequent pregnancy with another Rh-positive fetus, maternal antibodies will cross placenta, enter fetal bloodstream and attack RBCs causing hemolysis and fetal anemia; Rhogam is given to mother to prevent development of these antibodies, but it cannot reverse the reaction once it occurs

2) Erythroblastosis fetalis is the most severe hemolytic reaction; it causes severe anemia, cardiac decompensation, edema, ascites, hypoxia, and may result in fetal death

b. ABO incompatibility

1) If mother has blood type O and is carrying a fetus with blood type A, B, or AB, fetal RBCs enter maternal bloodstream through breaks in maternal–fetal circulation late in pregnancy and after separation of placenta at delivery, causing maternal antibody formation; in a subsequent pregnancy with another fetus with that blood type, maternal antibodies will cross placenta, enter fetal bloodstream and attack fetal RBCs causing hemolysis and anemia; this reaction tends to be less severe than with Rh incompatibility

! c. Jaundice begins within first 24 hours of life

D. Assessment

1. Determine mother's blood type and Rh factor; if mother is Rh-negative or type-O blood, determine infant's blood type and Rh factor
2. Evaluate results of Coombs' tests
   ! a. Indirect Coombs' determines presence of maternal antibodies (sensitization) in maternal blood; a positive test indicates presence of antibodies
   ! b. Direct Coombs' determines presence of maternal Rh antibodies in fetal blood; cord blood is generally used; a positive test indicates presence of antibodies
3. Golden amniotic fluid indicates severe hemolytic disease
4. ! Assess for jaundice by gently pressing on sternum or forehead; in dark-skinned infants, assess sclera, palms of hands, and soles of feet
5. Evaluate results of bilirubin levels
   a. Bilirubin can be assessed transcutaneously with a bilimeter
   ! b. Total serum bilirubin levels greater than 13 to 15 mg/dL indicate hyperbilirubinemia
6. Enlarged liver and spleen
7. Anemia
8. Concentrated, dark urine

E. Priority nursing diagnoses: Deficient Fluid Volume (red blood cell); Risk for Injury (brain damage); Disturbed Thought Processes (mental retardation)

F. Interventions

1. Early and frequent feedings to stimulate peristalsis
2. **Phototherapy** (exposure of infant to bright light)
   ! a. Cover closed infant's eyes when under phototherapy light; remove eye covers every two hours when under light to assess for conjunctivitis and when not under phototherapy to promote bonding
   b. Infant should be undressed to maximize amount of circulating blood exposed to phototherapy light; genitalia can be covered to prevent soiling
   ! c. Change infant's position every two hours and assess for skin breakdown
   d. Assess for loose green stools as bilirubin is excreted through intestines
   e. Increase fluid intake to prevent dehydration
   ! f. Assess temperature every two hours and monitor for hypo- or hyperthermia
   g. Monitor bilirubin levels
3. **Exchange transfusion**
   a. Used to quickly decrease high bilirubin level by exchanging infant's circulating blood volume with donor blood; also removes anti-Rh antibodies and fetal RBCs coated with antibodies from infant's bloodstream and corrects anemia
   ! b. Only use Rh-negative blood to decrease risk of a transfusion reaction
   ! c. Warm blood to room temperature to prevent cardiac arrest
   d. Give calcium gluconate, when ordered, after each 100 mL
   ! e. Assess vital signs before procedure, every 15 minutes during procedure and post-procedure

f. Record time, amount of blood withdrawn, time and amount injected, medications given
g. Assess for dyspnea, listlessness, bleeding, cyanosis, bradycardia or arrythmias, hypoglycemia

G. Evaluation

1. Infant's bilirubin levels decrease to within normal range
2. Infant does not demonstrate any long-term effects of hyperbilirubinemia

IX. HYPOGLYCEMIA

A. Etiology

1. Definition: blood glucose (BG) less than 40 mg/dL in a term newborn
2. Glucose levels are assessed with a heel-stick
3. Newborns at risk: infants of diabetic mothers (IDM), small for gestational age, premature, and infants experiencing cold stress, hypothermia, or delayed feedings
4. Poor prognosis if hypoglycemia is not treated
5. Blood glucose usually stabilizes within 48 to 72 hours

B. Assessment

1. ! Tremors, jitteriness
2. Lethargy
3. Decreased muscle tone
4. Apnea
5. Anorexia

C. Priority nursing diagnosis: Imbalanced Nutrition: Less Than Body Requirements

D. Interventions

1. ! Check BG on all infants at risk by 1 hour of age (30 minutes if IDM), and any symptomatic newborn as ordered
2. ! Treat hypoglycemia by breastfeeding immediately or feeding D_5W or $D_{10}W$, either orally or intravenously; do not attempt to feed a lethargic infant orally because of an increased risk of aspiration
3. If treated for hypoglycemia, reassess BG level before next feeding

X. INFANT OF A DIABETIC MOTHER (IDM)

A. Etiology

1. Hormones secreted during pregnancy (HPL) increase maternal resistance to insulin, increasing insulin requirements; in diabetic clients, pancreas cannot secrete additional insulin needed during pregnancy and BG levels increase
2. Maternal insulin cannot cross placenta but glucose can; fetal glucose levels rise; fetal pancreas responds by secreting more insulin, which metabolizes additional glucose and acts as a growth hormone; increased insulin needs decreased surfactant production

B. Assessment

1. ! Large for gestational age; birth trauma more likely
2. Assess for effects of shoulder dystocia
3. Enlarged internal organs: cardiomegaly, hepatomegaly, splenomegaly
4. ! Hypoglycemia
5. Hypocalcemia
6. Hyperbilirubinemia
7. Respiratory distress syndrome (RDS)
8. ! False-positive L/S ratio
9. Increased risk for congenital anomalies, particularly cardiac and spinal defects

C. Priority nursing diagnoses: Impaired Gas Exchange; Risk for Injury; Imbalanced Nutrition: Less Than Body Requirements

D. Interventions

1. Assess for birth trauma
2. Assess BG level at 30 minutes and 1, 2, 4, 6, 9, 12, and 24 hours after birth
3. Treat hypoglycemia per orders

E. Evaluation

1. Newborn experiences minimal or no episodes of hypoglycemia, hypocalcemia, or hyperbilirubinemia
2. Newborn exhibits adequate respiratory function and gas exchange

XI. SUBSTANCE ABUSE

A. Fetal alcohol syndrome (FAS)

1. Etiology
   a. Alcohol crosses placenta and interferes with protein synthesis
   b. Increased risk of congenital anomalies, mental deficiency, intrauterine growth restriction (IUGR)

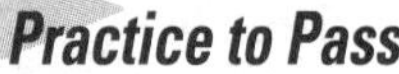

Practice to Pass

How could chronic diabetes cause a baby to be small for gestational age (SGA)?

2. Assessment
   a. Small for gestational age
   b. Facial features: epicanthal folds, maxillary hypoplasia, long and thin upper lip
   c. Irritable, hyperactive
   d. High-pitched cry
   e. Breastfeeds or bottle-feeds poorly (breastfeeding needs monitoring to make certain mother is not consuming alcohol, which can be transmitted through milk)
   f. Persistent vomiting
3. Interventions
   a. Reduce environmental stimuli
   b. Swaddle to increase feeling of security

   c. Administer sedatives as ordered to decrease side effects of withdrawal
   d. Maintain nutrition and hydration
4. Priority nursing diagnoses: Imbalanced Nutrition: Less Than Body Requirements; Disturbed Sensory Perception
5. Evaluation: newborn maintains adequate respirations, gains weight, demonstrates normal newborn reflexes, and shows no evidence of CNS hyperirritability

B. Neonatal abstinence syndrome (NAS)

1. Etiology
   a. Repeated intrauterine absorption of drugs from maternal bloodstream causes fetal drug dependency
   b. Increased risk of spontaneous abortion, preterm labor, stillbirth
   c. Degree of drug withdrawal depends on type and duration of addiction and maternal drug levels at delivery
2. Assessment

   a. Hyperactivity, jitteriness
   b. Absence of "step" reflex and "head-righting" reflex
   c. Shrill, persistent crying
   d. Frequent yawning and sneezing; nasal stuffiness
   e. Respiratory distress
   f. Sweating

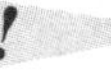

   g. Feeding difficulties (regurgitation, vomiting, and diarrhea), increased need for non-nutritive sucking
   h. Developmental delays
3. Priority nursing diagnoses: Ineffective Airway Clearance; Ineffective Protection; Impaired Gas Exchange; Imbalanced Nutrition: Less Than Body Requirements

4. Interventions
   a. Position infant on side to facilitate drainage of mucus
   b. Suction prn to maintain patent airway
   c. Decrease environmental stimuli, swaddle for comfort
   d. Monitor I&O, daily weight
   e. Obtain meconium and/or urine for drug screening as ordered
   f. Administer medications as ordered
      1) Paregoric elixir may be used to wean infant, but is controversial as it contains alcohol
      2) Chlorpromazine (Thorazine) and diazepam (Valium) are used to decrease hyperirritability; Valium predisposes to hyperbilirubinemia and is contraindicated in jaundiced newborns
      3) Phenobarbital is used to decrease hyperirritability and hyperbilirubinemia
   g. Pacifier may be used to allow non-nutritive sucking
5. Evaluation: newborn maintains adequate respirations, gains weight, demonstrates normal newborn reflexes, and shows no evidence of CNS hyperirritability

Case Study

A 29-week-gestation newborn is 6 hours of age. You are the nurse assigned to care for him in the neonatal intensive care unit.

1. What additional information do you need before planning care for this newborn?
2. What are the priorities for the newborn's care at this time?
3. The parents are concerned because they have heard oxygen can cause blindness in preterm infants. How would you respond?
4. Discuss how you can meet the newborn's psychosocial and developmental needs.
5. The mother asks if she can still breastfeed. How should you respond?

For suggested responses, see pages 306–307.

POSTTEST

POSTTEST

1 The parents of a 28 weeks' gestation neonate ask the nurse, "Why does he have to be fed through a tube in his mouth?" What is the nurse's best response?

1. "It allows us to accurately determine the baby's intake since he is so small."
2. "The baby's sucking, swallowing, and breathing are not coordinated yet."
3. "The baby's stomach cannot digest formula at this time."
4. "It helps to prevent thrush, an infection that could affect the baby's mouth."

2 Which nursing diagnosis should have highest priority for the nurse who is caring for a preterm newborn?

1. Ineffective Thermoregulation related to lack of subcutaneous fat
2. Grieving related to loss of "perfect delivery"
3. Imbalanced Nutrition: Less Than Body Requirements related to immature digestive system
4. Risk for Injury related to thin epidermis

3 A nurse is caring for a 12-hour-old newborn. The nurse notes a yellow tint to the baby's skin and sclera. What laboratory tests should the nurse anticipate being ordered? Select all that apply.

1. Serum glucose
2. Direct Coombs' test
3. Blood culture and sensitivity
4. Hemoglobin
5. Total bilirubin

4 A newborn is admitted with a diagnosis of transient tachypnea of the newborn (TTN). When planning nursing care for this baby, what nursing goal should the nurse formulate?

1. Promote adequate quantity of surfactant.
2. Promote absorption of fetal lung fluid.
3. Assist in removal of meconium from airway.
4. Stimulate respirations.

5 The nurse is assigned to a baby receiving phototherapy. Which assessment warrants further investigation by the nurse?

1. Loose, green stools
2. Yellow tint to skin
3. Temperature 97.2°F
4. Fine, red rash on trunk

6 A mother is crying while sitting by the isolette of her premature newborn who was born at 25 weeks' gestation. What is the most therapeutic communication by the nurse?

1. "It's important to try not to worry. Let's hope that everything will work out."
2. "Can you tell me some specific things that have gotten you upset?"
3. "Would you like me to call the hospital chaplain? This has helped many others."
4. "This must be hard for you. Can you share with me what has you most concerned at this time?"

7 A baby's mother is HIV-positive. Which intervention is most important for the nurse to include when planning care for this newborn?

1. Encourage the mother to breastfeed.
2. Administer zidovudine (ZDV) after delivery.
3. Cuddle the baby as much as possible.
4. Place the baby's crib in a quiet corner of the nursery.

8 The nurse is preparing to initiate bottle-feeding in a preterm infant. In which situation would the nurse withhold the feeding and notify the health care provider?

1. Apical heart rate 120–130
2. Axillary temperature 97.2°F–98.4°F
3. Yellow tint to skin and sclera
4. Respiratory rate 62–68

9 A newborn's mother has a history of prenatal narcotic abuse. Which interventions would be most appropriate for the infant of a substance abusing mother (ISAM) in the immediate postpartum period? Select all that apply.

1. Monitor the weight every eight hours.
2. Offer infant a pacifier.
3. Assess blood glucose levels.
4. Allow breastfeeding if alcohol is the addiction.
5. Keep the infant in high-Fowler's position.

10 The nurse is caring for a preterm infant who is at risk for an intraventricular hemorrhage (IVH). Which assessment is most critical for this infant? Select all that apply.

1. Increasing head circumference
2. Sudden drop in hemoglobin
3. Pink skin with blue extremities
4. "Waxy" skin color with rapid onset
5. Intake and output

➤ *See pages 276–278 for Answers and Rationales.*

POSTTEST

ANSWERS & RATIONALES

Pretest

1 **Answer: 2, 5** **Rationale:** Nasal flaring and chest retractions could be signs of respiratory distress and require immediate intervention. Blue hands and feet, a minimal response to verbal stimulation and apical heart rate of 140–156 are normal findings for a neonate at two hours of age. **Cognitive Level:** Analyzing **Client Need:** Physiological Adaptation **Integrated Process:** Nursing Process: Diagnosis **Content Area:** Maternal-Newborn **Strategy:** Critical words are *neonate two hours after delivery* and *be concerned about*. This indicates the need to look for abnormal signs that indicate a problem. **Reference:** Ladewig, P. A., London, M. L., & Davidson, M. R. (2010). *Contemporary maternal-newborn nursing care* (7th ed.). Upper Saddle River, NJ: Pearson Education, p. 608.

2 **Answer: 3** **Rationale:** Maintaining a patent airway is the highest priority when providing care for a newborn. A newborn's condition will deteriorate rapidly without a patent airway. Pain is an important safety need, but airway, breathing, and circulation take priority. Nutrition is important to maintain life but is not the highest priority diagnosis for the high-risk newborn. Deficient Knowledge relates to the parents and has the lowest priority because it is psychosocial in nature. **Cognitive Level:** Analyzing **Client Need:** Physiological Adaptation **Integrated Process:** Nursing Process: Diagnosis **Content Area:** Maternal-Newborn **Strategy:** Remember ABCs. Maintaining an open airway would be the priority. **Reference:** Ladewig, P. A., London, M. L., & Davidson, M. R. (2010). *Contemporary maternal-newborn nursing care* (7th ed.). Upper Saddle River, NJ: Pearson Education, pp. 608–609.

3 **Answer: 1** **Rationale:** This newborn is at risk for sepsis caused by prolonged rupture of membranes and maternal fever. A primary sign of sepsis in the newborn is temperature instability, particularly hypothermia. An irregular respiratory pattern is normal. Jitteriness may be a sign of hypoglycemia. Excessive bruising is often related to a difficult delivery with an increased risk of hyperbilirubinemia. **Cognitive Level:** Analyzing **Client Need:** Physiological Adaptation **Integrated Process:** Nursing Process: Assessment **Content Area:** Maternal-Newborn **Strategy:** The focus of the question is the risk for neonatal sepsis. The correct answer would be the option that contains abnormal assessment data related to infection in the newborn. Eliminate incorrect options because they are not related to sepsis. **Reference:** Ladewig, P. A., London, M. L., & Davidson, M. R. (2010). *Contemporary maternal-newborn nursing care* (7th ed.). Upper Saddle River, NJ: Pearson Education, pp. 482, 783–787.

4 **Answer: 2** **Rationale:** Neonatal abstinence syndrome, or drug withdrawal, causes hyperstimulation of the neonate's nervous system. Nursing interventions should focus on decreasing environmental and sensory stimulation during the withdrawal period. Pacifiers allow for nonnutritive sucking by the infant. **Cognitive Level:** Applying **Client Need:** Physiological Adaptation **Integrated Process:** Nursing Process: Implementation **Content Area:** Maternal-Newborn **Strategy:** Recall that neonatal abstinence syndrome is accompanied by hyperstimulation of the central nervous system. The correct answer would be the option that contains a strategy to reduce stimulation. **Reference:** Ladewig, P. A., London, M. L., & Davidson, M. R. (2010). *Contemporary maternal-newborn nursing care* (7th ed.). Upper Saddle River, NJ: Pearson Education, pp. 724, 729, 731.

5 **Answer: 1** **Rationale:** A newborn can become infected with gonorrhea as he or she passes through the birth canal. Gonorrhea can cause permanent blindness in the newborn, called ophthalmia neonatorum. All babies' eyes are treated with an antibiotic prophylactically after birth. The eyes require antibiotic prophylaxis, not lubrication. Thrush would result from a yeast infection rather than gonorrhea. There is no risk for breastfeeding because of gonorrhea. **Cognitive Level:** Applying **Client Need:** Physiological Adaptation **Integrated Process:** Nursing Process: Planning **Content Area:** Maternal-Newborn **Strategy:** The focus of the question is providing safety for the newborn of a mother with a gonococcal infection. The correct answer would be the option that contains a true statement to prevent spread of infection from mother to infant. **Reference:** Ladewig, P. A., London, M. L., & Davidson, M. R. (2010). *Contemporary maternal-newborn nursing care* (7th ed.). Upper Saddle River, NJ: Pearson Education, pp. 738–739.

6 **Answer: 2** **Rationale:** Newborns experiencing macrosomia are more likely to experience birth injuries during delivery. Nursing care after delivery should focus on assessing for signs of birth injuries and intervening if appropriate. The risks related to ineffective thermoregulation are the same as for other infants born at term. A mature newborn has sufficient surfactant for gas exchange. Teaching would be a priority for the parents, but is a psychosocial need and takes precedence once the infant's physiological needs are attended to. **Cognitive Level:** Analyzing **Client Need:** Physiological Adaptation **Integrated Process:** Nursing Process: Diagnosis **Content Area:** Maternal-Newborn **Strategy:** The core issue of the question is an abnormally large infant. The correct answer would be the option that contains a true statement of a risk for this newborn. **Reference:** Ladewig, P. A., London, M. L., & Davidson, M. R. (2010). *Contemporary maternal-newborn nursing care* (7th ed.). Upper Saddle River, NJ: Pearson Education, pp. 517–518.

7 **Answer: 3** **Rationale:** Reflecting on what the client said offers the client an opportunity to share feelings. It is important to avoid giving false reassurance. It is important to avoid asking clients "why" they feel

the way they do. Talking about personal experiences is nontherapeutic and does not address the client's concerns. **Cognitive Level:** Applying **Client Need:** Psychosocial Integrity **Integrated Process:** Communication and Documentation **Content Area:** Maternal-Newborn **Strategy:** The focus of the question is therapeutic communication. The correct answer would be the option that validates the client's feelings. **Reference:** Ladewig, P. A., London, M. L., & Davidson, M. R. (2010). *Contemporary maternal-newborn nursing care* (7th ed.). Upper Saddle River, NJ: Pearson Education, p. 721.

8 **Answer: 2 Rationale:** Infants of diabetic mothers are at risk for hypoglycemia after delivery. A primary sign of hypoglycemia is jitteriness. The newborn is not showing any signs of hypoxia so oxygen would not be appropriate. Putting the newborn under a warmer or on a monitor would not harm the infant, but they are not the priority interventions at this time. **Cognitive Level:** Analyzing **Client Need:** Physiological Adaptation **Integrated Process:** Nursing Process: Implementation **Content Area:** Maternal-Newborn **Strategy:** Knowledge of the care of the newborn of a diabetic mother will aid in answering the question correctly. Recall that blood glucose is the primary test to assess diabetic control. **Reference:** Ladewig, P. A., London, M. L., & Davidson, M. R. (2010). *Contemporary maternal-newborn nursing care* (7th ed.). Upper Saddle River, NJ: Pearson Education, pp. 704–707.

9 **Answer: 4 Rationale:** This newborn has a low temperature and the nurse must intervene quickly to prevent complications related to hypothermia. Wrapping the baby in warm blankets and covering the head will help prevent heat loss through conduction, convection, and radiation and is the most important initial intervention. It is unnecessary to notify the health care provider at this time. Observing the infant for two hours delays care and is unsafe. Reassessment of temperature does not do anything to raise the infant's temperature at this time. **Cognitive Level:** Applying **Client Need:** Physiological Adaptation **Integrated Process:** Nursing Process: Implementation **Content Area:** Maternal-Newborn **Strategy:** The focus of the question is an abnormal finding indicating cold stress. The correct answer would be the option that counteracts this problem and safely warms the newborn. **Reference:** Ladewig, P. A., London, M. L., & Davidson, M. R. (2010). *Contemporary maternal-newborn nursing care* (7th ed.). Upper Saddle River, NJ: Pearson Education, pp. 637–638.

10 **Answer: 2 Rationale:** This newborn has signs of jaundice, which include a yellow tint to the sclera and skin. Jaundice is considered pathologic if it occurs within the first 24 hours of life, when it is most often caused by Rh or ABO incompatibility. It would be important to assess both the mother's and newborn's blood type and Rh factor to determine if this could be causing the jaundice. A bilirubin level should also be obtained. A blood glucose level would be important if the infant showed signs of hypoglycemia. The most recent infant blood pressure is not relevant. The length of time membranes ruptured prior to delivery would affect the risk of maternal infection. **Cognitive Level:** Analyzing **Client Need:** Physiological Adaptation **Integrated Process:** Nursing Process: Assessment **Content Area:** Maternal-Newborn **Strategy:** This question requires further assessment of jaundice, an abnormal finding in a newborn at this age. The correct answer would be the option that contains information related to pathologic jaundice. **Reference:** Ladewig, P. A., London, M. L., & Davidson, M. R. (2010). *Contemporary maternal-newborn nursing care* (7th ed.). Upper Saddle River, NJ: Pearson Education, p. 771.

Posttest

1 **Answer: 2 Rationale:** Neonates generally are not able to effectively coordinate sucking, swallowing, and breathing until 34–36 weeks' gestation. If fed orally before that time, they are at greater risk of aspiration. Typically they will be fed through a gavage tube until they are able to drink from a bottle or breastfeed. Intake can be accurately assessed with oral and gavage feedings but this is not the primary reason. The stomach of a preterm infant can digest small amounts of formula or breast milk. Thrush is an oral yeast infection commonly caused during passage through the birth canal and gavage feedings will not prevent it from occurring. **Cognitive Level:** Applying **Client Need:** Physiological Adaptation **Integrated Process:** Communication and Documentation **Content Area:** Maternal-Newborn **Strategy:** The wording of the question indicates that the correct option is also a true statement. Recall the preterm neonate's capabilities regarding nutritional intake to choose the correct answer. **Reference:** Ladewig, P. A., London, M. L., & Davidson, M. R. (2010). *Contemporary maternal-newborn nursing care* (7th ed.). Upper Saddle River, NJ: Pearson Education, pp. 714–715.

2 **Answer: 1 Rationale:** Newborns compensate for hypothermia by metabolizing brown fat. This process requires glucose and oxygen. Preterm newborns are at risk for hypoglycemia and respiratory distress, so hypoglycemia can further increase their needs for oxygen and glucose and cause serious complications. The other diagnoses are appropriate but not the highest priority. **Cognitive Level:** Analyzing **Client Need:** Physiological Adaptation **Integrated Process:** Nursing Process: Diagnosis **Content Area:** Maternal-Newborn **Strategy:** Remember ABCs. The correct answer would be the option that contains a true statement that could negatively impact breathing and circulation. Cold stress can contribute to respiratory distress. **Reference:** Ladewig, P. A., London, M. L., & Davidson, M. R. (2010). *Contemporary maternal-newborn nursing care* (7th ed.). Upper Saddle River, NJ: Pearson Education, p. 709.

3 **Answer: 2, 4, 5 Rationale:** Jaundice in an infant less than 24 hours of age is often caused by Rh or ABO incompatibility. A direct Coombs' test determines the presence of maternal antibodies in the baby's blood. Hemoglobin will provide additional crucial information about possible red blood cell destruction. Total bilirubin is a helpful

test to determine the amount of circulating bilirubin that can lead to increased jaundice. A serum glucose test would be useful if the infant was showing signs of hypoglycemia. Blood culture and sensitivity would be useful for the infant suspected of being septic. **Cognitive Level:** Applying **Client Need:** Physiological Adaptation **Integrated Process:** Nursing Process: Planning **Content Area:** Maternal-Newborn **Strategy:** The focus of the question is jaundice. Eliminate incorrect options because they do not provide data related to this abnormal condition. **Reference:** Ladewig, P. A., London, M. L., & Davidson, M. R. (2010). *Contemporary maternal-newborn nursing care* (7th ed.). Upper Saddle River, NJ: Pearson Education, pp. 772–773.

4 **Answer: 2 Rationale:** Transient tachypnea of the newborn (TTN) is caused by delayed absorption of fetal lung fluid. Nursing care is focused on supporting oxygenation needs to allow the newborn's body to reabsorb the fluid. Inadequate surfactant is related to prematurity and respiratory distress syndrome. Meconium in the airway results in meconium aspiration syndrome and is usually associated with fetal asphyxia. TTN causes tachypnea so stimulating respirations is not appropriate. **Cognitive Level:** Applying **Client Need:** Physiological Adaptation **Integrated Process:** Nursing Process: Planning **Content Area:** Maternal-Newborn **Strategy:** Recall that transient tachypnea is associated with amniotic fluid in the newborn lungs. Eliminate incorrect options because they are not related to this problem. **Reference:** Ladewig, P. A., London, M. L., & Davidson, M. R. (2010). *Contemporary maternal-newborn nursing care* (7th ed.). Upper Saddle River, NJ: Pearson Education, pp. 759–760.

5 **Answer: 3 Rationale:** Infants should be unclothed while receiving phototherapy to increase the circulating blood volume exposed to the phototherapy light. However, this increases the risk of temperature instability and infant temperature should be monitored carefully. Any temperature below 97.6°F is considered hypothermia and requires immediate attention. Loose, green stools and a yellow tint to the skin are expected findings with hyperbilirubinemia. A fine, raised red rash may appear on the infant's skin as a side effect of the phototherapy and does not require intervention. **Cognitive Level:** Analyzing **Client Need:** Physiological Adaptation **Integrated Process:** Nursing Process: Assessment **Content Area:** Maternal-Newborn **Strategy:** The focus of the question is an abnormal finding in the present treatment of jaundice. Eliminate incorrect options because they are normal findings in a newborn with jaundice being treated with phototherapy. **Reference:** Ladewig, P. A., London, M. L., & Davidson, M. R. (2010). *Contemporary maternal-newborn nursing care* (7th ed.). Upper Saddle River, NJ: Pearson Education, pp. 773–777.

6 **Answer: 4 Rationale:** Reflection allows the client to verbalize his or her feelings. The nurse should not give the client false hope. Clients often do not know why they feel the way they do and it is not helpful to ask them to determine this. Some clients may find comfort in a religious leader, but care should be taken not to stereotype the client's religious beliefs. **Cognitive Level:** Applying **Client Need:** Psychosocial Integrity **Integrated Process:** Communication and Documentation **Content Area:** Maternal-Newborn **Strategy:** The focus of the question is therapeutic communication. The correct answer would be the option that validates the client's feelings and invites further communication by the client. **Reference:** Ladewig, P. A., London, M. L., & Davidson, M. R. (2010). *Contemporary maternal-newborn nursing care* (7th ed.). Upper Saddle River, NJ: Pearson Education, pp. 791–794.

7 **Answer: 2 Rationale:** Administering zidovudine (ZDV, formerly AZT) to the mother prenatally and intrapartally, as well as to the infant immediately after delivery, decreases the prenatal risk of transmission of HIV by 60–70%. Breastfeeding is contraindicated in an HIV-positive mother because the virus can be passed through breast milk. Cuddling the infant is important, but not the highest priority in this situation. Decreasing environmental stimulation is not indicated. **Cognitive Level:** Applying **Client Need:** Physiological Adaptation **Integrated Process:** Nursing Process: Implementation **Content Area:** Maternal-Newborn **Strategy:** The core focus of the question is reduction of HIV transmission from mother to infant. The correct option contains a true statement to reduce the risk of transmission of the disease to the newborn. Eliminate options that are either unrelated to HIV transmission or that would increase risk of transmission. **Reference:** Ladewig, P. A., London, M. L., & Davidson, M. R. (2010). *Contemporary maternal-newborn nursing care* (7th ed.). Upper Saddle River, NJ: Pearson Education, pp. 669, 737–738.

8 **Answer: 4 Rationale:** Any sustained respiratory rate greater than 60 breaths/minute increases the risk of aspiration in the infant. Oral feedings should be withheld on infants experiencing tachypnea to decrease the risk of aspiration. An apical heart rate of 120–130 is a normal finding. Although an infant temperature of 97.2°F is considered hypothermia, it would not be a contraindication to oral feedings. Jaundice may be considered abnormal but it alone would not be an indication to withhold an oral feeding. **Cognitive Level:** Analyzing **Client Need:** Physiological Adaptation **Integrated Process:** Nursing Process: Implementation **Content Area:** Maternal-Newborn **Strategy:** The focus of the question is identification of abnormal findings that would contraindicate feeding. The correct answer would be the option that contains an abnormal finding related to a condition that could be exacerbated by feeding. **Reference:** Ladewig, P. A., London, M. L., & Davidson, M. R. (2010). *Contemporary maternal-newborn nursing care* (7th ed.). Upper Saddle River, NJ: Pearson Education, pp. 757–758.

9 **Answer: 1, 2, 3, 4 Rationale:** Infants experiencing neonatal abstinence syndrome (NAS) have needs immediately after birth that change as the hours pass. These infants need frequent weights as intake may be diminished due

to withdrawal symptoms. It may be helpful to the infant to be offered opportunity for nonnutritive sucking, such as with a pacifier to soothe and quiet the infant. These infants are at high risk for glucose abnormalities, making glucose monitoring important. Breastfeeding is allowed if the mother is addicted to alcohol but she must not breastfeed after alcohol ingestion. It is unnecessary to keep the infant in high-Fowler's position. **Cognitive Level:** Applying **Client Need:** Physiological Adaptation **Integrated Process:** Nursing Process: Implementation **Content Area:** Maternal-Newborn **Strategy:** The focus of the question is a newborn experiencing abstinence syndrome, a condition associated with hyperstimulation. The correct answer(s) would be options that reduce stimulation and quiet the infant. **Reference:** Ladewig, P. A., London, M. L., & Davidson, M. R. (2010). *Contemporary maternal-newborn nursing care* (7th ed.). Upper Saddle River, NJ: Pearson Education, pp. 735–737.

10 **Answer: 1, 2, 4** **Rationale:** A frequent sign of IVH is an increase in head circumference, since the cranial bones have not fused and can separate as the bleed accumulates in the cranium. A sudden drop in hemoglobin can be indicative of IVH. A change in skin color to a 'waxy' appearance can occur with drop in hemoglobin. Pink skin with blue extremities is not indicative of an IVH. Intake and output are routine measurements that are not directly helpful in this situation. **Cognitive Level:** Analyzing **Client Need:** Physiological Adaptation **Integrated Process:** Nursing Process: Assessment **Content Area:** Maternal-Newborn **Strategy:** The focus of the question is intraventricular hemorrhage. Evaluate each option and choose those that are consistent with blood loss into the cranium. **Reference:** Ladewig, P. A., London, M. L., & Davidson, M. R. (2010). *Contemporary maternal-newborn nursing care* (7th ed.). Upper Saddle River, NJ: Pearson Education, p. 716.

References

Davidson, M., London, M., & Ladewig, P. (2012). *Olds' maternal newborn nursing & women's health across the lifespan* (9th ed.). Upper Saddle River, NJ: Pearson Education.

Ladewig, P., London, M., & Davidson, M. (2009). *Contemporary maternal-newborn nursing care* (7th ed.). Upper Saddle River, NJ: Pearson Education.

Perry, S. E., Hockenberry, M. J., Lowdermilk, D. L., & Wilson, D. (2010). *Maternal child nursing care* (4th ed.). St. Louis, MO: Mosby.

Ricci, S. (2009). *Essentials of maternity, newborn, and women's health nursing* (2nd ed.). Philadelphia, PA: Lippincott Williams & Wilkins.

Issues of Loss and Grief in Maternity Nursing 14

Chapter Outline

Objectives

- Describe the parent's response to loss of a pregnancy.
- Describe the parent's response to infertility.
- Discuss parental grieving for the loss of the expected child.
- Discuss nursing interventions to foster healthy grieving in parents.

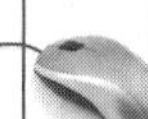

NCLEX-RN® Test Prep

Use the accompanying online resource, NursingReviewsandRationales, to test yourself with hundreds of NCLEX®-style practice questions.

Review at a Glance

anticipatory grieving grieving done prior to and in preparation for actual death

bereavement subjective responses experienced after death of a loved one

fetal anomaly abnormality of fetus, can be genetic or nongenetic causation, may be detected prior to or not until after delivery

grief total response to emotional experience of a fetal loss; experienced by parents, siblings, grandparents, and other close friends and relatives

incongruent grieving when partners are in different stages of grief, can create additional stress within family due to perceived lack of support or understanding

infertility inability to conceive after 12 months of unprotected intercourse

intrauterine fetal demise (IUFD) fetal death from any cause that occurs in utero prior to onset of labor

maceration changes undergone by a dead fetus as it is retained in utero; characterized by reddening and loss of skin, as well as distortion of features over time

mourning behavioral process through which grief eventually becomes resolved; influenced by culture, religion/spiritual practices, and customs; experienced by parents of infant who has died as well as siblings, grandparents, other close friends, and relatives

neonatal death death of a live-born fetus from any cause within first month of life

regrieving renewed sense of grief that occurs at anniversaries of a fetal loss

stillbirth birth of a dead infant at greater than 20 weeks' gestation

sudden infant death syndrome (SIDS) infant death without apparent cause after autopsy, death scene investigation, review of symptoms or illnesses infant had prior to dying, and any other pertinent medical history

PRETEST

PRETEST

1 The client who experienced a perinatal demise states, "Sometimes I feel like I left my baby somewhere, and can't remember where she is. Then I remember that she isn't alive." The nurse interprets that this client is experiencing which of the following?

1. Anticipatory grieving
2. Disorientation
3. Reorganization
4. Searching and yearning

2 The father of a stillborn infant tells the nurse he wants to hold the child. What is the nurse's best response?

1. Encourage him to discuss this with his wife first.
2. Dress the infant in a t-shirt and diaper and let him hold the infant.
3. Tell him that it would be better not to hold the infant.
4. Give him the photographs of the infant that the nurse took instead.

3 The nurse determines that teaching about sudden infant death syndrome (SIDS) has been effective when the client makes which statement?

1. "No definite cause of death is found at autopsy."
2. "Infants who sleep on their backs are more at risk for sudden infant death syndrome."
3. "Bottle-feeding causes sudden infant death syndrome."
4. "Genetic disorders are the cause of SIDS."

4 The nurse interprets which of the following as somatic complaints of a postpartal woman who is grieving for her deceased infant? Select all that apply.

1. Tingling on the back of the neck and hearing a baby's cry
2. Heaviness in the chest and fatigue
3. Increased taste sensitivity and deep sleep
4. Stiffness in the legs and arms
5. Weight loss and decreased appetite

5 The client being seen for a postpartal exam after delivering a stillborn girl six weeks ago asks the nurse, "When will I feel normal again?" The nurse's reply reflects the understanding that grief work takes approximately how long?

1. Two to three months
2. About one year
3. Four to six months
4. Not more than eight months

6 The maternal newborn nurse interprets that anticipatory grieving is likely to occur in a client who has experienced which of the following situations?

1. Sudden infant death syndrome (SIDS)
2. Ectopic pregnancy
3. Placental abruption during labor
4. Fetal anomaly identified during pregnancy

7 Which of the following tokens of remembrance would be appropriate for the nurse to provide to parents who are grieving the death of their infant?

1. Lock of hair, footprints
2. Baptism or naming
3. Visit from chaplain
4. Sympathy card from staff

8 The family is experiencing a fetal loss. Which statement indicates that the nurse's teaching about family involvement in the birthing process needs clarification?

1. "We can have our child baptized."
2. "We can decide not to stay on the postpartal unit after the birth."
3. "We will be able to name our infant."
4. "We should have the funeral through the mortuary the hospital uses."

9 The nurse is making assignments for the next shift. The nurse assigns the same nurse to the family experiencing a fetal loss as cared for them yesterday because continuity of care will have which benefit?

1. Decrease the family's need to interact with many others.
2. Increase support for the family.
3. Prevent the family from needing to ask questions.
4. Facilitate dependence on the nurse.

10 The nurse who is reviewing all subjective and objective prenatal assessment data interprets that which data is an indicator of intrauterine fetal death?

1. Diminished fetal activity over a three-day period
2. A bluish discoloration in the vaginal and cervical mucosa
3. Absence of fetal heart tones and fetal movement
4. Mother saying "the baby is just not moving today"

➤ *See pages 290–292 for Answers and Rationales.*

PRETEST

I. GRIEVING

A. ***Grief***: total response to emotional experience related to loss; manifested emotionally, somatically, and cognitively; associated with overwhelming distress or sorrow
B. ***Bereavement***: subjective responses experienced by a survivor of loss
C. ***Mourning***: behavioral process through which grief is eventually resolved; influenced by culture, religion, and customs; takes over one year

II. PERINATAL SITUATIONS IN WHICH GRIEF IS EXPECTED

A. ***Infertility***

1. Definition: lack of pregnancy after 12 months of unprotected intercourse
2. Etiology: male factors, female factors, genetic factors, or unknown causation (see also Chapter 2)
3. When pregnancy has not happened spontaneously and infertility treatment has been sought, couples are experiencing physical, emotional, and financial stress
   a. Physical stresses result from need to self-administer oral or injected medications, side effects of these medications, and need to adhere to schedules for intercourse, and lengthy course of treatment (possibly years)
   b. Emotional stresses result from loss of spontaneity in sexual relationship, threatened self-esteem to one or both partners if inability to conceive is regarded as a lack of femininity or virility, having to discuss personal aspects of sexuality during fertility counseling and treatment, uncertainty whether infertility treatment will be successful, possible feelings of loss of control or defectiveness, ambiguity and perceived social stigma as a couple, and possible tension between couple if one becomes angry and then experiences guilt or shame over these feelings when partner is perceived as "cause" for infertility
   c. Financial stresses result from high cost and limited insurance coverage of infertility medications and procedures, cost of appointments, and possibly time lost from work
4. Infertility can be perceived as a loss of previous relationship with spouse, family and friends, status or prestige, self-confidence or security, and loss of possibility of future children; any of these losses can trigger typical grief reaction
5. Achieving pregnancy through treatment for infertility brings a sense of optimism to parents as their dream of parenting becomes a possibility, but new fears emerge about ability to carry pregnancy to term
6. When pregnancy ends through fetal death, parents must grieve fetal loss as well as deal with recent sense of optimism; this complex set of emotional issues is difficult for parents to resolve

B. First trimester fetal loss

1. Twelve percent of diagnosed pregnancies in women younger than age 20 and 26% (or double) in women older than age 40 end in spontaneous abortion
2. Ectopic pregnancies (those occurring outside of the uterus) occur in 2% of U.S. pregnancies
3. Elective termination of pregnancy can also trigger a grief response and may be combined with guilt

C. *Fetal anomaly*

1. Parents often grieve loss of their "perfect child" when their baby is born with a congenital anomaly
2. Intensity of grief may be affected by type and severity of anomaly
3. Prenatally detected anomalies will allow for **anticipatory grieving**, which begins prior to actual loss or death

D. *Neonatal death*

! 1. Definition: death within first month of life
2. Etiology: typically related to congenital defects (genetic and nongenetic), sepsis, prematurity, or sudden infant death syndrome

E. *Sudden infant death syndrome (SIDS)*

! 1. Sudden death of an infant under 1 year of age that remains unexplained after a complete investigation (autopsy, examination of death scene, and review of symptoms or illnesses infant had prior to dying and any other pertinent medical history)
! 2. Higher incidence in nonwhite races, smokers, illegal drug users, and infants who sleep on their abdomens

F. *Stillbirth* or *intrauterine fetal demise (IUFD)*

! 1. Fetal demise in utero after 20 weeks' gestation
2. Etiology: placental abruption and knots or entanglement in umbilical cord are common causes (1% of all births have knots in cord); however, most often cause of stillbirth is unknown; fetal death can occur prenatally or during intrapartal period
3. Most mothers spontaneously begin labor within two weeks after intrauterine fetal demise; if spontaneous labor does not ensue, fetus can be coated in fibrin from maternal circulation, leading to disseminated intravascular coagulopathy (DIC)
! 4. First symptom of fetal death is absence of fetal movement
5. Stillborn infants will have dark red, peeling skin (**maceration**), soft and swollen-looking heads with overriding of fetal skull bones (Spalding's sign), and a mouth that hangs open; the longer the fetus has been dead, the worse the maceration will become

III. PHASES OF BEREAVEMENT

! **A. Responses of survivors of loss proceed through four phases (Table 14-1)**

B. Shock and numbness

1. Characterized by a feeling that "this is all a bad dream"; parents may have difficulty making decisions during this time
2. This phase predominates during first two weeks following loss

C. Searching and yearning

1. Parents search for answers and yearn for their infants; parents are preoccupied with thoughts about what happened, guilt about what they may have done or not done that caused death, and the death itself; mothers may also experience irrational perceptions, such as phantom fetal movement, hearing a baby crying, and a feeling of heaviness in their arms, which may lead them to think they are "losing their minds"; this is a normal response as they psychologically search for their baby
2. This phase begins within a week of loss and peaks between two weeks and four months after loss, and is longest phase of bereavement

Practice to Pass

One week after delivering a stillborn infant, the mother tells you that every time the doorbell rings she briefly thinks it is someone from the funeral home with her baby and they're going to tell her they made a mistake and her baby is just fine. What should your priority intervention be?

Table 14-1 Phases of Bereavement

Phase of Bereavement	Onset and Length	Symptoms
Shock and numbness	First two weeks after loss	Disbelief, difficulty making decisions
Searching and yearning	Within one week of loss, peaks at two to four months	Preoccupation with causes of death and feelings of guilt
Disorientation	First week after loss, recurs for months to years	Depression, appetite loss, decreased activities of daily living, regrieving on anniversaries
Reorganization	Up to 18 months to 2 years	Numbness diminishes, loss becomes real, able to cope and take care of themselves

D. Disorientation

1. Primary sign or symptom is depression; mourner may take on a sick role to legitimize their depression and avoid criticism; may lose appetite and not perform personal cares
2. This phase occurs during first week after loss, and will intensify and subside at intervals for months to years

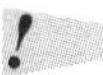

3. **Regrieving** is a common phenomenon, especially during anniversary of child's birth and death, holidays, and any other time that reminds parents of that child; this typically occurs for years after loss, and perhaps for lifetime of the parents; parents never "get over" loss of a child

E. Reorganization

1. During this stage, numbness wears off and reality of loss becomes apparent; parents are better able to cope with new challenges, take better care of themselves, and can feel sadness that is not immobilizing
2. Can take 18 months to 2 years to achieve full resolution

IV. NURSING CARE DURING PERINATAL GRIEF

A. Assessment of factors affecting grief reaction (see Table 14-2)

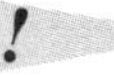

1. Male–female differences
   a. In many cultures, women tend to express more symptoms of grief, such as crying, anger, and guilt, than men
   b. Pregnancy may initially be less real to father because he does not directly experience changes of pregnancy; this may affect his reaction to an early pregnancy loss
2. Previous losses
   a. A history of a previous pregnancy loss will affect manner in which parents react to subsequent losses; once bereavement phases have been experienced and grief is resolved, grieving is a more familiar emotional territory
   b. Parents who have had difficulty conceiving may experience additional grief: failure of long-desired pregnancy and optimism for the future it brought, as well as loss of the child
   c. Other concurrent losses, such as divorce or death of another family member, may contribute to intensity of grief
   d. Pregnancy loss is often first death in the family that the parents experienced, so death rituals and grief work may be unfamiliar

Table 14-2 Factors Affecting Grief Reaction

Factor	Grief Reaction
Male–female differences	Men: internalize their grief, want to get back to routine; early pregnancy may not seem real yet Women: more expressive, cry more, and want to talk about the loss more; early pregnancy more real because of subjective changes in the body, and more likely to be grieved than in men
Previous losses	Previous pregnancy loss will have an effect Treatment for infertility will make grieving more complex Concurrent losses (i.e., divorce, death of another family member) intensify the grieving Pregnancy loss often the first death the couple has experienced
Timing of death	Anticipatory grief if death is anticipated (i.e., diagnosis of lethal fetal anomaly) Most often death sudden and unexpected
Coping style	Couple's ability to evaluate, plan, and adjust to new situations will influence length of grief and progression through bereavement phases
Cultural influences	Determine appropriate mourning behaviors (verbalization, facial expressions, clothing, who is present) Religious/spiritual or cultural rituals and ceremonies may be held Autopsy and when infant should be buried affected Naming may be prohibited
Support systems	Family, friends, religious community, social agencies assist grief work; stable relationship as a couple helpful

3. Timing of death
   a. When parents know fetus has died prior to delivery, they will experience anticipatory grieving
   b. In most cases, death is sudden and unexpected

!

4. Coping styles
   a. Parents' ability to evaluate, plan, and adjust to new situations will affect their ability to cope with a loss
   b. Positive coping mechanisms should be encouraged
   c. Reliance on alcohol or prescription sedatives should be discouraged to facilitate acceptance of loss as real

!

5. Cultural influences
   a. Verbalization and behavioral demonstrations of grief are determined by cultural norms, ranging from open wailing to stoic quietness; facial expressions and public crying will vary
   b. Clothing color and style to be worn by parents and dead infant may be culturally determined
   c. Presence of extended or nuclear family and or friends may be culturally determined
   d. Naming of infant may be culturally determined
   e. Religious or spiritual practices may include placing amulets, medallions, or other symbols on or near infant; rituals and ceremonies may be desired
   f. Timing of burial, autopsy, and organ donation may be culturally determined
6. Support systems
   a. Intact and available support systems, such as family, friends, and religious, community or social agencies, can assist the parents in their grief work
   b. A relationship in which the parents are supportive of each other is helpful

Practice to Pass

A Muslim woman has just given birth to a stillborn boy. What information do you need to plan culturally appropriate care for this family? Where can you obtain the information that you need?

Table 14-3 Signs and Symptoms of Grief

Somatic	Gastrointestinal Respiratory Cardiovascular Neuromuscular	Anorexia, weight loss, nausea/vomiting, overeating Sighing, hyperventilation Palpitations, chest heaviness Vertigo, headaches
Behavioral	Feelings Preoccupation with deceased infant Interpersonal relationships Crying Activities of daily living	Guilt, sadness, anger and hostility, apathy, helplessness Daydreams, fantasies, nightmares, arms ache to hold infant Withdrawal, decrease in sex drive, incongruent grieving Public or private Loss of concentration and poor memory, fatigue and exhaustion, insomnia or increased sleep time, decreased interest in grooming and dressing
Siblings	Up to age 6 Age 6–12 Over age 12	Death viewed as temporary and reversible, may think their negative thoughts caused the death View death as inevitable and irreversible Think of death abstractly
Grandparents	Similar somatic and behavioral symptoms that parents experience	

B. Assessment of signs and symptoms of grief (see Table 14–3)

1. Somatic (physiologic)
   a. Gastrointestinal
      1) Anorexia and weight loss, may persist for several months
      2) Nausea or vomiting, especially in shock and numbness phase
      3) Overeating
   b. Respiratory
      1) Hyperventilation, especially early in grieving and at time of disclosure of death
      2) Deep sighing respirations
   c. Cardiovascular
      1) Cardiac palpitations or "fluttering" in chest
      2) "Heavy" feeling in chest
   d. Neuromuscular
      1) Headaches, may persist as grief work continues
      2) Vertigo, especially with thoughts of deceased and when death is first discovered

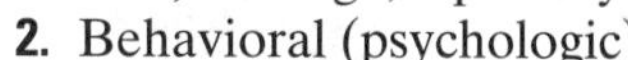

2. Behavioral (psychologic)
   a. Feelings
      1) Guilt over having somehow caused the death
      2) Sadness, can be overwhelming
      3) Anger and hostility toward self, partner, health care providers
      4) Apathy and inability to make decisions
      5) Helplessness
   b. Preoccupation with lost infant
      1) Daydreams and fantasies can manifest as hearing a baby cry
      2) Nightmares (often about forgetting the baby someplace); these may be recurrent
      3) "Empty arms" and a longing to hold baby

c. Interpersonal relationships
   1) Decreased sexual interest, partner may not feel the same
   2) Withdrawal from social activities
   3) **Incongruent grieving**: partners may be in different phases of bereavement, leading to perceptions that the other is either malingering or unfeeling
d. Crying: public and private, can be stimulated by minor occurrence
e. Activities of daily living
   1) Loss of concentration and motivation are common, and may interfere with job performance
   2) Fatigue and exhaustion, may or may not be associated with insomnia
   3) Sleep changes: insomnia, poor quality sleep, or increased amount of time spent sleeping
   4) Loss of interest in grooming and dressing leading to a disheveled appearance

Practice to Pass

The parents of a stillborn infant tell you that they are going to tell their 5-year-old son that his brother "went to sleep and is in heaven now." How should you respond?

3. Siblings
   a. A child's reaction to death of a sibling depends on surviving child's developmental level and response of parents to loss
   b. The universal fear of childhood is fear of separation and abandonment, and child may fear that parents may also die
   c. Through 6 years of age, children view death as temporary and reversible; children in this age group may feel guilty that their negative thoughts may have caused death
   d. Children 6 to 12 years of age view death as inevitable and irreversible
   e. By 12 years of age, most children can think abstractly like an adult about death
4. Grandparents
   a. Grandparents also grieve loss of their grandchild and may experience many of same signs and symptoms that parents do
   b. Grandparents also report a feeling of helplessness as they watch their child grieve

C. **Priority nursing diagnoses**: Anxiety; Anticipatory Grieving; Dysfunctional Grieving; Interrupted Family Processes; Compromised Family Coping; Situational Low Self-Esteem; Ineffective Coping; Spiritual Distress

D. **Planning and implementation with grieving parents**: nurse can respond in a variety of ways as shown in Table 14-4

Table 14-4 Responding to Grieving Parents

What to do	Call the child by name Cry with the family Attend the funeral or memorial service Remember the family on their baby's due date, birthday, and death date anniversaries
Remembrances you can give the family	Photographs Lock of hair Footprints and handprints Baby ID band Clothes the baby was photographed in
What you can say	"I'm sorry." "This must be hard for you." "How are you doing with all of this?"
What NOT to say	"At least it wasn't older." "It was God's will." "You can have other children." "At least you have other children." "Time will heal."

Practice to Pass

A client is 34 weeks' gestation and has come to the clinic because she has not felt the baby move today. When she arrives, the client says "I'm really afraid there's something wrong with my baby." How should you respond?

1. Nonhelpful responses
   a. Maintaining state of denial
      1) Not acknowledging pregnancy or loss
      2) Using tranquilizers, sedatives, and other drugs makes the experience "dream-like" for mother and may prolong denial and, therefore, the grieving process
      3) Encouraging parents not to cry or talk about their loss
   b. Isolation
      1) Not going into client's room
      2) Placing client on a non-maternity unit against couple's wishes
   c. Prohibiting contact between infant and parents
      1) Not encouraging parents to see and hold their child encourages fantasies about what child really looks like
      2) These fantasies are always more frightening than reality
2. Helpful responses

   !

   a. Environment
      1) Parents should be allowed to choose whether they want to stay on postpartal unit or another unit away from nursery
      2) Provide a quiet, private setting to allow parents to say hello and good-bye to their infant at same time
   b. Supportive relationship
      1) Utilize an empathic manner when working with family
      2) Provide consistency in nursing staff assignments and support from nurse

   !

   c. Information
      1) Parents should be told child's prognosis as soon as possible
      2) Information may need to be repeated as parents will be in a state of shock and not hear all that is said the first time

   !

   d. Encouraging expression of emotions
      1) Verbalizing thoughts and feelings provides an outlet for intense feelings associated with grief
      2) Telling and reliving the experience is necessary to gain understanding and mastery over a frightening situation

   !

   e. Seeing and touching
      1) Parents should be informed of appearance of their infant so they can make a decision whether or not to see and touch their child
      2) Many parents are reluctant to see and touch their baby initially, but most of them state they are glad they did
      3) Parents should be encouraged to spend as much time as they want with their infant; many parents will want to see their infant more than one time, if given the opportunity; this is the only chance they will ever have to see their child
      4) Infant should be dressed like other infants on unit (usually a diaper and t-shirt) and wrapped in a baby blanket; nurse should stay in room or close by for support

   !

   f. Remembrances
      1) Nurse should take pictures of infant both dressed in baby clothes and without clothes for parents; pictures should be offered to parents; if parents refuse pictures, they should be told pictures will be kept on unit in case parents change their mind; pictures help parents accept their child's death and move forward in grieving process
      2) A lock of hair, one of baby's identification bracelets, and handprints and footprints can also be obtained and given to parents
   g. Open visitation should be encouraged

Practice to Pass

A client delivered a stillborn infant three hours ago. You bring the infant to her so she can see and touch him. She asks if she can give her baby a bath. How should you respond?

h. Autopsy
   1) Knowing why infant died may help parents resolve guilt that is common after a child dies
   2) Permission to do an autopsy should be obtained after parents have had a chance to deal with reality of the death
   3) Some religious faiths prohibit autopsy

i. Religious or spiritual practices or ceremonies
   1) Families may wish to have baby baptized or participate in other religious or spiritual sacraments, ceremonies, or rituals
   2) A visit from hospital chaplain should be offered to family, or clergy from family's religious community should be contacted by hospital staff, if desired by parents
   3) Death of a child is often the first experience that parents have with death; hospital staff should contact funeral home of parents' choice and make beginning arrangements; someone knowledgeable about the options available should discuss them with parents

j. Anticipatory guidance
   1) Parents should be contacted periodically to provide support; this is especially important at anniversary of due date (with early pregnancy losses) and birth and death dates
   2) Support groups may help parents cope with death of their child; provide written information on support groups to family prior to discharge

E. Evaluation

1. Family members express their feelings about death of child
2. Family participates in decision to see, hold, or engage in other ceremonies or rituals regarding their baby
3. Family knows what community resources are available, if they choose to use them
4. Family moves through grieving process

Case Study

A client experienced a complete placental abruption during labor and delivered a stillborn infant following an emergency cesarean section. The client is married and has two other children, ages 10 and 6.

1. The couple is reluctant to see their infant. How would you explain this infant's appearance to them?
2. What should be considered when assigning this client to a room after delivery?
3. The parents state they are not sure how to explain this to their other children. What should you tell them?
4. You overhear the client's mother tell her, "I'll bet you'll be feeling better in no time." What should you do?
5. Two weeks later the client calls and states she feels like she's "going crazy" because she occasionally hears a baby cry, but when she looks for the baby she never finds it. How should you respond?

For suggested responses, see page 307.

POSTTEST

1. A woman is undergoing induction of labor for an intrauterine fetal death. The nurse considers that which plans should be made for the woman's partner?

   1. Should be included for support and to facilitate the partner's acceptance of the fetal death as real
   2. Should be included to decrease misunderstanding of medical procedures by the mother
   3. Should be excluded to prevent the additional emotional strain of the birth on the partner
   4. Should be excluded because another child can be conceived soon and help to forget this death

2. Which statement indicates to the nurse that the client is expressing somatic symptoms of the grieving process?

   1. "If our doctor hadn't insisted on doing that extra blood work our baby would be alive now."
   2. "I told God I'd never again smoke another cigarette if our baby could just be born alive."
   3. "I feel nauseated and don't want to eat. Please take the tray out of my room."
   4. "My mother can't stop crying. She says she feels like she failed me by letting this happen to me."

3. The plan of care for a pregnant client who experienced an unexplained intrauterine fetal demise during her last pregnancy should include which of the following? Select all that apply.

   1. Education about the causes of intrauterine fetal demise for both parents
   2. Encouragement to think positively and not dwell on the previous fetal loss
   3. Support for increased fears as this fetus reaches the gestational age of the previous fetal loss
   4. Facilitation of grieving of the lost fetus through carrying a photo and a lock of hair at all times
   5. Asking open-ended questions to determine how the parents are coping and identify any concerns

4. The client who had a stillborn infant at term has come to the clinic for her postpartal exam accompanied by her husband. What should the nurse anticipate at this time?

   1. Both parents will express their grief in the same way.
   2. The parents will use similar coping mechanisms.
   3. The parents will be in the same grief work stage.
   4. The parents will have differences in how they are grieving.

5. The mother of a stillborn infant tells the nurse that she feels like she is missing a part of herself. The nurse understands that this is not related to which of the following?

   1. Parents simultaneously grieving and resolving their attachment to the lost infant
   2. The unborn child having been incorporated into a mother's physical and emotional being
   3. A significant loss of self-esteem that often occurs with both parents after perinatal loss
   4. Mothers of stillborns finding a way to justify their desire to become pregnant again

6. The pregnant client has been told that the fetus has a neural tube defect. Which strategy by the nurse will facilitate anticipatory grieving during the pregnancy?

   1. Quietly and consistently encourage the family to terminate the pregnancy.
   2. Protect the family from information about what effects the defect will have on their child.
   3. Promote inner strength and avoiding asking for help from others after the child is born.
   4. Educate the client as to realistic expectations of the medical care the child will receive after birth.

7 The family has just received the amniocentesis report that their daughter has trisomy 21 (Down syndrome). The nurse concludes that which statement made by the father is the most common initial response?

1. "There has to be some mistake. This is someone else's results."
2. "If I pay for it myself, will you redo the test?"
3. "This can't be right. One of you must have made a mistake reading the results."
4. "This is difficult, but we'll get through it together."

8 The client has just given birth to full-term twins. One twin was stillborn. The nurse concludes that this family will need to do which of the following?

1. Simultaneously grieve the loss of one infant while becoming attached to the other.
2. Be passive in accepting the death in order to form an attachment to the living infant.
3. Control their emotions to prevent undue stress for the surviving twin.
4. Minimize the time spent with the dead infant to facilitate attachment to the survivor.

9 The nurse plans to facilitate bereavement after a fetal demise in utero by doing which of the following?

1. Protecting the parents from having to see the dead fetus
2. Encouraging culturally determined naming and burial practices
3. Encouraging the client to tell the older children nothing
4. Avoiding the financial stress of an autopsy

10 The client has given birth to a full-term stillborn male as a result of placental abruption. The grandparents have come to visit. The nurse anticipates that the grandparents will do which of the following?

1. Role model acceptance about the fetal loss
2. Experience a more intense grief reaction than the parents
3. Avoid talking about the dead fetus
4. Go through the same grief phases as the parents

➤ *See pages 292–293 for Answers and Rationales.*

ANSWERS & RATIONALES

Pretest

1 **Answer: 4 Rationale:** During the searching and yearning phase of grieving, parents yearn for their deceased infant, are preoccupied with thoughts of the lost infant, and will have physical manifestations such as aching arms, or looking for the infant. The client does not have anticipatory grieving as the loss has already occurred. The client shows no evidence of being disoriented to person, place, or time. The client has not yet reached a state of reorganization after the infant's demise. **Cognitive Level:** Applying **Client Need:** Psychosocial Integrity **Integrated Process:** Nursing Process: Diagnosis **Content Area:** Maternal-Newborn **Strategy:** The core focus of the question is the searching and yearning phase of grieving. Eliminate incorrect options that do not contain true statements about this phase of grieving. **Reference:** Ladewig, P. A., London, M. L., & Davidson, M.R. (2010). *Contemporary maternal-newborn nursing care* (7th ed.). Upper Saddle River, NJ: Pearson Education, pp. 525–526, 788–789.

2 **Answer: 2 Rationale:** Holding a stillborn helps the family to accept the infant's death as real, and thus facilitate the grieving process. There is no reason for the father to discuss this with the wife first. It is a false statement to tell the father that it would be better not to hold the infant. Giving photographs provides a lasting memory, but this should be done in addition to letting the father hold the child. **Cognitive Level:** Applying **Client Need:** Psychosocial Integrity **Integrated Process:** Nursing Process: Implementation **Content Area:** Maternal-Newborn **Strategy:** The focus of the question is facilitation of the grief work. The correct answer would be the option that contains a nursing action to encourage the client (father) to validate the death of the infant and facilitate his grief work. **Reference:** Ladewig, P. A., London, M. L., & Davidson, M. R. (2010). *Contemporary maternal-newborn nursing care* (7th ed.). Upper Saddle River, NJ: Pearson Education, pp. 525–526, 788–789.

3 **Answer: 1 Rationale:** Autopsy rules out other causes of death, but in cases of SIDS, autopsy findings are normal.

Infants who sleep on the abdomen are more at risk for SIDS. There is no association of bottle-feeding with SIDS. SIDS is not caused by a genetic disorder. **Cognitive Level:** Applying **Client Need:** Physiological Adaptation **Integrated Process:** Teaching and Learning **Content Area:** Maternal-Newborn **Strategy:** Specific knowledge of SIDS and the underlying findings will aid in choosing the correct answer. **Reference:** Ladewig, P. A., London, M. L., & Davidson, M. R. (2010). *Contemporary maternal-newborn nursing care* (7th ed.). Upper Saddle River, NJ: Pearson Education, pp. 653, 725–726.

4 **Answer: 2, 5 Rationale:** Somatic complaints during the grieving process include sighing, weight loss, decreased appetite, restless sleep, fatigue, choking, shortness of breath, throat or chest tightness, abdominal pain, weakness in the legs, or generalized weakness. Tingling on the back of the neck, hearing a baby's cry, increased taste sensitivity, deep sleep, and stiffness in the arms and legs are not somatic complaints during the grieving process. **Cognitive Level:** Applying **Client Need:** Psychosocial Integrity **Integrated Process:** Nursing Process: Assessment **Content Area:** Maternal-Newborn **Strategy:** The focus of the question is somatic symptoms of grief. The correct answers would be options that contain a true statement of a physical (somatic) symptom of grief. **Reference:** Ladewig, P. A., London, M. L., & Davidson, M. R. (2010). *Contemporary maternal-newborn nursing care* (7th ed.). Upper Saddle River, NJ: Pearson Education, pp. 525–526, 788–789.

5 **Answer: 2 Rationale:** The stages of grief must be worked through in order to resolve a fetal loss. This process takes about a year for most people. The other options represent less accurate, briefer timeframes. **Cognitive Level:** Applying **Client Need:** Psychosocial Integrity **Integrated Process:** Teaching and Learning **Content Area:** Maternal-Newborn **Strategy:** Knowledge of the normal period of grief and loss will help to choose the correct response. Recall that adjustment to loss can be a slow process to help guide your selection. **Reference:** Ladewig, P. A., London, M. L., & Davidson, M. R. (2010). *Contemporary maternal-newborn nursing care* (7th ed.). Upper Saddle River, NJ: Pearson Education, pp. 525–526, 788–789.

6 **Answer: 4 Rationale:** Anticipatory grieving is grieving that starts prior to the actual loss. When a fetal anomaly is identified by ultrasound during the pregnancy, the parents begin to grieve the loss of the perfect child prior to the child's birth. The other events have already occurred and so these clients would be grieving. **Cognitive Level:** Analyzing **Client Need:** Psychosocial Integrity **Integrated Process:** Nursing Process: Assessment **Content Area:** Maternal-Newborn **Strategy:** The core focus of the question is anticipatory grief, which by definition begins before the loss occurs. Eliminate options that are similar in representing sudden and unexpected situations that result in fetal loss. The likely correct answer is different from the other options. **Reference:** Ladewig, P. A., London, M.L., & Davidson, M.R. (2010). *Contemporary maternal-newborn nursing care* (7th ed.). Upper Saddle River, NJ: Pearson Education, pp. 525–526, 788–789.

7 **Answer: 1 Rationale:** Tokens of remembrance such as a lock of hair, photos, or a card with the infant's footprints or handprints help the parents accept the reality of their infant's death and facilitate the grieving process. Baptism, naming, a visit from a chaplain, or a sympathy card from staff may bring comfort to the family, but are not tokens of remembrance. **Cognitive Level:** Applying **Client Need:** Psychosocial Integrity **Integrated Process:** Nursing Process: Planning **Content Area:** Maternal-Newborn **Strategy:** Critical words in this question are *tokens of remembrance*, physical objects belonging or connected to the lost child. Eliminate incorrect options as they do not represent a physical reminder of the child that died. **Reference:** Ladewig, P. A., London, M. L., & Davidson, M. R. (2010). *Contemporary maternal-newborn nursing care* (7th ed.). Upper Saddle River, NJ: Pearson Education, pp. 525–526, 788–789.

8 **Answer: 4 Rationale:** Parents have options for nearly all decisions regarding their delivery and postpartal care, including whether or not to use sedatives during labor, naming the infant, rituals or religious rites or sacraments, and which funeral home to plan or hold the funeral or memorial service. The hospital staff can facilitate the mortuary's involvement, but should not recommend one over another or tell the family that the hospital endorses one. **Cognitive Level:** Applying **Client Need:** Psychosocial Integrity **Integrated Process:** Teaching and Learning **Content Area:** Maternal-Newborn **Strategy:** Recall nursing care of parents who have experienced a loss to aid in answering the question correctly. Because the stem of the question contains the critical words "needs clarification," the correct option will be a statement that is incorrect. **Reference:** Ladewig, P. A., London, M. L., & Davidson, M.R. (2010). *Contemporary maternal-newborn nursing care* (7th ed.). Upper Saddle River, NJ: Pearson Education, pp. 525–526, 788–789.

9 **Answer: 2 Rationale:** Continuity of care increases support through trust and familiarity. A new nurse assigned to this family would not know and understand the details of the loss, and would have to take extra time in obtaining a history that could otherwise be used to assess for coping with the loss. Continuity of staff assignment is not intended to decrease interactions with others, prevent the family from needing to ask questions, or facilitate dependence on the nurse. **Cognitive Level:** Applying **Client Need:** Psychosocial Integrity **Integrated Process:** Nursing Process: Planning **Content Area:** Maternal-Newborn **Strategy:** The focus of the question is facilitation of grief work for the client. The correct answer would be the option that supports the family in the time of loss. **Reference:** Ladewig, P. A., London, M. L., & Davidson, M. R. (2010). *Contemporary maternal-newborn nursing care* (7th ed.). Upper Saddle River, NJ: Pearson Education, pp. 525–526, 788–789.

10 **Answer: 3** **Rationale:** The only definitive sign of fetal death is absence of fetal heart tones and no fetal activity on the ultrasound. Diminished fetal activity over recent days is suspicious, but is not an indicator of intrauterine fetal death. A bluish discoloration in the vaginal and cervical mucosa has no significance. Lack of fetal movement for a single day is not an indicator of intrauterine fetal death. **Cognitive Level:** Analyzing **Client Need:** Physiological Adaptation **Integrated Process:** Nursing Process: Assessment **Content Area:** Maternal-Newborn **Strategy:** The focus of the question is objective data to determine fetal death. Recall that only absence of fetal heart tones and fetal movement as diagnosed by ultrasound are absolute signs. **Reference:** Ricci, S. (2008). *Essentials of maternity, newborn and women's health nursing* (2nd ed.). Philadelphia, PA: Lippincott Williams and Wilkins, pp. 634–635.

Posttest

1 **Answer: 1** **Rationale:** Involvement in the labor and birth process will help facilitate moving out of the denial stage, and help facilitate that the death of their child was real. The partner is often a good source of support for the mother during the pain of labor. **Cognitive Level:** Applying **Client Need:** Psychosocial Integrity **Integrated Process:** Nursing Process: Planning **Content Area:** Maternal-Newborn **Strategy:** The focus of the question is the needs of the family experiencing a childbearing loss. Eliminate incorrect options because they do not facilitate validation of the death or provide support to the grieving family. **Reference:** Ladewig, P. A., London, M. L., & Davidson, M. R. (2010). *Contemporary maternal-newborn nursing care* (7th ed.). Upper Saddle River, NJ: Pearson Education, pp. 528–529.

2 **Answer: 3** **Rationale:** Somatic symptoms of grief can be expressed in any physiologic system of the body. Common gastrointestinal symptoms include nausea, vomiting, anorexia, weight loss, or overeating. The other options do not include physiologic symptoms. **Cognitive Level:** Applying **Client Need:** Psychosocial Integrity **Integrated Process:** Nursing Process: Assessment **Content Area:** Maternal-Newborn **Strategy:** Critical words are *somatic symptoms of the grieving process*, which refers to physical expressions of grief. The correct answer would be the option that contains a physical symptom. **Reference:** Venes, D., & Ridge, H. (Eds.) (2009). *Taber's cyclopedic medical dictionary* (21st ed.). Philadelphia, PA: F.A. Davis, p. 2154.

3 **Answer: 3, 5** **Rationale:** Parents report increased stress around the time of the previous fetal loss during subsequent pregnancies. The nurse should provide support as indicated. The nurse should ask open-ended questions to determine the parents' stress level, how they are coping and to discover any client concerns. Educating the client about causes of intrauterine fetal demise serves no purpose and may increase anxiety about the current pregnancy. Encouraging the client to think positively and not dwell on losses is nontherapeutic and does not acknowledge any client concerns. Clients grieve in various ways and carrying a photo and lock of hair at all times may not be needed or desired. **Cognitive Level:** Applying **Client Need:** Psychosocial Integrity **Integrated Process:** Nursing Process: Planning **Content Area:** Maternal-Newborn **Strategy:** Knowledge of parents' reaction during subsequent pregnancies will aid in answering the question correctly. **Reference:** Ladewig, P. A., London, M. L., & Davidson, M. R. (2010). *Contemporary maternal-newborn nursing care* (7th ed.). Upper Saddle River, NJ: Pearson Education, pp. 525–533.

4 **Answer: 4** **Rationale:** The parents will often be in different stages of grief, using different coping mechanisms, and expressing their grief differently. Women tend to be more verbal in their grieving, while men tend to be more internalizing with their grief. The nurse's role is to facilitate communication between the parents and let them know that these differences are both normal and expected. **Cognitive Level:** Applying **Client Need:** Psychosocial Integrity **Integrated Process:** Nursing Process: Assessment **Content Area:** Maternal-Newborn **Strategy:** Three options are similar because the same experience is occurring for both parents; these options should be eliminated. It is more likely that the dissimilar option is the correct answer. **Reference:** Ladewig, P. A., London, M. L., & Davidson, M. R. (2010). *Contemporary maternal-newborn nursing care* (7th ed.). Upper Saddle River, NJ: Pearson Education, pp. 525–532.

5 **Answer: 4** **Rationale:** Loss of self-esteem is reported by both parents after fetal loss. During pregnancy, the fetus is incorporated into the pregnant woman's view of self both physically and emotionally, and a fetal loss is often viewed as a loss of a body part similar to an amputation. Parents form an attachment to the unborn child during pregnancy, and must terminate this attachment when the child is stillborn while also grieving the death of their child. Stating she feels like she is missing a part of herself is not a method of justifying a desire to become pregnant again. **Cognitive Level:** Applying **Client Need:** Psychosocial Integrity **Integrated Process:** Nursing Process: Assessment **Content Area:** Maternal-Newborn **Strategy:** Critical words are *she is missing a part of herself* and *is not related to*, which means that the answer is not correctly related to grief and loss. **Reference:** Ladewig, P. A., London, M. L., & Davidson, M. R. (2010). *Contemporary maternal-newborn nursing care* (7th ed.). Upper Saddle River, NJ: Pearson Education, pp. 525–533.

6 **Answer: 4** **Rationale:** Anticipatory grieving is grief work that takes place prior to the actual loss. In this case, the family will grieve the loss of a perfect child. Providing factual information on what the child will look like and what medical interventions will be necessary, along with support, facilitate this grief work. The nurse has no right to impose personal views on the client and family. Actual information helps the family grieve the loss of a "perfect" child. Support from others will facilitate grief work.

Cognitive Level: Applying **Client Need:** Psychosocial Integrity **Integrated Process:** Nursing Process: Implementation **Content Area:** Maternal-Newborn **Strategy:** The focus of the question is nursing action to promote effective family coping and grief work. The correct answer would be the option that contains common nursing roles of educator and counselor. **Reference:** Ladewig, P. A., London, M. L., & Davidson, M. R. (2010). *Contemporary maternal-newborn nursing care* (7th ed.). Upper Saddle River, NJ: Pearson Education, pp. 525–533.

7 **Answer: 1 Rationale:** The most common initial response is a statement that indicates shock and numbness and includes denial, the first stage of the grieving process. Offering to pay to have the test redone represents bargaining. Stating that the results can't be right has an element of denial, but stating that someone made a mistake has an element of blame, which is not a common initial response. Stating that the couple will get through it together represents acceptance, which is too early for the client's situation. **Cognitive Level:** Applying **Client Need:** Psychosocial Integrity **Integrated Process:** Nursing Process: Diagnosis **Content Area:** Maternal-Newborn **Strategy:** The focus of the question is the first stage of grieving (denial). The correct answer would be the option that contains a true statement regarding this stage. Eliminate incorrect options because they contain statements representative of later stages of grief. **Reference:** Ladewig, P.A., London, M. L., & Davidson, M. R. (2010). *Contemporary maternal-newborn nursing care* (7th ed.). Upper Saddle River, NJ: Pearson Education, pp. 525–533, 788–789.

8 **Answer: 1 Rationale:** The loss of one twin with the survival of the other creates a complex psychological situation. The family must go through the grief work associated with the fetal loss while simultaneously beginning attachment with the surviving infant. These mothers are at higher risk for a pathological grief reaction because of the complexity of the task. The parents do not need to be passive in accepting the death. The parents do not need to control their emotions. It is beneficial for the parents to spend time with the dead infant to help the loss be more real and begin the grieving process. **Cognitive Level:** Analyzing **Client Need:** Psychosocial Integrity **Integrated Process:** Nursing Process: Diagnosis **Content Area:** Maternal-Newborn **Strategy:** The core focus of the question is a family simultaneously experiencing joy and loss at the time of birth. The correct answer is the option that provides support for effective coping with both experiences. **Reference:** Ladewig, P. A., London, M. L., & Davidson, M. R. (2010). *Contemporary maternal-newborn nursing care* (7th ed.). Upper Saddle River, NJ: Pearson Education, pp. 525–526, 788–789.

9 **Answer: 2 Rationale:** Naming the child and having the newborn baptized or participating in other religious ceremonies or rituals also facilitates grief work and acceptance of the loss. Parents need to see and hold their infant to accept the reality of the child's birth and death. Older children must have the death explained to them in developmentally appropriate terms. Autopsy can sometimes provide an answer to the cause of the fetal death, and should be undertaken, if the parents request it or if law requires it. **Cognitive Level:** Applying **Client Need:** Psychosocial Integrity **Integrated Process:** Nursing Process: Planning **Content Area:** Maternal-Newborn **Strategy:** The focus of the question is facilitation of effective coping at the time of fetal loss. Eliminate incorrect options as they avoid the death and hinder the grief process. **Reference:** Ladewig, P. A., London, M. L., & Davidson, M. R. (2010). *Contemporary maternal-newborn nursing care* (7th ed.). Upper Saddle River, NJ: Pearson Education, pp. 205, 341, 525–526, 788–789.

10 **Answer: 4 Rationale:** Grandparents grieve the loss of the grandchild as well as feel pain at the suffering of their child in response to the loss. The grandparents may not be role models about how to accept fetal loss, especially if they have no experience with it. The grandparents' grief reaction is not likely to be more intense than that of the parents. The grandparents are not expected to avoid talking about the dead fetus. **Cognitive Level:** Applying **Client Need:** Psychosocial Integrity **Integrated Process:** Nursing Process: Assessment **Content Area:** Maternal-Newborn **Strategy:** The client includes the entire family system in this question. The correct answer would be the option that contains a true statement about the grief experience for all family members. **Reference:** Ladewig, P. A., London, M. L., & Davidson, M. R. (2010). *Contemporary maternal-newborn nursing care* (7th ed.). Upper Saddle River, NJ: Pearson Education, pp. 525–526, 788–789.

References

Davidson, M., London, M., & Ladewig, P. (2012). *Olds' maternal newborn nursing & women's health across the lifespan* (9th ed.). Upper Saddle River, NJ: Pearson Education.

Ladewig, P., London, M., & Davidson, M. (2009). *Contemporary maternal-newborn nursing care* (7th ed.). Upper Saddle River, NJ: Pearson Education.

Perry, S.E., Hockenberry, M.J., Lowdermilk, D. L., & Wilson, D. (2010). *Maternal child nursing care* (4th ed.). St. Louis, MO: Mosby.

Ricci, S. (2009). *Essentials of maternity, newborn, and women's health nursing* (2nd ed.). Philadelphia: Lippincott Williams & Wilkins.

Appendix

➤ Practice to Pass Suggested Answers

Chapter 1

Page 5: *Answer*—This nurse should be terminated as individual and institutional standards of care as well as national standards of care were violated. Through an educational program the nurse would have learned the proper way to administer medications: checking each medication against the physician's order at least three times, giving medications to one client at a time, and then charting the medications that had been administered. The institution's policies and procedure were violated, as within the policy would be a procedure for correct administration of medications. These policies and procedures are developed for the clients' safety and well-being and would be reviewed by national organizations that accredit hospitals and other health care institutions. The nurse violated national standards, as reasonable and diligent practice of the registered nurse within all regions would take more care in administering and documenting medications.

Page 10: *Answer*—While the decision to forego surgery may be considered negligent in the eyes of the law and unwise and inappropriate from a medical perspective, it is ethically justifiable. The nurse could refer the issue to the institution's ethics committee or use an ethical decision-making framework (MORAL) to guide discussions between the interested parties, the parents and health care professionals.

Page 12: *Answer*—The nurse manager will need to help the nursery nurses identify their own cultural beliefs, personal biases, attitudes, stereotypes, and prejudices. Then the nurses will need to learn about the cultures of the clients. As the nurses become more familiar with the cultural ways of their clients, the nurses can become more sensitive to the clients and share the goal of overcoming many of the cultural conflicts.

Page 15: *Answer*—The nurse needs to recognize that the client may not be the primary care provider for the infant when they go home, especially if the client will be returning to school. The nurse should include the grandmothers in the teaching, acknowledging their expertise and letting them share it with the client. The nurse could use the opportunity to educate the grandmothers and the client about current childbearing and childrearing practices to promote the health of all family members.

Page 20: *Answer*—Explain to your friend the different levels of care available for expectant mothers and the philosophical differences between physicians and advanced practice nurses. Since this is her first pregnancy and if she is low risk, you might encourage her to see someone who will provide a great deal of education throughout the pregnancy and encourage her and the family to be actively involved in the process.

Chapter 2

Page 34: *Answer*—The basal body temperature is most accurate when taken upon awakening from the longest period of sleep a woman gets in a day *prior* to arising. The client should be instructed to follow her usual sleep–wake routine, and take her temperature every day before she gets out of bed, regardless of what time she awakens.

Page 35: *Answer*—A hysterosalpingogram utilizes an iodine-based dye, which is then instilled into the uterus and fallopian tubes. Iodine allergy is a risk factor for anaphylactic reaction. The nurse's role is to verbally inform the physician performing the examination of the allergy, and to make certain it is clearly marked on the chart and on the client's allergy wristband.

Page 35: *Answer*—Lack of sperm in the ejaculate does not always indicate lack of sperm production. Blockage of the vas deferens or epididymis will prohibit the sperm from being ejaculated. A testicular biopsy will be performed to detect the presence of sperm deeper within the epididymis. If sperm are found, they can be obtained via needle aspiration, and then fertilization can be facilitated via intrauterine insemination, GIFT, in vitro fertilization, or sperm insertion into the ova. If no sperm are present, the couple will need to use donor sperm through artificial insemination to achieve pregnancy.

Page 36: *Answer*—Infertility treatments can create stress for a couple through a number of factors: cost of the treatments, time away from work for appointments, necessity of having intercourse at prescribed times, need for the male to masturbate for semen analysis or sperm samples, anticipatory grieving for the inability to conceive spontaneously, family and social pressures to have children, and medications used to induce ovulation that can create moodiness in women. Marital difficulties may manifest themselves as impotence, lack of interest in sexual intercourse, communication difficulties, and many others. The role of the nurse is to assess the couple's communication with each other, the need for further information regarding infertility treatments, and the need for professional counseling. Many couples find that attending a support group for infertile couples helps a great deal, and the nurse should provide the couple with information on such groups. Most important is to acknowledge that the stress response of both of the individuals and the couple together is normal and expected during the stressful time of infertility treatments.

Page 36: *Answer*—Ovulation induction medications are given on a daily basis beginning around day five of the menstrual cycle. Daily ultrasound examinations that require an office visit may be necessary beginning around mid-cycle to monitor ovarian follicle production and maturation, and for timing of hCG administration to stimulate final maturation. Egg retrieval is performed when several follicles are mature, after which the client must rest for about two hours. Embryo reinsertion is performed 42 to 72 hours later; zygotes are reinserted 18 to 24 hours later. In either case, the client should restrict her activities to bedrest for 12 to 24 hours after the procedure is performed. No further clinic visits will be needed for about 14 days, when pregnancy testing or ultrasound examination will be undertaken if menses do not begin.

Chapter 3

Page 46: *Answer*—A teaching plan for a client with low literacy skills can be effectively modified through the use of less printed instructions and greater use of models and diagrams with reinforcement through verbal instructions. Clients should be given the opportunity to see and handle the method selected for contraception, demonstrating the correct usage, and verbally restating pertinent information to verify understanding.

Page 49: *Answer*—Fertility awareness methods of contraception are based on identification of the fertile period, which surrounds the time of ovulation, and the avoidance of unprotected intercourse during this period to prevent pregnancy. Ovulation usually occurs about 14 days prior to the next menses and physical signs can be used in addition to a menstrual calendar to indicate the release of the ovum. Primary indicators of ovulation include basal body temperature and changes in the cervical mucus. Basal body temperature typically drops just prior to ovulation, then rises and remains elevated until two to three days prior to the next menses. Cervical mucus becomes thin, clear, watery, slippery, and stretchable at the time of ovulation. Secondary indicators of ovulation include increased libido, abdominal bloating, mid-cycle abdominal pain or mittelschmerz, breast or pelvic tenderness, a feeling of pelvic or vulvar fullness, slight dilatation of the cervical os, and the softer cervix is located higher in the vagina.

Page 53: *Answer*—Because the diaphragm covers the cervix and remains in place for up to four hours prior to intercourse and at least six hours following coitus, the risk of infection is a possibility. By teaching the woman to remove the diaphragm at least once in a 24-hour period, the incidence of toxic shock syndrome can be reduced. Use of the diaphragm should also be avoided during the menstrual period or when any abnormal vaginal discharge is present. If the client experiences any warning signs of toxic shock syndrome such as elevation of temperature >100.4°F, diarrhea and vomiting, weakness and faintness, muscle aches, sore throat, or sunburn-type rash, the woman should contact the health care provider immediately.

Page 57: *Answer*—The nurse should first determine what type of oral contraceptive pill, progestin-only or combination estrogen–progestin, the woman is taking and which week in the menstrual cycle the woman is in. If the woman is using progestin-only pills, every pill is an active pill. She should take the next pill at the regular time and use a back-up method for the remainder of the cycle. If the woman is using combination pills and is in week one or two of the cycle, she should take two pills a day for two days, finish the cycle, and use a back-up method. If she is in the third week of the cycle and uses combination pills, she should take one pill a day until Sunday, start a new pack of pills on Sunday, and use a back-up method for one week.

Page 62: *Answer*—The nurse should inquire what method of contraception the woman is currently using or has used in the past and with what degree of success in preventing pregnancy. The nurse should explore if the woman is dissatisfied with the method itself, is experiencing side effects, and what the woman's plans are for future childbearing. If the woman desires no further pregnancies, it may be appropriate to discuss permanent sterilization through tubal ligation or vasectomy for the male partner. If pregnancy is desired in the future, alternative methods of contraception should be explored.

Chapter 4

Page 71: *Answer*—It requires two recessive genes to develop PKU. Therefore, a mother with PKU carries these two genes. Although the father does not have PKU, he may be a carrier having one of the recessive genes. If he is a carrier, the possible combinations of genes are PKU/no PKU, no PKU/PKU, PKU/PKU, and no PKU/no PKU. There is a 50% chance of having a child with PKU and a 50% chance that the child will be a carrier. If the father is not a carrier, the possible genetic combinations are all PKU/no PKU. No children will have PKU, but all will be carriers.

Page 71: *Answer*—Humans possess 23 pairs of chromosomes for a total of 46 chromosomes. Each parent contributes 23 chromosomes that are paired during the union of the sperm and ovum. Trisomy 21 is a chromosome condition seen when the 21st chromosome has three chromosomes rather than the usual two. The third chromosome often forms before fertilization even occurs. The ovum may have two chromosomes 21 instead of one because the cells did not separate as expected. When this ovum joins with a sperm, the extra chromosome is included.

Page 72: *Answer*—The nurse educates the client by defining and describing anencephaly in a sensitive manner. The nurse validates client understanding of the seriousness of the condition and expectations for the pregnancy. She reviews the client's options and possible outcomes for each option while being sensitive to the client's social, cultural, and religious beliefs. Questions are asked and answered in a nonjudgmental manner. Decisions regarding the pregnancy belong to the client only. The nurse maintains confidentiality.

Page 72: *Answer*—If the couple is trying to achieve a pregnancy it is important that the clients understand the viability of sperm and ova. An ovum released during ovulation is capable of being fertilized for 24 hours. Sperm survive for 48 to 72 hours in the female genital tract but are most capable of fertilization 24 hours after ejaculation. To achieve fertilization, the couple should have intercourse no earlier than 24 hours prior to ovulation and no later than 24 hours after ovulation.

Page 73: *Answer*—Monozygotic twins are often called identical twins. They are identical in that they have the same genetic code. Since chromosomes determine gender, they will always be the same sex and have similar physical characteristics. Identical twins occur at random when a fertilized ovum separates very early in the pregnancy to form two identical zygotes. They may share placentas and amniotic sacs. Dizygotic twins are not identical and are also called fraternal twins. They occur when the mother releases two ova during ovulation and they are fertilized by two different sperm. They carry different genetic codes so they may be different sexes and physical characteristics. They are related genetically the same way any sibling is related. They usually have separate placentas and amniotic sacs. The tendency to have dizygotic twins does run in families.

Page 81: *Answer*—The ductus arteriosus connects the pulmonary artery to the aorta in the fetus to allow blood to bypass the fetal lung. The lung receives little circulation in the fetus because it is not a unit for gas exchange. If the ductus arteriosus remains patent in the newborn there is a potential for the infant's circulation to continue bypassing the lung. Once out of the uterus, the infant depends on the lungs as a unit of gas exchange. If blood bypasses the lungs, this cannot take place.

Page 83: *Answer*—The embryo is a stage of development from two to eight weeks' gestation characterized by cell multiplication and specialization. All of the body's tissues and organs are formed during this time, although they are immature. The embryo may not have a human external appearance. The fetal stage is from eight weeks' gestation until birth. This is a time of growth and maturation of tissues and organs. The fetus takes on a very human appearance.

Chapter 5

Page 93: *Answer*—The nurse should begin by assessing what the mother is thinking and feeling. Questions such as, "What are you feeling now that you have seen your baby?" or "You seem upset; how are you feeling about your pregnancy?" might help to clarify the situation. The nurse can affirm the mother's feelings by telling her that most women have ambivalent feelings toward pregnancy, even if the pregnancy is planned. Explaining to the mother that pregnancy is a developmental challenge resulting in stress and anxiety for the woman and her family will help her realize that her response is not abnormal or unusual.

Page 95: *Answer*—The nurse should begin by assessing what the woman knows about prenatal care, as she may be uninformed or have been misinformed by relatives or friends, as well as her reasons for not planning to participate in prenatal care. Then the nurse can take the opportunity to teach her the purposes of prenatal care including assessment of well-being of both mother and baby; screening, prevention, or management of any problems that may develop; and opportunities for education related to childbirth, nutrition, management of the discomforts of pregnancy, and parenting. Barriers to prenatal care such as money, transportation, and childcare can be explored with the mother. The nurse may be able to make referrals to help the mother overcome any barriers that are impacting her care.

Page 96: *Answer*—The nurse can share information on what classes are available and the content of these classes. By assessing the mother's goals and expectations for this pregnancy, the nurse may be able to direct the mother or other members of her family to a class that is helpful. New information since her last delivery may be available, or specialized classes, such as those designed for siblings or grandparents, may be useful.

Page 97: *Answer*—According to her menstrual history, the client is about eight weeks' pregnant. This means it is probably too early to hear the fetal heartbeat with a Doppler device or fetoscope or to palpate fetal movement. The only way to positively diagnose pregnancy at this point is to visualize the fetus by ultrasound. This can be done as early as two to three weeks after conception.

Page 99: *Answer*—The nurse should begin by explaining that when the client lies on her back, the weight of the pregnant uterus presses on major blood vessels and decreases the amount of blood returning to the heart. This compromises oxygen supply to both the mother and the fetus, should be avoided, and probably explains the feeling of faintness. The nurse should suggest that the mother try positioning herself with pillows for back support, between her legs, and/or for her upper arm when she sleeps on her side. If the mother must sleep on her back, she could try elevating her upper body or putting a pillow under her right hip.

Page 100: *Answer*—Assuming the client's weight was within normal limits before she became pregnant, the nurse should begin by affirming the woman's concerns about her weight. The client and the nurse should review the client's dietary history and preferences and then work together to develop a plan for lunches and snacks that include increased amounts of fruits and vegetables with decreased fried foods. This might involve bringing lunch and snacks from home or making better food choices at restaurants.

Page 102: *Answer*—The nurse should begin by assessing former and current family roles and expectations. The nurse can help the mother determine what support systems are available and what types of help would best relieve the situation. The nurse can then help the mother develop a plan for getting needed help from her husband, extended family, or other sources.

Chapter 6

Page 112: *Answer*—"The problem was probably caused by your mother's blood type or Rh status and both these factors are hereditary. Your blood type and Rh will be checked in the laboratory work that is done at the first prenatal visit. If it is determined that you have Rh negative blood or a blood group which places your baby at increased risk for problems, these findings will be explained to you and follow-up assessments will be done."

Page 114: *Answer*—Several of the TORCH infections cause severe problems for the fetus but only minor signs or symptoms in adults and it is possible to have the infection without knowing it. Routine testing of all pregnant women can help to identify women who have had an infection, women with a current infection and no symptoms, or women at risk for an infection because of lack of immunity.

Page 115: *Answer*—"Testing your urine at every visit is an important assessment of your health during pregnancy and can tell us if problems are developing. If we found sugar in your urine, it could mean you are developing gestational diabetes. If we found protein in your urine, it could indicate preeclampsia with hypertension. White blood cells or nitrites in the urine can indicate an infection."

Page 117: *Answer*—The human immunodeficiency virus (HIV) is transmitted through exchange of body fluids including semen, blood, or vaginal secretions and can be passed in this manner from any person to another. Women are the group of people showing the greatest rise in incidence, and transmission is usually through heterosexual contact. Testing of pregnant women is especially important, since the woman may not know she is infected. The virus can cross the placenta and infect the baby or it can be passed to the newborn in breast milk. Early diagnosis of the disease is not only important to the woman, but treatment during pregnancy decreases the incidence of the baby contracting the infection before birth.

Page 121: *Answer*—"This test provides information about how your baby's heart rate reacts when the baby is active and gives an indication of the current well-being of the baby. Typically, when a baby is active, moving, and receiving enough oxygen, the heart rate will speed up. The contractions of labor provide an additional source of stress to the baby. Because this test does not involve uterine contractions, it does not give any information about how well the baby will tolerate labor."

Chapter 7

Page 136: *Answer*—The narcotic antagonist properties of Stadol will block the effects of the methadone causing narcotic withdrawal symptoms in the addicted client. A better choice for this client would be epidural analgesia.

Page 137: *Answer*—Standard blood and body fluid precautions should be implemented with all clients. The nurse should avoid contact with maternal blood by wearing gloves and using other protective devices as needed. The mother should be instructed to wash her hands after pericare and before caring for her infant. She should be advised to formula-feed her baby to avoid passing the virus through breast milk.

Page 142: *Answer*—The nurse should be supportive without offering false hope. The client should be given accurate information with time allowed for questions and expression of feelings. Communication techniques such as empathy, reflection, and providing information about the grief process are most appropriate after perinatal loss. The loss should not be minimized in any way.

Page 146: *Answer*—The client needs to be evaluated closely for possible placental abruption. She should be placed on a fetal monitor and baseline FHR, variability, and any accelerations or decelerations noted. Uterine activity should be palpated as well as monitored. The client should be instructed to report any abdominal pain or vaginal bleeding. Ultrasound may be used to identify an abruption.

Page 146: *Answer*—Test the fluid with nitrazine paper; amniotic fluid will change color from yellow to blue because of alkaline pH. Amniotic fluid also shows the characteristic ferning pattern on a slide with dried fluid.

Chapter 8

Page 158: *Answer*—This is a late deceleration, which is always ominous. Nursing interventions are aimed at increasing oxygenation of the fetus through facilitating utero-placental transport. If the client is in a supine position, she should be repositioned to the left lateral position to improve utero-placental perfusion. If the client is hypotensive, increase the IV fluid rate or start an IV. Oxygen should be administered by mask at 7 to 10 liters per minute. If the contractions are being augmented or induced, decrease uterine stimuli by turning off or decreasing the oxytocin. Findings should be documented, fetal monitoring should be continuously maintained and assessed, and the health care provider notified.

Page 159: *Answer*—The intrauterine pressure catheter (IUPC) detects the strength of uterine contractions, measured in mm of Hg just like blood pressure. IUPCs are used when inducing labor or when labor is not progressing as quickly as expected to determine if augmentation of contractions is needed. External contraction monitoring could also be used but it cannot accurately measure contraction strength and may not accurately detect contractions if the fetus is transverse, the client is either very thin or obese, or the woman or fetus frequently change positions.

Page 160: *Answer*—The attitude, or relationship of fetal parts to one another, of the fetus in a frank breech position demonstrates flexion of the hips with extension of the knees. The lie is longitudinal with the cephalocaudal axis of the fetus parallel to the cephalocaudal axis of the mother. Presentation refers to the part of fetus entering the pelvis first. In this case, the breech, or buttocks are presenting first. The position, RSA, indicates the fetal sacrum is presenting with the back of the fetus toward the right anterior portion of the maternal pelvis.

Page 164: *Answer*—The nurse should teach the client that episiotomies are sometimes performed in the case of fetal distress or when the health care provider suspects that lacerations may occur. Because each birth is unique, it is not possible to predict in advance which clients will need episiotomies or sustain lacerations during delivery. The nurse should reassure the client that the health care provider will try to prevent serious lacerations and will perform an episiotomy only if necessary. The client also needs reassurance that should she need an episiotomy or experience a laceration, adequate anesthesia will be provided so that the repair will not be painful.

Page 166: *Answer*—Nonpharmacologic methods of pain relief appropriate for this client include hydrotherapy through soaking in a tub or sitting or standing in the shower; breathing techniques; relaxation techniques, which may be facilitated through massage; listening to relaxing music, imagery, or visualization; position changes as dictated by the location of the client's pain or walking; and therapeutic touch or support from the presence of the nurse or other support person. Pharmacological options appropriate for this stage of labor would include intrathecal narcotics or epidural placement. It is critical to ascertain that informed consent has been obtained before intrathecal or epidural analgesia is performed, so that the client is aware of the potential side effects. It is too early for IV administration of a narcotic agent because labor progress may be slowed.

Chapter 9

Page 177: *Answer*—It is best to tell the client that forceps may leave a red mark or a bruise on the face that will go away in a few days. Sometimes there is slight swelling and often the baby's head will seem misshapen because it molds or conforms to the shape of the birth canal. Clients who have not been forewarned may be worried about the appearance of their baby right after delivery.

Page 179: *Answer*—As you begin the assessment, visualize the fetus lying in the abdomen. In a breech presentation, the examiner should find a much firmer, rounded fetal pole in the fundus (the fetal head), as opposed to the softer irregular shape of the feet and buttocks. The fetal head floating in the uterine fundus is also ballottable (bounceable or easily moveable between the examiner's hands). During the third and fourth maneuvers (palpating the lower uterine segment and determining engagement of the presenting part), the examiner will note a softer, irregular, and wider fetal pole as opposed to the firm and rounded fetal head. An additional finding to help confirm suspicion of breech presentation is the location of fetal heart tones above the umbilicus (in an upper quadrant).

Page 181: *Answer*—Using lay terminology, tell the client that the fetal monitor indicates that something needs to be done to improve blood supply to the placenta so there will be more oxygen available to the baby. Lying on the side improves blood circulation to the placenta and to the baby, so there is a better oxygen supply. It is better to lie on either side, rather than on the back, but the left side has been shown to be the best position for good circulation to the baby.

Page 187: *Answer*—"If your baby's birth can be delayed about three or four weeks, it would be best. Even though all the baby's organs are formed, they are still not functioning at a mature level. This is especially true of the lungs. Many babies who are born before 37 weeks have problems with breathing (respiratory distress). Every day that your baby stays inside you helps make sure that he or she is developed enough to live outside your body without help."

Page 188: *Answer*—As with any precipitate birth, do not leave the patient alone. Call for help. If time allows, obtain a towel or blanket and put on sterile gloves. Feet and/or buttocks may appear at the introitus and can deliver through an incomplete cervix, setting the stage for entrapment of the fetal head. Therefore, allow the delivery to proceed slowly. Observe for cord prolapse. Encourage the woman to pant or blow to decrease the urge to push. If the client is more comfortable on her side, allow her to stay in that position until the fetal abdomen begins to deliver. At that point, reposition the mother and raise the infant's trunk and legs upward to facilitate delivery of the head. The infant's head must be delivered quickly to prevent asphyxia. Applying slight pressure above the symphysis may help speed delivery of the head. The major risks of vaginal delivery of a breech infant are cord prolapse, head entrapment, and birth injury.

Page 191: *Answer*—The most common causes of emergency cesarean section are dystocia or difficult labor, which is most often caused by the baby's head being too large for the size of the bony pelvis (cephalopelvic disproportion), fetal distress, and breech presentation. None of these factors can be controlled by the mother; therefore, avoiding an emergency cesarean section may not be possible. The only thing that a woman can do is to maintain her health throughout the prenatal period and to preserve her strength and well-being during labor. The outcome, a healthy baby, is more important than the method of delivery. It is important to learn about cesarean delivery in case your baby needs to be delivered in this way.

Chapter 10

Page 203: *Answer*—It is not unusual for a client's white blood cell count to rise as high as 30,000/mm^3 during the first few days after delivery. However, the nurse should always assess for signs of infection such as fever, increased uterine pain or tenderness, foul-smelling lochia, or frequency, burning, and urgency with urination.

Page 203: *Answer*—It is true that women who are breastfeeding are less likely to ovulate and may have more difficulty conceiving while breastfeeding, but they can still become pregnant again. Although it is used as a birth control method in some Third World countries, breastfeeding is only considered effective if the woman breastfeeds exclusively and nurses throughout the night. It is not generally recommended for women in the United States as a method of birth control because other reliable and safe methods are readily available.

Page 205: *Answer*—The nurse must be careful to avoid contact with blood and body fluids. Because there is a chance of exposure to lochia and other body fluids while assessing the perineum, gloves should be worn during this part of the assessment.

Page 206: *Answer*—The nurse should first assess the front of the perineum with the client on her back and her legs apart. Then the nurse should have the client turn onto her side and stand behind the client to examine the back portion of the perineum and anus. The client should draw the upper leg toward the chest and the nurse should lift the upper buttock to improve visualization.

Page 207: *Answer*—Breast milk production is based on supply and demand. The more the breasts are stimulated, the more milk they will produce. The mother will need to drink additional fluids and will have additional nutritional needs of 200 to 500 kcal per baby. The mother may choose to nurse both babies at the same time to allow herself more rest between feedings or she may feed one baby at a time in sequence. Mothers who breastfeed simultaneously may wish to experiment with positions and often need help getting the babies to latch on or be removed from the breast. Cultural considerations are also important to the care of this client. Warm fluids may be more acceptable than cold to restore balance and food preferences should be respected. Hmong women find expressing or pumping the breasts unacceptable, but combining breast- and bottle-feeding is a common feeding practice.

Chapter 11

Page 218: *Answer*—In assessing the client, her birth history indicates she is at risk for several complications. She delivered a large-for-gestational age infant that could cause overstretching of the uterus resulting in uterine atony. Lacerations of the genital tract are associated with forceps-assisted births. Macrosomia and operative delivery both increase the likelihood of hematoma, which can result from birth trauma. All three of the identified risk factors increase the likelihood of early postpartum hemorrhage for this client.

Upon physical assessment, the nurse might find a boggy uterus, expelled clots, and visible, bright red bleeding. If a laceration were present, the bleeding would appear as a steady stream or trickle in the presence of a firm uterus. Bleeding from a hematoma is not readily visible as blood is collected in the tissues and can be located anywhere in the genital tract that has been subjected to trauma during birth. The client may complain of extreme pain or pressure, and may be unable to void.

Page 222: *Answer*—Following delivery, subinvolution is the failure of the uterus to return to its normal size. Subinvolution of the placental site due to retained placental tissue is the most frequent cause of late postpartum hemorrhage occurring within one to two weeks after childbirth. Symptoms may include fundal height greater than expected, lochia that fails to progress from rubra to serosa to alba normally, and lochia rubra that persists longer than two weeks. Women may also report scant brown lochia or irregular heavy vaginal bleeding. If infection is a cause, there may be leukorrhea, backache, or foul-smelling lochia.

Page 226: *Answer*—Preventing mastitis is easier than treating it. Mothers should be instructed in correct breastfeeding techniques before discharge. The nurse or lactation consultant should assist new mothers with breastfeeding as soon as possible following delivery.

In this case, the client probably has a low-grade fever that is coinciding with her breast milk coming in. The difference between breast fullness and engorgement should be defined. With engorgement, the breasts are hard, painful, and appear taut and shiny. Nursing is difficult for the infant and painful to the mother. To relieve engorgement the client should hand-express some of the milk. A warm, moist cloth can be placed over the breast and the woman can massage her breast to stimulate let down or use a manual pump to express some of the milk. This relieves the pressure, which will allow the infant to latch on to the breast more successfully. The mother should be encouraged to wear a well-fitting and supportive nursing bra 24 hours a day to prevent discomfort from the increased weight of the breast.

The client should be provided instructions on symptoms of mastitis, which appear suddenly and include fever greater than 100.4°F, headache, flu-like symptoms, and warm, reddened, painful areas of the breast, usually in the upper outer quadrant accompanied by enlarged and tender axillary lymph nodes. The client should contact her health care provider immediately if she suspects mastitis. Ten percent of all cases of mastitis will result in a breast abscess requiring incision and drainage. Mastitis should be treated with a 10-day course of antibiotics and nonsteroidal anti-inflammatory drugs (NSAIDs) as needed, increased fluid intake, rest, local applications of heat and cold, and the breasts should be emptied frequently either by nursing or pumping.

Page 228: *Answer*—Thromboembolic disease may occur during the antepartum period, but it is considered more of a postpartum problem. Risk factors include history of thromboembolic disease, varicosities, anemia, obesity, increased maternal age, high parity, and anesthesia or surgery with resultant venous stasis. The client should be assessed for signs of pain, edema, color and temperature changes, and peripheral pulses. Absence or differences in peripheral pulses should also be noted and may be indicative of altered circulation. The client should be instructed not to massage her leg or get out of bed until the nurse discusses the client's condition with her health care provider.

Page 230: *Answer*—Adjustment reaction with depressed mood (baby blues) is accompanied by feeling overwhelmed, unable to cope, fatigued, anxious, irritable and oversensitive. Episodic tearfulness without an identifiable reason is a key feature. Symptoms of postpartum psychosis include agitation, hyperactivity, insomnia, labile mood, confusion, irrationality, difficulty remembering or concentrating, poor judgment, delusions, and hallucinations. Postpartum major mood disorder, or postpartum depression, is characterized by sadness, frequent crying, insomnia, appetite change, difficulty concentrating and making decisions, feelings of worthlessness, obsessive thoughts of inadequacy as a person and parent, lack of interest in usual activities, and lack of concern about personal appearance. Persistent anxiety contributes to the woman's feeling out of control, and irritability and hostility toward others, including the newborn, may be evident.

Chapter 12

Page 240: *Answer*—"Those small white spots are called milia. They are plugged sebaceous or sweat glands and are normal in newborns. They will disappear without treatment in a few weeks."

Page 241: *Answer*—Posture: breech deliveries and a dislocated hip may affect the ability to perform the leg and hip maneuvers required for the gestational age assessment. A fractured clavicle will not allow the arm and shoulder maneuvers. Sole creases: assessment must be performed within the first few hours after birth. After two hours, the edema of tissues present in most newborns begins to resolve and creases appear; these creases do not have the same predictive value as those assessed before resolution of newborn edema. Breast bud tissue: there may be accelerated development in a large-for-gestational age newborn and there may be less tissue development in a small-for-gestational age newborn.

Page 242: *Answer*—Newborns usually assume a flexed position as it allows less body surface to be exposed to the environment, thereby preserving body heat. The infant has also been in a flexed position while in the uterus and prefers to maintain a position that is familiar and comfortable.

Page 244: *Answer*—When mothers choose not to bottle-feed, the American Academy of Pediatrics recommends the infant be given only formula for the first six months and then formula plus the addition of solid food for the remainder of the first year of life to reduce the possibility of the infant developing allergies. Cow's milk is more difficult for the newborn to digest because the protein molecules are much larger, resulting in vomiting or diarrhea.

Page 246: *Answer*—The mother can listen for audible swallowing by the third or fourth day, check the infant for one wet diaper the first day, two wet diapers the second day, and so on until the infant is having seven or more wet diapers per 24-hour period. As the breast milk supply increases, so will the amount of wet diapers. Mother can inspect the infant's mouth after a feeding to look for signs of colostrum (a white-yellowish thick substance). If the newborn is quiet for 1 ½ hours after a feeding, this can indicate satiation. The mother can try to express colostrum or milk from her breast to validate lactation and provide reassurance that nutrition is available for her infant.

Chapter 13

Page 255: *Answer*—The initial response should always be to look at the infant first, because occasionally the monitor is not accurately measuring the saturation. If the infant is pink and active, assess the probe site and possibly reposition it. However, if the infant is not pink, begin the steps of resuscitation: airway, breathing, and compressions. Remember to treat the client, not the machine.

Page 264: *Answer*—If meconium is present in the amniotic fluid, the infant is at risk for meconium aspiration syndrome (MAS). The infant's airway should be thoroughly suctioned prior to delivery of the shoulders. The infant should be placed under a radiant warmer and the vocal cords visualized with a laryngoscope. If there is meconium present it should be suctioned out. When the cords are clear of meconium, respiratory effort can be stimulated and resuscitation can proceed if necessary.

Page 268: *Answer*—HIV has been isolated in the breast milk of mothers who are HIV-positive. The risk of transmission to the newborn is not clear. Mothers in the United States have access to nutritious formula supplements, which are not readily available in many underdeveloped countries. For this reason, the Center for Disease Control (CDC) has recommended that HIV-positive women in the US should not breastfeed. In underdeveloped countries, the risk of severe malnutrition and death is significant for infants who are not breastfed. It is felt that even though there is a risk the infant will contract HIV from the breast milk of an HIV-positive woman, the risk of severe malnutrition is even greater. Therefore, HIV-positive women in these countries are encouraged to breastfeed.

Page 269: *Answer*—This means that if this infant were in an open crib, he most likely would be experiencing hypothermia. Hypothermia is a common sign of early sepsis and should be evaluated closely.

Page 272: *Answer*—Clients with chronic diabetes are at risk for vascular disease. This can include the blood vessels of the uterus, which would decrease the blood flow to the placenta during pregnancy, resulting in decreased growth in the fetus and an infant who is small for gestational age (SGA).

Chapter 14

Page 282: *Answer*—Reassure the mother that what she is experiencing is normal and is indicative of the searching and yearning phase of bereavement. Although disturbing, this will pass as the client moves toward reorganization.

Page 284: *Answer*—You need to explore Muslim requirements and customs regarding infant death. If the client speaks English, gently ask her or a family member if there are specific timelines to be adhered to regarding burial, if autopsy is desired, and what you need to do when you care for the infant. If the client does not speak English, obtain the services of a trained medical interpreter. Consulting a sourcebook on nursing care in other cultures can also be helpful, but the nurse must avoid assuming what is presented is true for all families. Clarify the accuracy of the information with this specific family before intervening to ensure cultural competence.

Page 286: *Answer*—Children under 6 do not understand the abstract nature of death yet. Additionally, they may believe that negative feelings they had about the new baby caused the fetal death. Comparing death to sleeping can be confusing to young children, and should be avoided so that the child does not fear going to sleep himself because he might also die.

Page 287: *Answer*—Respond therapeutically, asking "Tell me what you think might be wrong." Then either obtain a doppler and listen for fetal heart tones or ask the health care provider to listen for fetal heart tones. If listening is inadequate to verify fetal heart tones, an ultrasound may be used to document the heart beat and fetal movement.

Page 288: *Answer*—Allow the parents of a stillborn to perform whatever cares they desire, including bathing, dressing, applying lotion, combing the hair, etc. Provide for privacy for the clients while they bathe their infant, and encourage the parents to explore the fingers, toes, and body just as parents of a live-born child will do.

➤ Case Study Suggested Answers

Chapter 1

1. Because the child was not conceived with the hope that the stem cells would genetically match their son, there are not as many ethical issues as there would be with a planned conception. An ethical framework could be used to identify the ethical concerns and address the issues.
2. Hindus consider organ donation and the giving of blood and blood products acceptable practices, therefore, harvesting stem cells to donate to another would also be an acceptable practice. The specific views and values of the family involved need to be explored to validate the acceptability of this practice.
3. Sons are very significant to Asian Indians. The son is the one to inherit, to provide for the parents in their old age, and to participate in the ritual of death and mourning that guarantees the passage of the parent into Heaven. The birth of a son, especially as a first born, significantly improves his mother's status within the family.
4. In many cultures, the extended family plays a significant role during the postpartal period. A grandmother will generally come for an extended stay to help with the running of the household.
5. The nurse should realize that the issue of stem cell harvesting and birth of a daughter could have significant cultural meaning. As the client is being admitted, the nurse should explore the couple's cultural beliefs, sharing them with other staff, and supporting the couple's plans. This might also be an opportunity for the nurse to develop cultural awareness about Asian Indian Hindu families.

Chapter 2

1. You will obtain a full medical and surgical history. Has she ever had any surgery (especially abdominal or pelvic surgery)? Does she have any medical problems? Has she ever had to be hospitalized, and if so, why? Has she had pelvic infections such as PID or sexually transmitted infections such as gonorrhea or chlamydia? Has she had recent weight loss or gain? What medications, vitamins, and herbs does she take? Does she have any allergies? When did her menses begin, and what is her cycle frequency, length, and flow? What contraceptive methods has she used, when did she use them, and has she had any problems with the methods?
2. You will obtain a full medical and surgical history. Has he ever had any surgery? Does he have any medical problems? Has he ever had to be hospitalized, and if so, why? Has he had sexually transmitted infections such as gonorrhea or chlamydia? Has he had recent weight loss or gain? What medications, vitamins, and herbs does he take? Does he have any allergies? In addition, you will need to ask if he has ever had trauma to his scrotum and/or genitals, whether he had mumps, and if so, when?

3. You should describe the need to detect abnormalities in either member of the couple, which may require discussion about their sexual practices, physical examination, blood testing, semen analysis, hysterosalpingogram, and postcoital examination.
4. How often is the couple having intercourse, and when in the menstrual cycle? What positions do they use? Does the husband have any difficulty with either premature ejaculation or impotence?
5. Women after the age of about 35 tend to ovulate less regularly, and are more likely to have anovulatory menstrual cycles. Therefore, she is more likely to be prescribed ovulation induction medications. For unknown reasons, IVF is less successful in women after their mid-30s. However, by no means does her age indicate that the couple will not be able to become pregnant.

Chapter 3

1. While oral contraceptives are a safe and effective method, they are not indicated for every woman. A woman with a history of thromboembolic or cardiovascular disorders, breast cancer, or estrogen-dependent neoplasms should not use combination pills. Combination oral contraceptives are also contraindicated for women who are currently pregnant, lactating of less than six weeks' duration, smoking more than 20 cigarettes per day, are over 35 years old, have focal headaches with neurological symptoms, have had recent leg surgery or prolonged immobility, have hypertension greater than 160/100, or diabetes mellitus of more than 20 years duration with vascular disease.
2. The advantages of birth control pills include menstrual periods which are more regular and predictable, a decrease in menstrual flow and premenstrual symptoms, and provide a safe, effective contraceptive method that can be used until menopause for women who do not smoke.
3. Disadvantages include no protection against sexually transmitted infections, the need to remember to take a pill each day at the same time, decreased effectiveness of the birth control pill when taken with some other drugs (anticonvulsants, antifungals, or antibiotics), and decreased effectiveness of insulin or oral anticoagulants when taken with oral contraceptives. If progestin-only pills are used, they are more likely to cause irregular bleeding or amenorrhea, and if the client conceives, the risk of ectopic pregnancy is increased.
4. Most clients are advised to begin the cycle of pills on the Sunday following the first day of the menstrual period and take one pill at the same time each day. A back-up method of contraception is usually advised for the first month until the contraceptive effect of the oral contraceptives is established. If pills are missed, the client is advised to contact the health care provider for specific instructions based on the type of oral contraceptive provided, the number of pills missed, and the time in the cycle. Clients should always be advised that a mechanical method of contraception should be used to provide protection against sexually transmitted infections.
5. The client should be taught the acronym ACHES to represent the warning signs related to the use of oral contraceptives. These include abdominal pain; chest pain, cough, and/or shortness of breath; headaches, dizziness, weakness, or numbness; eye problems, such as blurring or change in vision, and problems with speech; and severe leg, calf, and/or thigh pain. If any of these signs develop, the client should be instructed to contact the health care provider immediately.

Chapter 4

1. The preembryonic period spans two weeks, the time from fertilization until the zygote is embedded in the uterus. There are three significant events of the preembryonic period, cellular multiplication, travel through the fallopian tube into the uterus, and implantation. The fertilized ovum, or zygote, divides rapidly in a process called cleavage. It takes on a mulberry-like shape and is called a morula. The morula has a solid inner mass called the blastocyst and an outer layer that will become the placental tissue. It takes three to four days for the blastocyst to make its journey from the fallopian tube to the uterus. It floats in the uterus for another four to five days. The uterus prepares for pregnancy with each monthly menstrual cycle. The uterine lining after ovulation is thick and vascular. Uterine glands secrete nourishment used by the blastocyst before it implants. The blastocyst burrows into this rich lining, now called decidua, seven to nine days after fertilization. The outer layer of the blastocyst develops fingerlike projections that imbed in the decidua. These projections are called villi that later become the placenta. Once implanted, the blastocyst begins the process of differentiation by developing three layers of tissue from which all body tissue is derived. All of these events occur in the first two weeks after fertilization, a time prior to when most women have not even had a missed period or realize they are pregnant. If the pregnancy is lost during this time, the woman most likely will not realize she is even pregnant.
2. Weeks two through eight are called the embryonic stage. During this time, cells are changing to become the various organ systems that make up the human. This process is called organogenesis. Because organogenesis occurs very rapidly, the embryo is extremely vulnerable to anything that interferes with this process. Should that occur, a birth defect or miscarriage may result. Such interferences are called teratogens. They include chemicals, radiation, and microorganisms. Since organogenesis begins before most women realize they are pregnant, it is important that women avoid potential teratogens if they are attempting to become pregnant.

3. While many congenital anomalies are genetic, others may be caused by teratogens in the first eight weeks of pregnancy, or, as in many cases, there may be no identifiable cause. As childbearing age increases, the risk of having a child with a chromosome anomaly such as Down syndrome increases. Genetic testing procedures and genetic counseling are available for parents concerned about genetic disease. The nurse informs the class how to receive a referral if desired.
4. The fetus has the potential to survive outside of the womb after 23 weeks' gestation, provided the infant receives intensive care. At this time the lung's small air sacs, called alveoli, are beginning to form. This is also the time when the capillaries are close enough to the lung to allow oxygen exchange. While survival is a possibility it is still unlikely since every body system is immature.
5. First trimester: All body organs are formed but immature. The fetus has a human appearance. The heart is beating and the fetus is moving. Facial features are present although the eyelids are fused. Genitalia are identifiable. Length is 3.2 inches and weight is 1.6 ounces.

   Second trimester: The fetus has the potential for life outside of the womb with intensive care. Its length is 11.2 inches and weight is 1 pound, 10 ounces. The fetus has hair on its head, eyelashes, and eyebrows. It is covered with downy hair called lanugo and a cheesy protective coating called vernix caseosa. Fetal movement is clearly felt by the mother. The skin is red and wrinkled with little fat deposit. Testes are not descended. The eyelids are closed but will open shortly.

   Third trimester: After 38 weeks the fetus is considered term. The length is 18 to 21 inches. The weight is 6 pounds, 10 ounces to 7 pounds, 15 ounces. The fetus has the appearance of a newborn consistent with race. Lanugo and vernix caseosa are mostly gone. Fat deposits give the body a plump appearance. Fingernails and toenails are present.

Chapter 5

1. The nurse should assess for factors possibly affecting the GI system such as the client's dietary intake, especially with regard to fruits and vegetables, fiber, and spicy foods; use of stool softeners, laxatives, or antacids; and timing of food intake. Factors affecting lower-extremity swelling such as rest and activity patterns should be assessed.
2. With regard to GI function, the nurse should inspect the anus for the presence of hemorrhoids. Lower extremities should be assessed for varicose veins. The client should also be assessed for signs and symptoms of gestational hypertension and/or preeclampsia such as elevated blood pressure, protein in the urine, and swelling other than in the lower extremities.
3. Nursing diagnoses could include Mild Anxiety, Body Image Disturbance, Constipation, Risk for Aspiration, or Altered Comfort.
4. The nurse should assure the client that all of these symptoms, while not life threatening, can affect her function and comfort, are commonly associated with pregnancy, and can be treated. To manage heartburn, the client could avoid lying down after eating, avoid fatty or fried foods, eat smaller and more frequent meals, and take a low-sodium antacid, if needed. To minimize constipation and the development of hemorrhoids, the woman could increase her fluid intake to at least 2000 mL per day; increase her intake of fruits, vegetables, and fiber; participate in daily exercise; allow sufficient time for bowel function; and use stool softeners, if needed. To decrease or prevent ankle edema, the client could avoid prolonged standing or sitting, dorsiflex the feet frequently, avoid tight bands or garters around the legs, and elevate the feet and legs during frequent rest periods.
5. The nurse should encourage the client to call the health care provider's office if these symptoms are not relieved by the measures suggested. When the woman returns for her next prenatal visit, these problems should be assessed and, if needed, further management should be considered.

Chapter 6

1. Because the mother's age is greater than 35 years, her fetus is at increased risk for Down syndrome (trisomy 21).
2. This client should be offered a triple test or quadruple test, an amniocentesis, or chorionic villus sampling for genetic testing that would indicate chromosomal problems such as Down syndrome.
3. Chorionic villus sampling can be done earlier in gestation. This provides information more quickly, decreases the amount of time the client has to wait or worry about the results, and provides for earlier and safer options for pregnancy termination, if the client so desires.
4. Having chromosomal information can decrease worry concerning the condition of the fetus and result in a less stressful pregnancy. If there is a problem, being aware of it may affect decisions regarding delivery site, health care providers needed for mother or baby, and postpartal plans. It also provides a period of adjustment for the family prior to delivery.
5. Potential maternal complications from amniocentesis include hemorrhage, infection, preterm labor, abruptio placentae, inadvertent damage to the intestines and/or bladder, and amniotic fluid leakage or embolism. Potential fetal complications include death, hemorrhage, infection, and direct injury from the needle. Complications occur in less than 1% of cases. Potential maternal complications from chorionic villus sampling include vaginal spotting or bleeding, miscarriage, rupture of membranes and chorioamnionitis. Limb anomalies of the fetus have been reported when the procedure is done before 10 weeks' gestation but this complication is very rare.

Chapter 7

1. Other assessments for the severe preeclamptic client include temperature every four hours unless membranes are ruptured; hourly blood pressure, pulse and respirations, deep tendon reflexes (DTRs) with clonus assessment, assessment of edema, intake and urine output with assessment for proteinuria, and assessment of the presence of headaches, visual changes or epigastric pain. The fetus needs to be continuously monitored.
2. The severe preeclamptic client is at risk for seizures (eclampsia), pulmonary edema, abruption of the placenta, HELLP syndrome, DIC, hepatic hematoma with possible rupture, cerebrovascular accident (CVA), and possible acute renal tubular necrosis.
3. The client with severe preeclampsia should be given IV magnesium sulfate to decrease the likelihood of seizures, and possibly antihypertensive medications. Since this client is at 42 weeks' gestation, she will probably also have oxytocin (Pitocin) to induce labor since delivery is the only cure for preeclampsia.
4. This fetus is at risk for intrauterine growth retardation (IUGR) resulting in a small-for-gestational age (SGA) infant, and chronic hypoxia because of the underlying vasospasm creating damage to the placental vasculature. The infant is also almost postterm (greater than 42 weeks) and may have meconium-stained amniotic fluid. This fetus may not have the reserves and placental resources needed to tolerate labor.
5. The client and her family should be given honest, simple explanations about the condition, the plan of care, and all interventions. Family may be asked to limit visitors and noise to decrease central nervous system irritability.

Chapter 8

1. During the active phase of the first stage of labor and with intact membranes, the maternal temperature is assessed every four hours unless it is elevated >99.6°F. Blood pressure, pulse, and respirations are assessed every hour, if normal. Fetal status is being continuously monitored electronically. The nurse should review the monitor tracing and document her findings in the client's record every 30 minutes if the client is low-risk or every 15 minutes if the client is high-risk or nonreassuring findings are determined.
2. With a posterior position the hard occiput of the fetus is against the maternal sacrum, which causes pressure and pain in the low back. Additionally, the woman may feel discomfort in the region of the symphysis pubis from the cervical dilatation that is occurring.
3. Nonpharmacologic methods to promote comfort for a woman in active labor with intact membranes and a posterior position include: positioning the client in anything except a supine or semi-Fowler's position to keep the weight of the fetus off her low back. Walking, hydrotherapy, music, relaxation, visualization, and breathing techniques may be helpful. Reassurance and support may also increase comfort. Pharmacologic options that could be offered include IV narcotics, intrathecal narcotics, and epidural block. The client's desires, beliefs, and cultural preferences should be assessed when planning for increased comfort during labor.
4. The contractions can be expected to become stronger and last longer. In transition, contractions may also become more frequent. As delivery becomes more imminent, anxiety, irritability, and restlessness may increase and the woman may experience a normal but intense sensation of pressure with contractions. The client may find it more difficult to understand directions; experience hiccupping, belching, nausea, or vomiting; perspire more; or experience rectal pressure or the uncontrollable urge to bear down. During the second stage, the woman may feel relief and a regained sense of control when she can push in response to the urge to bear down with contractions. As the fetus descends and the perineum distends, the client may feel pain and a burning sensation. Following delivery, nausea and vomiting usually cease, the woman may be hungry or thirsty, and may experience a shaking chill associated with the end of the physical exertion of labor. The client should be reassured that she will not be left alone and that the nurse will be available to provide comfort and support in coping with the stress of labor.
5. Some health care providers advocate electronic monitoring only for pregnant women at high risk for complications. Others recommend continuous monitoring for all women in labor as a means to provide a constant and objective assessment of the fetal response to the stress of contractions. Even though the client's pregnancy has been uneventful, there is no guarantee that labor and delivery will also proceed normally. Constant surveillance can detect changes in fetal well-being earlier so interventions can be implemented more effectively.

Chapter 9

1. Assess the contraction frequency, duration, and intensity, and compare this to previous contractions. A common cause of nonprogressive labor is hypotonic uterine dysfunction or poor contraction quality. In addition, assess fetal and maternal response to contractions to detect distress in the fetus and tension and anxiety in the mother. Maternal psyche can also impact labor progress.
2. The small triangular fontanel is the posterior fontanel. This means that the presentation is occiput and the position (toward mother's back and right side) is right occiput posterior (ROP).
3. Explain to the husband that there are several possible causes of prolonged labor. The most common reasons are decreased contraction quality, shape of the mother's pelvic bones, and the way the baby is positioned. You might say, "Your baby seems to be in a 'facing-upward'

position that is more difficult to deliver than the usual 'facing-downward' position. This is called a posterior position. It may take your wife a little longer to deliver, but there doesn't seem to be any signs of a health problem for the baby right now."

4. Reassuring the client and repositioning her on her left side (opposite the fetal back) may help with rotation of the fetal head from ROP to an occiput anterior (OA) position. Continue to assess contractions and maternal response to contractions. Encourage relaxation. Laboring in a position on hands and knees for several contractions, pelvic rocking, and assuming a tailor sitting position have been reported to be helpful for rotation and descent of the fetus.
5. Yes, the physician should be notified. Although there are no signs of fetal distress, the physician needs to know about the client's lack of progress, contraction status, and fetal position. Augmentation of labor with oxytocin (Pitocin) may be ordered to correct hypotonic uterine dysfunction. Continuous assessment of contractions, fetal heart rate, maternal response, and labor progress is warranted.

Chapter 10

1. Other important information to gather about this client would include: gravida, para, length of labor and type of delivery, how long membranes were ruptured before delivery, blood type and Rh, baseline vital signs, findings from last postpartal physical assessment, time of the last voiding, medications received during labor and delivery, and if she has received analgesia since birth.
2. If her vital signs are normal and stable, the client should first be assisted to sit on the side of the bed and then gradually adjust to a standing position. The nurse assists the woman to ambulate slowly to the bathroom making sure the woman has feeling and control of her legs prior to ambulation. It is normal for new mothers to experience a trickle of lochia the first time they stand after delivery, caused by pooling in the uterus and vagina, and the nurse should anticipate and teach the woman about this. If the client becomes weak or dizzy, she should be encouraged to sit down immediately. The nurse should stay with the client until she returns to bed.
3. Postpartum women may have difficulty voiding the first time after delivery. The sensation of a full bladder or the urge to void may be decreased and the woman may feel uncomfortable with another person present. The nurse should reassure the woman this is normal and that the nurse's presence is to protect the woman's safety, not to invade her privacy. The nurse should first try interventions to encourage voiding such as running water in the bathroom, putting the woman's hands in warm water, or pouring warm water over the perineum. The client could try again to urinate after a short time. If the client's bladder is distended, the uterus displaced, or six hours have elapsed since delivery, the client will need to be catheterized.
4. Clients may experience a mild elevation in body temperature shortly after delivery related to dehydration. Bradycardia after delivery is common to 50 to 70 beats per minute and the blood pressure is within normal range. The nurse should continue to monitor the vital signs and encourage oral fluids, unless contraindicated. The nurse may suspect the fever is related to dehydration, however, the client should also be assessed for signs of infection. If signs of infection are identified or the temperature reaches 101°F, the physician should be notified.
5. New parents typically want to see and hold their new baby immediately after delivery. Mothers often speak in quiet, high-pitched tones and call the baby by name. Eye contact is usually established with the en face position. Touch is typically progressive beginning with fingertip exploration of the extremities, then palmar contact with larger body areas, and finally the newborn is enfolded with the whole hand and arm and held closely cradled to the mother's body. The mother may identify characteristics of family members present in the infant. The mother should respond to newborn cues, attempt to meet the infant's needs, and show general concern for the baby's well-being.

Chapter 11

1. The client's risk factors for a postpartal infection, especially an infection of the abdominal wound or lining of the uterus, include the following:
   - Cesarean delivery places her at risk because it is an invasive procedure.
   - Prolonged rupture of membranes allows organisms from the non-sterile vagina to reach the uterus.
   - An unsuccessful course of labor predisposes the client to infection because of fatigue, possible use of internal monitoring, and increased likelihood of vaginal examinations to determine progress, or lack of progress, in labor.
2. Ongoing nursing assessments necessary to identify an infection include the following:
   - Monitoring vital signs every four hours, especially temperature
   - Wound assessment using REEDA to determine redness, edema, ecchymosis, discharge and approximation of skin edges
   - Monitoring laboratory results, especially WBCs, Hgb, and Hct
   - Assessment of lochia: observing for amount, color, and odor
   - Assessment of malaise, lethargy, chills: subtle signs of infection

3. The definition of postpartal infection is a fever of greater than 100.4°F that occurs on 2 out of 10 days after the first 24 hours following childbirth.
4. The first step is to identify the location of the infection and the organism causing the infection so that appropriate antibiotic therapy can be initiated. This information is usually obtained through cultures of any wound drainage, lochia, or urine prior to the administration of antibiotics.
5. Pertinent nursing diagnoses could include the following:
   - Hyperthermia related to postpartal infection
   - Pain related to the presence of infection
   - Knowledge Deficit related to lack of information about condition and its treatment
   - Risk for Impaired Parent–Infant Attachment secondary to woman's malaise and other symptoms of infection
   - Ineffective or Interrupted Breastfeeding related to delayed interaction with infant secondary to symptoms of infection

Chapter 12

1. The first assessment reveals that the client's blood pressure was elevated one hour after delivery. This may indicate the mother is experiencing pain and negatively impacts her desire to hold or feed her infant at this time.
2. Asking her an open-ended question about how she is feeling may reveal that she is experiencing pain or that she is disappointed or fatigued after her cesarean delivery. You explain to the mother that her comfort and readiness are essential to breastfeeding success. You reassure the mother that she can begin breastfeeding at a later time. You tell her that you will take the infant to the nursery but will bring him back to her when she is rested, more comfortable and you will be available to assist her when she is ready to initiate breastfeeding.
3. You should take the baby to the mother when she requests him. If she does not request the baby, the nurse should offer to do so at frequent intervals and provide information about his status while mother and baby are separated.
4. Begin with simple instructions and offer to stay with the mother and baby to provide assistance. Your initial focus should be a position of comfort to hold the infant and initiate breastfeeding if the mother is ready. Suggest the side-lying position which may be the most comfortable for a cesarean-delivered mother with an abdominal incision. Place the infant so that the mother can use the hand that does not have an intravenous infusion. Use pillows to position and support mother's body in good alignment and use a rolled-up baby blanket to keep the infant directly facing his mother, not rolling partially onto his back.
5. The priorities for promoting a positive breastfeeding experience for this mother and baby are flexibility, continued patient education, follow-up by telephone or a home visit, and referral to a lactation consultant or public health nurse, if indicated.

Chapter 13

1. Client history would include any pertinent prenatal or labor/delivery history (i.e., maternal diabetes, infectious diseases, prolonged rupture of membranes, fetal distress, etc.), Apgar scores, and birth weight. Current information would include respiratory status, oxygen therapy, oxygen saturation reading, and any other unexpected findings.
2. The initial priority of care for this infant is to establish and maintain an airway. Another high priority need for this infant is thermoregulation. Fluid balance, risk of infection, nutrition, and bonding are additional nursing problems appropriate for this patient.
3. Oxygen given in high doses over a prolonged period of time can increase the risk of retinopathy of prematurity (ROP). Oxygen should not be withheld from infants but administered cautiously, using the minimal amount to meet the infant's oxygenation needs. If the infant is not receiving enough oxygen, cells within the body will begin to die, including brain cells. This could result in permanent neurologic damage. It is also known that hypoxia increases the risk of necrotizing enterocolitis (NEC), which can be life threatening.
4. It is important to promote bonding. Encourage the parents to visit as much as possible. Parents can bring personal items for the baby, such as pictures, small toys, etc. Parents are often initially afraid to touch their preterm baby because they are afraid they will hurt the infant. Encourage parents to touch the baby, stroke the hand or foot, and hold the newborn, if the condition allows. When the baby is stable, parents can be encouraged to do "kangaroo care," where they put the unclothed baby on their bare chest to allow for skin-to-skin contact for short periods of time. Preterm infants need developmental stimulation, just like a term baby, but may need shorter periods of interaction. The baby should be positioned in a fetal position in the isolette or radiant warmer to provide a sense of security as well as limit loss of body heat.
5. The mother should be encouraged to breastfeed, although the baby will not be able to nurse until the suck/swallow reflex is established and the newborn is strong enough to nurse. Until that time, the mother should pump her breasts every two to three hours while awake, save the milk in small amounts in glass or plastic containers, and freeze it. The milk can then be given to the baby during tube feedings. This will also stimulate milk production in the mother. Breast milk is easier to

digest and contains valuable immunoglobulins which can help prevent infection in the baby.

Chapter 14

1. The infant will be pale and bluish. The muscle tone will be very floppy, making the baby feel limp like a rag doll. The mouth may droop open.
2. Ask the client if she would like to be on the postpartum unit, or on another unit. If on the postpartum unit, assign her to a room that is away from the nursery. Try to assign consistent caregivers to increase support to the family.
3. Children age 6 and under do not yet understand what death is, or that it is permanent, but may feel responsible for the death if they had negative feelings toward the expected infant. School-age children understand that death is inevitable and permanent. It is best to explain that the baby died while it was being born, giving details of the placental abruption only if the children ask about it or if the children are used to talking about body parts and functions.
4. Gently tell the client while the mother is still in the room that although she will recover from surgery over the next few weeks, her grieving will take up to two years to completely resolve. Give the client written information on the phases of bereavement, as well as on infant loss support groups.
5. Listen to the client's concerns. Provide empathy through therapeutic communication. Reassure the client that hearing a baby's cry after a fetal loss is a common and completely normal occurrence. It indicates being in the searching and yearning phase of bereavement. These sensations will gradually fade with time. Encourage the client to read the information on grieving that was given to her in the hospital or consider joining a support group.

Index

Page numbers followed by b indicate box; those followed by f indicate figure; those followed by t indicate table.